Principles of Assessment and Outcome Measurement for Allied Health Professionals: Practice, Research and Development

Principles of Assessment and Outcome Measurement for Allied Health Professionals: Practice, Research and Development

SECOND EDITION

Alison J. Laver-Fawcett

Associate Professor in Occupational Therapy
School of Science, Technology and Health
York St John University
England, UK

Diane L. Cox

Emeritus Professor of Occupational Therapy
University of Cumbria
Carlisle, UK

WILEY Blackwell

This edition first published 2021
© 2021 John Wiley & Sons Ltd

Edition History
Wiley (1e, 2007)

The right of Alison J. Laver-Fawcett and Diane L. Cox to be identified as the authors of this work has been asserted in accordance with law.

Registered Office(s)
John Wiley & Sons, Inc., 111 River Street, Hoboken, NJ 07030, USA
John Wiley & Sons Ltd, The Atrium, Southern Gate, Chichester, West Sussex, PO19 8SQ, UK

Editorial Office
9600 Garsington Road, Oxford, OX4 2DQ, UK

For details of our global editorial offices, customer services, and more information about Wiley products visit us at www.wiley.com.

Wiley also publishes its books in a variety of electronic formats and by print-on-demand. Some content that appears in standard print versions of this book may not be available in other formats.

Library of Congress Cataloging-in-Publication Data
Names: Laver-Fawcett, Alison J., author. | Cox, Diane L., author. |
    Laver-Fawcett, Alison J. Principles of assessment and outcome
    measurement for occupational therapists and physiotherapists.
Title: Principles of assessment and outcome measurement for allied health
    professionals : practice, research and development / Alison J.
    Laver-Fawcett, Diane L. Cox.
Description: Second edition. | Hoboken, NJ : Wiley-Blackwell, 2021. |
    Preceded by Principles of assessment and outcome measurement for
    occupational therapists and physiotherapists : theory, skills and
    application / by Alison J. Laver Fawcett. 2007. | Includes
    bibliographical references and index.
Identifiers: LCCN 2020051154 (print) | LCCN 2020051155 (ebook) | ISBN
    9781119633099 (paperback) | ISBN 9781119633327 (adobe pdf) | ISBN
    9781119633334 (epub)
Subjects: MESH: Needs Assessment | Outcome Assessment, Health Care |
    Occupational Therapy | Physical Therapy Modalities
Classification: LCC R697.A4 (print) | LCC R697.A4 (ebook) | NLM W 84.3 |
    DDC 610.73/7–dc23
LC record available at https://lccn.loc.gov/2020051154
LC ebook record available at https://lccn.loc.gov/2020051155

Cover Design: Wiley
Cover Images: © Gokcemim/DigitalVision Vectors/Getty Images

Set in 10.5/13pt STIXTwoText by Straive, Pondicherry, India
Printed and bound by CPI Group (UK) Ltd, Croydon, CR0 4YY

C9781119633099_140721

This book is dedicated to Alison's parents,
Diane and Philip Laver

Contents

Authors' Biography

Dr Alison J. Laver-Fawcett, PhD, DipCOT, OT(C), PgCAP, SFHEA

Alison qualified as an Occupational Therapist in 1986 from the then Dorset House School of Occupational Therapy in Oxford. She obtained a PhD in Psychology from the University of Surrey in 1995, and the output from her doctoral studies was the Structured Observational Test of Function (SOTOF; Laver and Powell 1995) which was published by NFER Nelson. Alison began her career in clinical posts in London working with people with learning disabilities and with mental health conditions in the Richmond, Twickenham, and Roehampton Health Authority and then with older people and Bolingbroke Hospital, Wandsworth Health Authority. In 1990, she became a Research Occupational Therapist in the Department of Geriatric Medicine at St George's Hospital. She has worked as an educator and researcher at universities in the United Kingdom (Canterbury Christchurch College, Teesside University, and York St John University), Canada (McMaster University), and the United States of America (Washington University School of Medicine). Alison spent eight years as a modernisation manager working on the evaluation and improvement of older people's mental health services in across several NHS services in North Yorkshire. She currently works as an Associate Professor at York St John University, where she has been teaching and conducting research since 2008. She has represented the College of Occupational Therapists as the UK delegate on the World Federation of Occupational Therapists Council (2009–2011) and is currently chair of the Research into Occupational Therapy and Occupational Science (ROTOS) Foundation and sits on the Occupational Therapy Europe Foundation Board. Her expertise is in test development and psychometric studies, service evaluation and improvement, and occupational therapy for older people, particularly with neurological conditions and dementia.

Prof. Diane L. Cox, PhD, MSc, DipCOT, CLTHE, FRCOT

Diane qualified as an Occupational Therapist in 1983, from the then Welsh School of Occupational Therapy, Cardiff. She worked in the NHS for 15 years, starting her early career working for Southmead Health Authority, Bristol. Diane then moved to London to work at The Middlesex Hospital in Central London, then to St Georges Hospital, in Tooting, London, and finally to Oldchurch Hospital in Romford, Essex. In 1998, Diane moved into Higher Education, initially at South Bank University, London, and then to the University of Cumbria (formally St. Martin's College). Her expertise is in long-term conditions, particularly the management of fatigue, and occupational science. Diane studied for an MSc in Research Methods part time at Kings College London from 1989 to 1991 and then completed a PhD part time in Occupational Therapy and Chronic Fatigue Syndrome from 1994 to 1999, also at Kings College London. These higher degrees were completed while working full time in the NHS. Diane is a Fellow of the Royal College of Occupational Therapists, a past Elizabeth Casson Memorial Lecturer, and previous trustee of the Elizabeth Casson Trust and at the time of co-writing the book the Chair of Council at the RCOT/BAOT. Diane became a Professor of Occupational Therapy in 2011. Diane has been a research ethics adviser to a number of national and European projects, sat on a number of national research funding bodies, and has led and been a co-applicant on a substantial number of funded research projects. Diane has supervised many occupational therapists to successful award their bachelor's, master's, and doctoral degrees. Diane has led occupational therapy programmes, managed departments, and been an ambassador for occupational therapy research. Diane took early retirement in December 2020 from her role as Director of Research and Knowledge Exchange, at the University of Cumbria, although she continues as an Emeritus Professor of Occupational Therapy with the university.

Authors Contributing to Case Studies

Dr Sally Payne, Professional Adviser, Royal College of Occupational Therapists, London; Claire Howells, Paediatric Occupational Therapist, Help 4 Psychology, Midlands

Chapter 2: This case study illustrates how an occupational therapy service assembled a toolkit of standardised assessments to gather information from a range of sources using a number of different methods. The first part of this study describes the service and the rationale for the measures that therapists selected to use. The second part shows how these assessments were applied in a clinical setting through the case of a teenage boy, whom we will refer to as 'Scott'.

Dr Alison J. Laver-Fawcett

Chapter 3: This case study is based on Alison's experience of working for a couple of years as an allied health professional (AHP) in a geriatric day hospital setting and on her research experience with people with stroke. It is not based on one particular case but is rather an imaginary case developed to illustrate the application of explicit thinking about purposes of assessment to a clinical setting.

Rachel Hargreaves, Tees, Esk and Wear Valleys NHS Foundation Trust

Chapter 5: The AHP completing the assessment and report has worked as an Occupational therapist, practising in a variety of clinical settings including Neurology and Mental Health Services for Working Age Adults and Older Adults. She has undertaken the Assessment of Motor and Process Skills (AMPS) training to be a calibrated assessor. AMPS is an assessment which she used in the Multi-Disciplinary Specialist Memory Clinic service and in the Community Mental Health Team for Older Adults.

Acknowledgement to Karen Innes, Independent Practitioner *who co-wrote the original case study on which this version is based with* Dr Alison Laver-Fawcett, United Kingdom

Chapter 6: This case study has been written to illustrate the AHP's (an Occupational Therapist) clinical reasoning related to the initial assessment of a client with whom she is likely to work with over many months. The case is provided to illustrate several of the different types of reasoning outlined earlier in this chapter. It is a detailed study, so that students and novice AHPs can see an example of how an AHP frames and explains her assessment approach. The AHPs' thinking is given in italics and is mostly provided in boxes to separate the reasoning from the description of what happened during the assessment process for this case.

Acknowledgement to Mr David Jelly, Physiotherapist, who wrote the original case study on which this version is based.

Chapter 11: This case study is focused on Mary, an 83-year-old woman living alone who fell in the night when she got up to go to the toilet. She was unable to get herself up and lay on the floor for four-and-a-half hours. She was found when one of her daughters, Anne, popped in to check on her the next morning. Mary was cold and shaken and complained of severe pain in her left forearm.

Kathryn Moyse, Royal College of Speech and Language Therapists, London, United Kingdom
Chapter 13: The Royal College of Speech and Language Therapists (RCSLT) is undertaking a programme of work on data collection and analysis with the aim of supporting the profession by delivering quality services. Although health and care policies across the United Kingdom reference the importance of data information and technology in delivering care (Health and Social Care Board 2016; NHS England 2019a,b; Scottish Government 2018; Welsh Government 2015), there remain numerous barriers for speech and language therapists (SLTs) in the United Kingdom, including the absence of tools to support data collection and analytics. In response to this challenge, the RCSLT Online Outcome Tool (ROOT) has been developed to support the speech and language therapy profession with collecting, analysing, and reporting on outcome measures data.

Dr Sue Pemberton, Yorkshire Fatigue Clinic, York, United Kingdom
Chapter 13: This case study presents the development of a local rehabilitation service for adults and young people with the condition Chronic Fatigue Syndrome/Myalgic Encephalomyelitis (CFS/ME) in collaboration between an independent provider and three Clinical Commissioning Groups. CFS/ME is a disabling condition that significantly impacts an individual's ability to live their daily life (NICE 2007).

Professor Carolyn Unsworth, Central Queensland University, Australia
Chapter 14: This case study presents information on a free outcome measure that is used internationally by AHPs, called the Australian Therapy Outcome Measures (AusTOMs). Scales have been developed for use by occupational therapists (OTs) Unsworth and Duncombe (2014), physiotherapists (PT) (Morris et al. 2014), and speech pathologists (SPs) (Perry and Skeat 2014) (see Figure 14.2) although other AHPs may also work with these disciplines to score clients using AusTOMs.

Eden Marrison, York Teaching Hospitals NHS Foundation Trust, York, United Kingdom
Chapter 15: This case study presents the methodology for conducting a face validity study. Patients with neurological diagnoses were assessed using the SOTOF and then interviewed to gather their experiences, views, and opinions regarding undertaking the assessment. A literature-based first stage content validity study (Marrison and Laver-Fawcett 2016) led to further development of SOTOF's dynamic assessment component. Face validity and content validity were previously evaluated (Laver and Powell 1995), and a further study was required following the changes made for the 2nd edition.

Foreword

I am honoured to have been invited to provide the foreword for this edition. The widened scope it provides, through extension of assessment and outcome measurement principles to a range of allied health professions (AHPs), builds on the value that was provided in the first edition for occupational therapists and physiotherapists.

The ability of AHPs to evaluate, improve, and evidence the impact of their contribution was detailed as a key priority within the first AHP strategy for England, AHPs into Action. However, we are yet to consistently evidence the impact of our interventions. This lack of information presents significant challenges in evidencing the operational contribution AHPs make at an organisational, local, or national level. This text provides comprehensive detail to enable the appropriate selection and utilisation of assessment and outcome measures that will support provision of this much-needed evidence.

The detail of each section makes it accessible for AHPs at any stage of their career. For the pre-registration AHP student, it introduces assessment and the use of outcome measures. For new registrants, it enables a greater depth of knowledge to inform practice. For expert practitioners and those looking to undertake research though to PhD studies, the book will support development of existing or new measures and associated concepts. It will also act as reference for AHP managers looking to evidence the impact of their services.

This book takes a pragmatic approach to a complex subject area. It skilfully walks the reader through the importance and practical application of assessment and measurement, highlighting the role of clinical reasoning and reflective practice within this. The detailed narrative is expertly annotated with case study examples throughout the text, bringing the subject to life and enabling an understanding of the practical application for the reader to augment their learning. Overall, this reference text has relevance across all levels of practice and will provide a source of information for both individuals and teams. I have pleasure in commending it.

Suzanne Rastrick
Chief Allied Health Professions' Officer (CAHPO)
for England, April 2021

Preface

Purpose: The purpose of this book is to enable allied health professional (AHPs) students, clinicians, educators, researchers, and managers to understand the complex art and science of assessment and outcome measurement processes.

Who Is This Book For?

For students, the book will introduce you to the process and purpose of assessment and outcome measurement for practice, research, and service evaluation; help you to understand levels of measurement, standardisation, and psychometric properties and help you to apply this knowledge to appraise and select the best assessments and outcome measures.

For educators, the book will assist in exploring with students the purpose and importance of assessment and outcome measurement, standardisation and psychometrics, key aspects of test development, and the reasoning required to select and apply assessments and measures in practice.

For practitioners, the book will familiarise you with assessment and outcome measure terminology and enable you to identify the properties of tests in order to select and confidently implement appropriate standardised tests and outcome measures in your practice, service evaluation, service development, and research.

For researchers, the book will assist you in developing a new assessment or outcome measure; creating a culturally sensitive version of an existing measure; undertaking a linguistically valid translation of a measure published in another language; collecting normative data; conducting psychometric studies to examine aspects of validity and reliability; and/or exploring the face validity or clinical utility of a measure.

For managers, the book will assist in identifying the importance of assessment and outcome measures for service evaluation and improvement, and to select and measure outcomes as required by commissioners and senior managers.

How Is This 2nd Edition Structured?

In this 2nd edition, there are a number of changes to enable you to locate the information you require for different aspects of assessment and outcome measurement, such as choice, development, and utilisation. The book is divided into four sections. The following pages provide a brief description of each section and the related chapters. Each chapter will start with key words, a chapter overview, and review questions.

Signposts are provided to help you to navigate to what you need and want to know. Worksheets are embedded in the relevant chapters for you to use on your own or for group learning. There are worksheets with relevance for students, clinicians, researchers, and/or managers. A completed worksheet could be used within your Continuing Professional Development portfolio as part of your evidence of learning and development, e.g. in the United Kingdom (UK) for Health and Care Professions Council (HCPC) registration requirements. Throughout the book, examples of standardised tests along with clinical examples, case vignettes, and case histories are used to help you see how to apply the principles and skills described in your practice, research, and/or service evaluation. Review questions and brief answers are provided to help you check whether you have understood the key concepts from each chapter.

Section 1: Assessment and Measurement in Practice

Chapter 1 focuses on the importance of accurate assessment in practice. Chapter 2 describes methods of assessment (including the advantages and disadvantages of informal versus standardised methods) such as self-report, proxy, and observational approaches. In Chapter 3, the different purposes of assessment in practice (such as descriptive, discriminative, predictive, and evaluative) are explored, and the timing of assessments (including initial, baseline, monitoring, and outcome) are considered. Chapter 4 addresses the question of 'what is measurement?' and provides definitions and examples of four levels of measurement (nominal, ordinal, interval, and ratio). Chapter 5 explains the process of test administration and makes suggestions for reporting and recording test results. Chapter 6 explains the importance of clinical reasoning and reflective practice in effective assessment and discusses different types of clinical reasoning (including diagnostic, interactive, pragmatic, procedural, narrative, and ethical reasoning).

Section 2: Concepts for Assessment and Measurement

Chapter 7 examines the importance of standardisation in research and the role of norm-referenced and criterion-referenced tests. Chapter 8 focuses on the topic of validity and concludes with an exploration of face validity and clinical utility. Chapter 9 examines reliability, including an explanation of the different types of reliability, statistics used to examine levels of reliability, and concepts such as responsiveness, test specificity, sensitivity, error of measurement, and floor or ceiling effects. Chapter 10 explains how to find, select, and critically appraise assessment and outcome measurements, along with a detailed example of a test critique.

Section 3: Assessment and Measurement for Service Evaluation and Improvement

Chapter 11 explores the application of models of function to AHP assessment and measurement, illustrated with several examples, including the World Health Organisation's (2002) International Classification of Functioning, Disability and Health. Chapter 12 gives advice on implementing the optimum assessment and measurement approach for your practice or service. Chapter 13 considers how to use assessment and outcome measures for evaluating your assessment practice, undertaking a service evaluation, and planning improvements to your assessment process.

Section 4: Developing and Evaluating Assessments and Outcome Measures

Chapter 14 explores test development, in particular, what to consider when developing a new test or undertaking additional work on an existing measure such as to improve cultural sensitivity or to translate it into another language. Chapter 15 explores methodology for examining different psychometric properties of measures.

As we were considering the structure and format for this new edition of the book, we had the opportunity to lead two professional Twitter dialogues through #OTalk (https://twitter.com/OTalk_). The first Twitter dialogue focussed on 'Assessment and Outcome Measures' (19 February 2019), and we thank the 40 participants in the chat for an engaging and fast-paced one-hour discussion with 400 tweets. The second was on 'Why Aren't All Therapists Using Standardised Assessments Routinely in Practice?' (21 May 2019), and we thank the 42 participants in that chat for an interesting and informative discussion with 515 tweets.

Table 1 highlights the recurring themes, and related needs and requirements, identified by participants in the Twitter chat. These themes, although predominantly drawn from occupational therapists, echo those identified within the literature by other AHPs, and we felt it would be useful to share them in this preface.

The participants' questions and recommendations about assessment are listed below and have been incorporated, as appropriate, throughout the book.

- Think
  - What do you need to know?
  - What is causing the person's problem?
  - What assessment tool will measure the person's difficulties?
  - What influences your choice of assessment or outcome measure?
- Select an assessment that is the most suitable and reliable for the needs of the individual.
- Be clear that you may need more than one assessment to consider a range of difficulties.
- Do not modify or 'tweak' the assessment, as it is no longer valid.
- Informal interviews and observations may help you build a rapport with the person; however, you need to be able to demonstrate therapy outcomes through your assessment and measures.
- Gain an understanding of the measure, consider how it was validated, and with which client groups.
- Learn how to administer, score, and interpret results. This can require time.
- Make use of supervision and peer support. Reflect, discuss, evaluate, and learn about a range of assessments. Practise by assessing your peer group.
- Balance demonstration of outcomes for commissioners and having quality interaction to demonstrate person-centred care.
- Have a 'go to' resource to identify appropriate assessment and measures such as Asher's book (2014) and McDowell's (2006).

Alison J. Laver-Fawcett and Diane L. Cox (March 2021).

TABLE 1 Assessment and outcome measures themes and requirements (@OTalk, Feb 2019).

Theme	Requirements and needs
Humans are complex	Need to use complex skills & knowledge in assessment
People's abilities, strengths, deficits, and occupation are different	Individualised person-centred assessments
Assessment results inform therapy goals	Person-centred approach
Information needed on the person and their social and physical environment (s)	Build a picture of person and environment
People's abilities and needs can change	A toolkit of assessments for different purposes
Identifying the person's priorities and needs	Asking questions to gain an understanding of the person
Information needed from other people and services in the person's life	Information gathering across their network
Need for reassessment and measuring change	Assessment that can be repeated and used as an outcome measure
Need for a baseline measurement	Measure change over time
Specificity and sensitivity of an assessment	Consider the expected level of change or maintenance of ability
Assessment to meet individual needs	Assessment tool right fit for that person or location (home, work, school, play)
"Hearing the individual's voice" – valuing their desired goals	Comprehensive assessment to consider past, present, and future
Reliability and Validity of the assessments and measures	Standardised assessments and outcome measures Suggestions included: • Therapy Outcome Measure (TOMS)/ AUS-TOMS • Goal Attainment Scaling (GAS) • Stroke Efficacy Scale
Enable engagement of the individual through narrative, self-report, and self-rating	Flexible approach and time to allow discussion
Type of assessment • Descriptive • Discriminative • Predictive • Evaluative • Combination	Link to International Classification of Function (ICF) (World Health Organisation, 2001)
Visual changes	Use of photographs and video – outcome and feedback to person

Acknowledgements

There are many people we would like to thank that have supported this 2nd edition of Alison's original 2007 book. We are grateful to both our universities, York St John University and University of Cumbria, for giving us the dedicated study time to enable the focussed writing.

We would like to thank the therapists who contributed case study examples integrated within the chapters, for sharing their practice, expertise, and insights. We would like to thank the therapists who contributed the case studies for the first edition, some of which have been updated and edited for this edition.

Alison and Diane met while working at the then Wandsworth Health Authority, now St George's NHS Foundation Trust, in the mid-1980s, and they have continued to work together on several projects and presentations since then. We are particularly grateful to Beryl Steeden, the then District Occupational Therapy lead, for having the vision to create a funded occupational therapy research post, which both Diane and Alison undertook, Diane looking at the development and impact of one of the first Cardiac Rehabilitation Programmes and Alison working on the development of the Structured Observational Test of Function (SOTOF).

We thank the @OTalk team for enabling us to lead two Twitter chats related to assessment and outcome measurement during the period when we were planning this 2nd edition and the therapists who participated in these Twitter dialogues.

Introduction

OVERVIEW

This introduction discusses and defines the key terminology to be used in the text, including assessment, evaluation, outcome, and measurement. It provides a review of definitions for key terms used in everyday therapy practice, research, and evaluation. It concludes by presenting the definitions of these key terms that have been developed or selected as a foundation for this text.

QUESTIONS TO CONSIDER

1. What are the differences between assessment, evaluation, and outcome measurement?
2. What key terms do you need to be familiar with?

This book is written for allied health professionals (*AHPs*). In exploring assessment and outcome measurement within these professions, it is critical to understand what AHPs are trying to achieve in their practice (Slade et al. 2018). The major goal of AHPs is to help people to maximise their potential by reducing the impact of any impairments and limiting the resulting disability and/or handicap. AHPs work with people, helping them obtain their highest levels of activity and participation to enhance their quality of life. When a person has a progressive or terminal illness, the goal may be to maintain function for as long as possible and reduce the negative impact of pathology on quality of life. Therefore, the major objective of assessment is to gain a clear picture of the individual to develop an intervention plan that will result in improved, or maintained, function, participation, and enhanced quality of life. AHPs strive to ensure that these interventions are effective, efficient, and economical, thus providing quality services to clients and their carers. AHPs need to use outcome measures to evaluate the effects of their interventions and to establish if therapy goals have been met.

As well as managing impairments, disabilities and participation restrictions, AHPs bridge the gap between the medical and nursing professions, advocate for patients and their families, and foster inter-professional teams and multidisciplinary care.

There are 14 Allied Health Professions (AHPs) working in a wide range of settings including hospitals, health centres, peoples' own homes, schools, residential facilities, supported housing, social enterprise, charities, industry, and work environments (NHS England 2019). Throughout this text, the term AHPs will mainly be

Principles of Assessment and Outcome Measurement for Allied Health Professionals:
Practice, Research and Development, Second Edition. Alison J. Laver-Fawcett and Diane L. Cox.
© 2021 John Wiley & Sons Ltd. Published 2021 by John Wiley & Sons Ltd.

used. The terms patient, client, service user, and person will be used interchangeably throughout the text to indicate a recipient of services.

- The word *patient* stems from the Latin word *pati*, which means 'to suffer' and is still used in medical settings such as inpatient hospital care (Turner 2002, p. 355).
- In community settings the term *client* is more frequently used, but like Turner (2002), we feel the derivation of this word from the Latin *cluere* which means 'to obey' or 'hear' does not reflect concepts of person-centred working, which are becoming more prominent in therapy literature (Mroz et al. 2015).
- An emphasis on the rights of people receiving healthcare, and the move away from viewing patients as passive recipients of care, has led to the use of the term *service user* (Turner 2002). A service user is defined as a person who uses healthcare and/or social care services from service providers (NHS England 2020).

Turner (2002) recommended that, as proponents of partnership and person-centred working, we should use the terms *people* and *person*, as opposed to client or patient. Where the context allows and the meaning is clear in this book, the term *person* will be used to denote the recipient of services (Edvardsson 2015). In some instances, the term *carer* will be used to differentiate between the person taking part in the assessment and intervention, and a person who provides care/support to the recipient of health or social care. The term will be used in the context of the Department of Health's (DoH 2001) definition of a carer as 'a person, usually a relative or friend, who provides care on a voluntary basis implicit in relationships between family members' (p. 153).

THE IMPORTANCE OF THE SELECTION AND APPLICATION OF TERMINOLOGY IN PRACTICE

It is important to begin a book on assessment and outcome measurement with clear definitions of the key terminology to be used within the text. However, this is far from a simple exercise. Assessment, evaluation, scales, outcome, measurement, and outcome measurement mean different things to different people (Stokes and O'Neill 1999). The selection and application of terms to describe AHP practices is important because the language that we use gives our practice a public face and enables us to share ideas and information. In the area of assessment and measurement, AHPs need to obtain a clear understanding of what is meant by regularly used terms in order to communicate effectively about the assessment process and outcomes with service users and their carers, other professionals, referral sources, discharge destinations, managers, and policy developers.

DEFINITIONS OF KEY TERMS

Assessment

There are numerous definitions of assessment in the health and social care literature. The Department of Health (DoH 2001) has defined assessment as 'a process whereby the needs of an individual are identified and quality of life is evaluated' (p. 151). The

English Oxford Living Dictionary (2019) defines 'assess' as 'fix amount of and impose (on person or community); ... estimate magnitude or quality of'. In healthcare, the term *to assess* refers to the professional identifying, describing, and/or validating information. Assessment can be a process by which data are gathered, hypotheses formulated, and decisions made for further action. As an AHP, you gather information to understand what is currently important and meaningful to the person (their wants and needs) and to identify past experiences and interests that may assist in the understanding of their current issues and problems (Christiansen et al. 2005). The Royal College of Physicians (2012) suggested that assessment includes both the 'collection of data and the interpretation of those data' to inform decision making (Table 1.1, p. 11). Some themes about the nature of assessment that emerge in health and social care literature are the following:

- Assessment is a process.
- Assessment involves multiple methods of obtaining and interpreting information/data.
- Information obtained through assessment enables AHPs to decide whether therapy is required, set a baseline for intervention, and evaluate the results of that intervention.
- Assessment is a process that encompasses evaluation and measurement of outcomes.

For the purposes of this book, assessment is defined as follows:

Definition of Assessment

Assessment is the overall process of selecting and using multiple data collection tools and various sources of information to inform decisions required for guiding the negotiation of outcomes, setting goals, and selecting appropriate interventions. Assessment involves interpreting information collected from informal methods, dynamic assessment, and/or standardised tests to make clinical decisions related to the person's needs and management. Assessment involves the evaluation of the outcomes of treatments/interventions.

Evaluation

Jacobs (1993) noted that 'often, the term assessment is incorrectly thought to be synonymous with evaluation' and goes on to describe that 'assessment encompasses evaluation as one of its ... phases' (p. 228). The word *evaluation* is a noun, and related words used by AHPs include: to evaluate (verb); and evaluative (adjective). Corr (2003) stated that 'a service might be very good, but without evaluation its value diminishes because there is no objective measure of it being "very good" ...' (p. 235). The Heath Foundation (2015) adopted the definition of evaluation as:

- The process of determining the merit, worth, or value of something
- Using systematic, data-based inquiries about whatever is being evaluated
- A process undertaken for purposes of improvement, decision making, enlightenment, persuasion.

Some ideas about evaluation that appear in the health and social care literature are the following:

- Evaluation involves examining or judging the amount or value of something.
- Evaluation can be viewed as a sub-component of a broader assessment process.
- Evaluation is undertaken to enable an AHP to make a clinical judgement about the person or a judgement about the value of the service provided.
- Evaluation of outcomes requires re-examination, so an AHP has to obtain the same information/data on two occasions to evaluate any change in the outcome of interest.
- Evaluation can involve expressing something numerically.

For the purposes of this book evaluation is defined as follows:

Definition of Evaluation

Evaluation is a component of a broader assessment process. Evaluation involves the collection of data to enable an AHP to make a judgement about the amount of a specific construct of interest (such as degree of range of movement, or level of independence in an activity of daily living). Evaluation can require an AHP to make a judgement about the value of an intervention for delivering the desired outcome for a person, or the value of a service for delivering outcomes of relevance to the service user population. Evaluation often involves data being collected at two time points to measure effect and can involve the translation of observations to numerical scores.

Scale

Within the literature, you will see the terms *scale, rating scales,* and *measurement scales.* The word *scale* appears in a lot of standardised health and therapy tests, for example, the Beck Scale for Suicide Ideation (Beck and Steer 1991). So, what do AHPs mean by the word *scale*? The *English Oxford Living Dictionary* (2019) defines a scale as 'a graduated range of values forming a standard system for measuring or grading something'. Therefore, a scale provides a means of recording something that might be defined in terms of levels, amounts, or degrees, and it may also involve numbers. *Scaling* is the measurement of a variable in such a way that it can be expressed on a continuum. Rating your preference for a product from 1 to 10 is an example of a scale. With *comparative scaling*, the items are directly compared with each other: for example, do you prefer the colour blue or red? In *non-comparative scaling*, each item is scaled independently of the others: for example: how do you feel about the colour red? (Streiner et al. 2015).

The Department of Health (2005) stated that 'a scale is a means of identifying the presence and/or severity of a particular problem, such as depression or difficulties with personal care. It is important that scales are used in support of professional judgement, and are valid, reliable and culturally sensitive. A scale is valid if it actually measures what it is supposed to measure. It is reliable if trust can be placed on it when used by different assessors or over time. A scale is culturally sensitive, if questions and the interpretation of responses are not prejudiced against people from specific cultures and backgrounds' (DoH 2005).

Ideas about scales that appear in health and social care literature are as follows:

- A scale provides a means of recording something that might be defined in terms of levels, amounts, or degrees.
- In healthcare settings, scales often are used to rate the presence or severity of a problem, for example, a symptom or the level of independence in a daily activity, such as personal care.
- Scales may also involve the use of numbers assigned as scores.

There is an accepted categorisation of scales into four levels of measurement. Stevens (1946) described a well-accepted and used model of four levels of measurement scales that differ in the extent to which their scale values retain the properties of the real number line. The four levels are called nominal, ordinal, interval, and ratio scales (see Chapter 4 for details).

For the purposes of this book, a scale and the term scaling are defined as follows:

Definition of Scale`

A scale provides a means of recording something that can be rated in terms of levels, amounts, or degrees. AHPs use scales to rate the presence or severity of a problem, such as a symptom, or to rate the person's level of independence in a needed or chosen occupation, activity or task. Scales can be categorised into one of four levels of measurement as defined by Stevens (1946): nominal, ordinal, interval, or ratio. Numbers are frequently assigned as scores in scales. How these numerical scores can be used and interpreted depends upon the level of measurement used in the scale.

Definition of Comparative Scaling

With comparative scaling, items being rated are directly compared with each other in some way, items might be rated in terms of which are the best, or the most difficult, or the most frequently occurring, or the preferred option (for example: Do you prefer coffee or tea?)

Definition of Non-comparative Scaling

With non-comparative scaling, each item in the scale is rated/scored independently of all the other items. This might be in terms of how well the item can be performed, or how frequently the item occurs, or how the person feels about that item. For example, how well can you get dressed? How often do you go out with friends?

Other terms used in a similar context are *instrument, index, indices, typology*, and *profile*. These terms appear in the literature and are also used in the titles of some standardised health and therapy tests. For example:

- *Barthel Index* (Mahoney and Barthel 1965)
- *Caregiver Strain Index* (Robinson 1983)
- *Capabilities of Upper Extremity Instrument* (Marino et al. 1998)
- *Functional Assessment of Multiple Sclerosis Quality of Life Instrument* (*FAMS*; Cella et al. 1996)
- *Physiotherapy Functional Mobility Profile* (Platt et al. 1998)
- *Abbreviated Functional Limitations Profile (UK) SIP68* (de Bruin et al. 1994).

An **instrument** is a tool or device that is used to perform a particular task, measuring something such as speed, height, or sound. An **Index** is a system by which changes in the value of something and the rate at which it changes can be recorded, measured, or interpreted. According to the *English Oxford Living Dictionary* (2019), an index is:

- 'Something that serves to guide, point out, or otherwise facilitate reference', for example 'an alphabetized list of names, places, and subjects treated in a printed work, giving the page or pages on which each item is mentioned'
- 'Something that reveals or indicates; a sign", for example, her facial expression was a fair index of her mood'
- 'An indicator or pointer, as on a scientific instrument'.

Indexes are similar to scales except that multiple indicators of a variable are combined into a single measure. The index of consumer confidence, for example, is a combination of several measures of consumer attitudes.

A **typology** is like an index except that the variable is measured at the nominal level (any numbers used in a nominal scale are mere labels that express no mathematical properties).

The word **indices** is the plural of index, and describes the compilation of multiple similar or related performance measures/metrics (Sackett et al. 1977). Indices are generally used to link related issues, to evaluate interrelated leading or lagging performance indicators, or to reduce the total number of measures to a manageable number.

The word **profile** has multiple definitions, but in relation to measurement it is defined by the *English Oxford Living Dictionary* (2019) as 'a graphical or other representation of information relating to particular characteristics of something, recorded in quantified form: record of a person's psychological or behavioural characteristics, and preferences'. For example, the *Nottingham Health Profile* (*NHP*; Hunt et al. 1985) is a patient-completed questionnaire to determine and quantify perceived health problems. It covers sleep, mobility, energy, pain, emotional reactions, social isolation, and specific aspects of daily life such as employment, household chores, social life, relationships, sex life, and hobbies; so the NHP provides a summary of the person's health profile.

Outcome

The term *outcome* is used often in health and social care, therapy and rehabilitation literature, so it is an important term to understand. An outcome is a measurable end result or consequence of a specific action, treatment, or intervention. Abrams et al. (2006) suggested that AHP services can only be considered valuable if they provide demonstrable benefits, and this is achieved by measuring outcomes to evaluate the effectiveness of the interventions provided.

An outcome can be the:

- consequence of some sort of action or occurrence,
- result of an intervention, or
- observed and/or measured change, for example in the person's function or symptom.

It is critical for AHPs to understand the differences between:

- a [person's] *desired outcome*,
- the *pre-determined outcomes* that a service is expected to deliver', for example, 'as described in a service level agreement or commissioning contract,
- the *negotiated outcome* between a [person] and therapist, as articulated in a goal, and
- the *actual outcome*, which is the measured effect of a specific intervention or the effects of a multidisciplinary or interagency management plan ...' (Laver-Fawcett 2013, p. 604).

For the purposes of this book, outcome is defined as follows:

Definition of Outcome

An outcome is the observed or measured consequence of an action or occurrence. In a therapeutic process, the outcome is the result of the therapeutic intervention.

Measurement

The verb 'to measure' has a few different meanings including:

- 'ascertain extent or quantity of (thing) by comparison with fixed unit or with object of known size
- ascertain size and proportions of (person) for clothes
- ... estimate (quality, person's character, etc.) by some standard or rule
- take measurements
- be of specified size
- have necessary qualification for' (Sykes 1983).

In the *National Clinical Guidelines for Stroke* (Royal College of Physicians 2012), measurement is defined as the 'comparison of data against some standard or "metric", in order to give the data an absolute relative meaning' (p. 11). Streiner et al. (2015) suggested '... the evidence of the value of an instrument is to demonstrate that measurements of individuals on different occasions, or by different observers, or by similar or parallel tests, produce the same or similar results' (p. 9).

Measurement and assessment are linked, but are not the same. Concepts about measurement in health and social care literature indicate the following:

- Measurement is a component of a wider assessment process.
- A measurement is the data obtained by measuring.
- The assessment provides a context for understanding the relevance of measures obtained.
- Measuring is used to ascertain the dimensions (size), quantity (amount), or capacity of an aspect of the person.

- Measurement involves assigning numbers to represent quantities of a trait, attribute, or characteristic or to classify objects.
- A measurement is obtained by applying a standardised scale to variables to provide a numerical score.

For the purposes of this book, measurement is defined as follows:

Definition of Measurement

A measurement is the data obtained by measuring. Measuring is undertaken by AHPs to ascertain the dimensions (size), quantity (amount), or capacity of a trait, attribute, or characteristic of a person that is required by the therapist to develop an accurate picture of the person's needs and problems in order to form a baseline for therapeutic intervention and/or to provide a measure of outcome. A measurement is obtained by applying a standardised scale to variables, thus translating direct observations or patient/proxy reports to a numerical scoring system.

Outcome Measures

Outcome measurement is essential to establish the effectiveness of an intervention or the overall effectiveness of a service. Skinner and Turner-Stokes (2006) reported that outcome measures were increasingly used in routine practice; however, outcome measures have yet to be universally embedded in AHP services (e.g. Duncan and Murray 2012). The thoughtful, strategic, and informed use of outcome measures will help AHPs to support and sustain their valuable contribution to patient care and also aid in demonstrating how AHPs fulfil governments' health and social care policies (Moore 2016). Outcome measurement should be a priority in clinical practice, and 'sufficient time should be allocated to enable outcome measurement to occur' (Duncan and Murray 2012, p. 6).

Cole et al. (1995) defined an outcome measure as 'a measurement tool (instrument, questionnaire, rating form etc.) used to document change in one or more patient characteristic over time' (p. 22) and stated that outcome measures are used to evaluate services. The Royal College of Occupational Therapists (2017) defined an outcome measure as a tool to measure or quantify change. An initial assessment provides the baseline against which a later measurement can be compared when considering the outcome for the service user. A robust outcome measure is required to take these pre- and post-intervention measurements in a standardised, valid, and reliable way. The desired outcome might be an improvement or the maintenance of some area of function; therefore, change is not always the object of intervention, and 'outcome measures need to be sensitive to protective and preventive effects as well as to improvements' (Heaton and Bamford 2001, p. 347). It is important to note that 'clinical outcome measures in general, document change over time but do not explain why the change has occurred' (Cole et al. 1995, p. vi). So, AHPs also need to include in their overall assessment process methods for exploring the mechanisms underlying a desired or observed change.

In summary, outcome measures:

- are used to document change in one or more trait, attribute, or characteristic over time,

- establish whether the desired outcome (the therapy goals or objectives agreed prior to therapeutic intervention) have been achieved, and
- need to be sensitive to the type and degree of anticipated change.

For the purposes of this book, an outcome measure and measurement are defined as follows:

Definition of Outcome Measure

An outcome measure is a standardised instrument used by AHPs to establish whether their desired therapeutic outcomes have been achieved.

Definition of Outcome Measurement

Outcome measurement is a process undertaken to establish the effects of an intervention on an individual or the effectiveness of a service on a defined aspect of the health or well-being of a specified population. Outcome measurement is achieved by administering an outcome measure on at least two occasions to document change over time in one or more trait, attribute, or characteristic to establish whether that trait/attribute/characteristic has been influenced by the intervention to the anticipated degree to achieve the desired outcome.

Figure I.1 illustrates how assessment is the whole data gathering and interpreting process, within which evaluation and outcome measurement is nested.

Table I.1 summarises the key terms of assessment, evaluation, outcome, and outcome measurement.

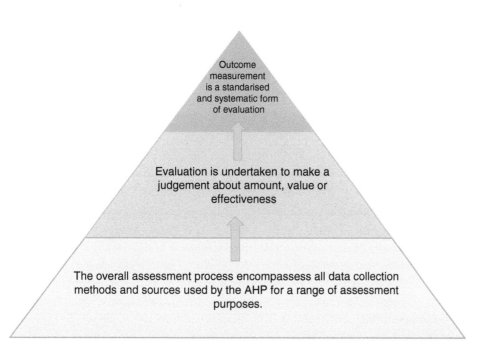

FIGURE I.1   Relationship between assessment, evaluation, and outcome measurement. *Source*: Adapted from Laver-Fawcett 2013; Figure 18.2, p. 605.

TABLE I.1   Definitions of assessment, evaluation, outcome and outcome measure.

Term	Definition
Assessment	Assessment is a process involving the selection and application of a range of informal and standardised methods: interview, observation, questionnaires, dynamic assessment, and document review. To collect information from relevant sources (the person, carers, and other staff) in order to provide a profile, understand the person's skills and needs, and inform the negotiation of outcomes, setting of goals, and selection of therapeutic interventions. Assessment involves the ongoing review of the person, their occupations and environments, and the evaluation of the outcomes of interventions and packages of care.
Evaluation	Evaluation is a component of a broader assessment process. Data is collected to inform judgements about amount, degrees, or levels of a specific construct, component, or characteristic such as level of independence or to make a judgement about the degree to which an intervention has achieved the planned outcomes for a person or a group of people. Evaluation usually requires data to be collected at two time points in order to measure change over time. Evaluation may involve the translation of observations to numerical scores.
Outcome	An outcome is the measured or observed consequence of an action. It is of paramount importance for AHPs to differentiate between 1. a person's *desired outcome*; 2. the *pre-determined outcomes* that a service is expected to deliver (as described in a service level agreement or commissioning contract); 3. the *negotiated outcome* between a client and AHP, as articulated in a goal; and 4. the *actual outcome*, which is the measured effects of a specific intervention or the effects of a multidisciplinary or inter-agency management plan for the person.
Outcome measurement	Outcome measurement is required to establish the effectiveness of an intervention for an individual or the effectiveness of an overall service for a population. Outcome measurement is undertaken by administering an outcome measure on at least two occasions to evaluate change over time in order to establish whether the intervention has achieved the anticipated outcome.

Source: Laver-Fawcett 2013, p. 604. © 2003, Cengage Learning, Inc.

REFERENCES

Abrams, D., Davidson, M., Harrick, J. et al. (2006). Monitoring the change: current trends in outcome measure usage in physiotherapy. *Manual Therapy* 11 (1): 46–53. https://doi.org/10.1016/j.math.2005.02.003 (accessed 7 September 2020).

Beck, A.T. and Steer, R.A. (1991). *Manual for the Beck Scale for Suicide Ideation (BBS)*. London: The Psychological Corporation.

de Bruin, A.F., Diederiks, J.P.M., de Witte, L.P. et al. (1994). The development of a short generic version of the sickness impact profile. *Journal of Clinical Epidemiology* 47: 407–418. https://doi.org/10.1016/0895-4356(94)90162-7 (accessed 8 September 2020).

Cella, D.F., Dineen, K., Arnason, B., Reder, A., Webster, K.A., Karabatsos, G., Chang, C., Lloyd, S., Mo, F., Stewart, J. and Stefoski, D. (1996). Validation of the functional assessment of multiple sclerosis quality of life instrument. *Neurology* 47(1): 129–139. doi:https://doi.org/10.1212/WNL.47.1.129 (accessed 7 September 2020).

Christiansen, C., Baum, C.M., Bass-Haugen, J., and Bass, J.D. (eds.) (2005). *Occupational Therapy: Performance, Participation, and Well-Being*. Thorofare, NJ: Slack Incorporated.

Cole, B., Finch, E., Gowland, C., and Mayo, N. (1995). *Physical Rehabilitation Outcome Measures*. London: Williams and Wilkins.

Corr, S. (2003). Evaluate, evaluate, evaluate. *British Journal of Occupational Therapy* 66 (6): 235. https://doi.org/10.1177/030802260306600601 (accessed 7 September 2020).

Department of Health (DoH); 2001) National Service Framework for Older People. London: Department of Health. https://www.gov.uk/government/publications/quality-standards-for-care-services-for-older-people (accessed 8 September 2020).

Department of Health (DoH) (2005). *Single Assessment Process (SAP) Annex E: Stages of assessment*. London: Department of Health.

Duncan, E.A. and Murray, J. (2012). The barriers and facilitators to routine outcome measurement by allied health professionals in practice: a systematic review. *BMC Health Services Research* 12 (1): 96. https://doi.org/10.1186/1472-6963-12-96 (accessed 8 September 2020).

Edvardsson, D. (2015). Notes on person-centred care: what it is and what it is not. *Nordic Journal of Nursing Research* 35 (2): 65–66. https://doi.org/10.1177/0107408315582296 (accessed 8 September 2020).

NHS England (2019). Allied Health Professions. https://www.england.nhs.uk/ahp (accessed 7 September 2020).

NHS England (2020). Involving people in their own care. https://www.england.nhs.uk/ourwork/patient-participation (accessed 8 September 2020).

English Oxford Living Dictionary (2019). https://en.oxforddictionaries.com (accessed 1 April 2019).

Health Foundation (2015). Evaluation: what to consider Commonly asked questions about how to approach evaluation of quality improvement in health care. www.health.org.uk/sites/default/files/EvaluationWhatToConsider.pdf (accessed 8 September 2020).

Heaton, J. and Bamford, C. (2001). Assessing the outcomes of equipment and adaptations: issues and approaches. *British Journal of Occupational Therapy* 64 (7): 346–356. https://doi.org/10.1177/030802260106400705 (accessed 8 September 2020).

Hunt, S.M., McEwen, J., and McKenna, S.P. (1985). Measuring health status: a new tool for clinicians and epidemiologists. *The Journal of the Royal College of General Practitioners* 35 (273): 185–188.

Jacobs, K. (1993). Occupational therapy performance areas: section 2B1 work assessments and programming. In: *Willard & Spackman's Occupational Therapy*, 8e (eds. H.L. Hopkins and H.D. Smith), 226–248. Philadelphia: Lippincott.

Laver-Fawcett, A. (2013). Assessment, Evaluation and Outcome Measurement. In: *Psychosocial Occupational Therapy: An Evolving Practice*, 3e (eds. E. Cara and A. MacRae), 600–642. Clifton Park, NY: Delmar Cengage Learning.

Mahoney, F. and Barthel, D. (1965). Functional evaluation: the Barthel index. *Maryland State Medical Journal* 14: 61–65.

Marino, R.J., Shea, J.A., and Stineman, M.G. (1998). The cpabilities of upper extremity instrument: reliability and validity of a measure of functional limitation in tetraplegia. *Archives of Physical Medicine and Rehabilitation* 79: 1512–1521. https://doi.org/10.1016/S0003-9993(98)90412-9 (accessed 8 September 2020).

Moore, A.P. (2016). Outcome measurement in clinical practice. In: *Managing Money, Measurement and Marketing in the Allied Health Professions* (eds. R. Jones and F. Jenkins), 131–141. London: CRC Press.

Mroz, T.M., Pitonyak, J.S., Fogelberg, D., and Leland, N.E. (2015). Client centeredness and health reform: key issues for occupational therapy. *American Journal of*

Occupational Therapy 69 (5): 1–8. https://doi.org/10.5014/ajot.2015.695001 (accessed 8 September 2020).

Platt, W., Bell, B., and Kozak, J. (1998). Functional mobility profile: a tool for measuring functional outcome in chronic care clients. *Physiotherapy Canada* 50 (1): 47–74.

Robinson, B.C. (1983). Validation of a caregiver strain index. *Journal of Gerontology* 38 (3): 344–348. https://doi.org/10.1093/geronj/38.3.344 (accessed 8 September 2020).

Royal College of Occupational Therapists (2017). *Research Guide: Measuring Outcomes*. London: Royal College of Occupational Therapists www.rcot.co.uk/sites/default/files/Research%20Guide%20-%20Measuring%20Outcomes%20June%20%202017.pdf (accessed 8 September 2020).

Royal College of Physicians and Intercollegiate Stroke Working Party (2012). *National Clinical Guideline for Stroke*, 4e. London: Royal College of Physicians https://www.strokeaudit.org/Guideline/Historical-Guideline/National-Clinical-Guidelines-for--Stroke-fourth-edi.aspx (accessed 8 September 2020).

Sackett, D.L., Chambers, L.W., MacPherson, A.S. et al. (1977). The development and application of indices of health: general methods and a summary of results. *American Journal of Public Health* 67 (5): 423–428. https://ajph.aphapublications.org/doi/abs/10.2105/AJPH.67.5.423 (accessed 8 September 2020).

Skinner, A. and Turner-Stokes, L. (2006). The use of standardized outcome measures in rehabilitation centres in the UK. *Clinical Rehabilitation* 20 (7): 609–615. https://doi.org/10.1191/0269215506cr981oa (accessed 8 September 2020).

Slade, S.C., Philip, K., and Morris, M.E. (2018). Frameworks for embedding a research culture in allied health practice: a rapid review. *Health Research Policy and Systems* 16 (1): 1–15. https://health-policy-systems.biomedcentral.com/track/pdf/10.1186/s12961-018-0304-2 (accessed 8 September 2020).

Stevens, S.S. (1946). On the theory of scales of measurement. *Science* 103: 677–680.

Stokes, E.K. and O'Neill, D. (1999). The use of standardised assessments by physiotherapists. *British Journal of Therapy and Rehabilitation* 6 (11): 560–565. https://doi.org/10.12968/bjtr.1999.6.11.13928 (accessed 8 September 2020).

Streiner, D.L., Norman, G.R., and Cairney, J. (2015). *Health Measurement Scales: A Practical Guide to their Development and Use*, 5e. Oxford: Oxford University Press.

Sykes, J.B. (1983). *The Concise Oxford Dictionary*, 7e. Oxford: Oxford University Press.

Turner, A. (2002). Patient? Client? Service user? What's in a name? *British Journal of Occupational* 65 (8): 355. https://doi.org/10.1177/030802260206500801 (accessed 8 September 2020).

SUGGESTED RESOURCES

NHS Health Research Authority (2019). Outcome Measures https://www.hra.nhs.uk/planning-and-improving-research/best-practice/outcome-measures (accessed 8 September 2020).

University of Birmingham (2020). Centre for Patient Reported Outcomes www.birmingham.ac.uk/research/activity/applied-health/research/prolearn/index.aspx (accessed 8 September 2020).

Ustun, T.B., Kostanjesek, N., Chatterji, S. et al. (2010). *Measuring Health and Disability: Manual for WHO Disability Assessment Schedule (WHODAS 2.0)* (eds. T.B. ÜstÜn, N. Kostanjsek, S. Chatterji and J. Rehm). Geneva: World Health Organization http://www.who.int/iris/handle/10665/43974 (accessed 8 September 2020).

ASSESSMENT AND MEASUREMENT IN PRACTICE

CHAPTER 1

The Importance of Accurate Assessment and Outcome Measurement

OVERVIEW

This chapter focuses on the requirement of allied health professionals (AHPs) to undertake thorough and accurate assessment and measurement. Developments and policy directions in health and social care practice in recent years include:

- a demand for evidence-based practice;
- a shift towards the use of standardised assessments;
- a requirement to measure outcomes and demonstrate effectiveness;
- a focus on person-centred practice;
- a demand for robust governance and audit activities;
- and the use of standards, care pathways, protocols, and guidelines.

The chapter discusses some of the advantages and limitations of standardised versus non-standardised tests. We also explore the complexity of assessment, including the challenges of measuring human behaviour and the impact of the environment, and reflect upon how such complexities influence what can be measured and the adequacy of these measurements.

QUESTIONS TO CONSIDER

What is the relationship between assessment, evaluation, and outcome measurement?

What is evidence-based practice?

How do you track down the best evidence?

What is the difference between a standardised and non-standardised assessment?

What is the difference between a standard, a guideline, and a protocol?

How does human function influence assessment and outcome measurement?

ASSESSMENT AS A CORE PART OF THE THERAPY PROCESS

Assessment is a core component of health and social care. We defined **assessment** in the *Introduction* as the overall process of selecting and using multiple data collection tools and various sources of information to inform decisions required for guiding therapeutic intervention during the whole therapy process. Assessment involves interpreting information collected to make clinical decisions related to the needs of the person, the appropriateness and nature of our interventions, and the evaluation of the outcomes.

Assessment is an essential part of a quality service and the health care process, and is central to the management of any disability. The health care process has been described as (Austin and Clark 1993, p. 21):

1. a needs analysis of the client;
2. identification of what service needs to be provided;
3. identification of the provider of the service;
4. provision of the service;
5. evaluation of the service provided.

Assessment is the first step in the health care process and provides the foundation for effective treatment. Assessment occurs again at the end of the health care process in the form of evaluation. Re-assessment is necessary at several stages during the process 'service provision' because without thorough and accurate assessment the intervention selected may be inappropriate and/or ineffective (see Figure 1.1).

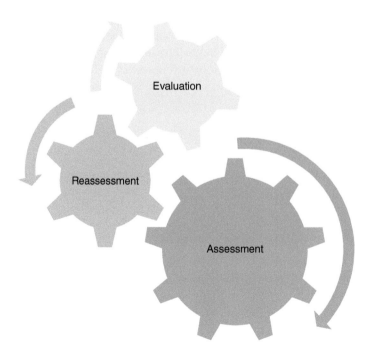

FIGURE 1.1   The relationship between assessment, reassessment and evaluation.

THE IMPACT OF HEALTH AND SOCIAL CARE POLICY ON ASSESSMENT PRACTICE

The organisational and policy context for health and social care has been under frequent change and reform, particularly over the past two decades. In recent years, the provision of health and social care has been exposed to a more market-oriented approach in which government fundholders, commissioners, and organisations that procure therapy services have become more concerned about 'value for money' and require assurances that the service provided is both clinically effective and cost-effective. The demand for cost-effective health care is obliging AHPs to be able to prove the efficacy and efficiency of their interventions. In the current policy context that focuses on cost-effectiveness, quality, standards, value, and evidence-based practice (EBP) the ability to demonstrate service outcomes has become increasingly important (Rycroft-Malone 2004; Rycroft-Malone et al. 2004). In 2014, Greenhalgh cautioned us to return to real evidence-based [medicine] practice, characterised by expert judgement and shared decision making (Greenhalgh, Howick, and Maskrey 2014).

An emphasis on clinical governance means that therapists are more overtly responsible for the quality of their practice and this is reflected in an increase of evidence-based practice (Veenstra et al. 2017). AHPs need to be aware of the reasons that drive their practice, it is only reasonable to be influenced by financial and political drivers when the resultant change in practice yields true benefits for service users. Unsworth (2000) noted 'pressures to document outcomes and demonstrate the efficacy of occupational therapy intervention arise from fiscal restraints as much as from the humanitarian desire to provide the best quality health care to consumers. However, measuring outcomes is important in facilitating mutual goal setting, increasing the focus of therapy on the client, monitoring client progress, as well as demonstrating that therapy is valuable' (p. 147).

THE DEMAND FOR EVIDENCE-BASED PRACTICE

Evidence-based practice is commonly referred to as EBP. AHPs should explicitly be working towards achieving EBP in all areas of their practice. EBP has developed from work on evidence-based medicine (EBM), EBP expands the concept of EBM to apply across all health care professionals. *So what is evidence-based medicine?* EBM has been defined as:

> *the conscientious, explicit, and judicious use of current best evidence in making decisions about the care of individual patients. The practice of evidence based medicine means integrating individual clinical expertise with the best available external clinical evidence from systematic research.*
>
> (Sackett et al. 1996, p. 71)

Sackett and his colleagues further described 'individual clinical expertise' as the 'proficiency and judgment that individual clinicians acquire through clinical experience and clinical practice'. They stated that a clinician's increasing expertise can be demonstrated in a number of ways 'especially in more effective and efficient diagnosis and in the more thoughtful identification and compassionate use of individual patients' predicaments, rights, and preferences in making clinical decisions about their care'.

SO WHAT IS EVIDENCE-BASED PRACTICE?

EBP focuses on making the best decisions for each client and using the best information available (Law and MacDermid 2014). The knowledge and use of evidence-based practice by AHPs in the United Kingdom (UK) can differ across the professions (Upton and Upton 2006). Driever (2002) and Rycroft-Malone et al. (2004) have suggested that evidence needs to be drawn from multiple sources such as standards, evaluation data, research, clinical experience, patient experience, values and circumstances, and the local practice context. Engaging in practices that are driven solely by research evidence and/or by organisational factors, are at odds with the intent of EBP as outlined by the founders, and could shape the AHP's practice, outside of a professions philosophy, and the client's needs (Gustafsson, Molineux, and Bennett 2014). To identify the best available external evidence AHPs need to seek relevant research, and should particularly seek patient-centred clinical research into the accuracy and precision of standardised tests and the efficacy of therapeutic interventions. When new evidence is acknowledged sometimes it can invalidate previously accepted tests and treatments. AHPs are beholden to replace old unsubstantiated practices with evidence-based practices that are more effective, more accurate, more efficacious, and safer (Sackett et al. 1996).

IMPLEMENTATION OF EVIDENCE-BASED PRACTICE

In practice, implementing EBP may be difficult. There are many potential barriers to its full implementation, including lack of time, lack of access to literature, and lack of skills in finding and interpreting research (Upton and Upton 2006). In a later study by Upton et al. (2012) they demonstrated that newly qualified practitioners have a good understanding and knowledge of EBP, although they need support to translate their knowledge into practice. Some of the strategies that have been suggested for supporting evidence-based practice (Law and MacDermid 2014) include:

- fostering a supportive environment in the workplace for EBP;
- providing continuing education to develop skills in literature searching, critical appraisal, and research methods;
- collaborating/participating in research evaluating therapy interventions;
- participating in or establishing a journal club;
- focusing on reading research articles that have a rigorous study design, or reviews that have been critically appraised;
- accessing evidence-based clinical guidelines.

In order to use evidence it is necessary to undertake a number of tasks, search for and locate the evidence related to a specific clinical question.

- Appraise the evidence collected.
- Store and retrieve the evidence when required.
- Ensure the body of evidence used to inform clinical decisions is kept updated.
- Communicate the findings from the evidence and use these findings in clinical practice (Belsey and Snell 2003).

Greenhalgh et al. (2014) suggested that any evidence must be individualised for the person. They reminded us that evidence-based practice relies on us being able 'to individualise evidence and share decisions through meaningful conversations in the context of a humanistic and professional clinician–patient relationship' (p. 5). Mickan et al. (2019) following a small-scale study suggested that 'a tailored small group EBP education intervention can enhance AHPs' self-efficacy to develop answerable questions, search the literature, critically appraise, apply and evaluate research evidence. Through practicing these behaviours and sharing new learning with their peers, allied health professionals can enhance their capability and motivation to use research evidence to potentially improve clinical practice' (p. 131).

SO HOW DO YOU TRACK DOWN THE BEST EVIDENCE?

In terms of databases, a good place to start is the **Cochrane Library** (https://www.cochranelibrary.com/about/about-cochrane-library#databases [accessed 2 April 2019]), which provides a collection of separate databases. These provide coverage of evidence-based reviews, controlled trials, and clinical answers. The databases are:

1. The Cochrane Database of Systematic Reviews (CDSR)
2. Cochrane Central Register of Controlled Trials (CENTRAL)
3. Cochrane Clinical Answers.

BMJ Best Practice (https://bestpractice.bmj.com/info/toolkit/discuss-ebm/what-is-the-best-evidence-and-how-to-find-it [accessed 2 April 2019]) suggest two further useful ways to find the best evidence available:

1. Pick the best systematic review
2. Read trustworthy guidelines.

PROSPERO is an international prospective register of systematic reviews (https://www.crd.york.ac.uk/prospero [accessed 2 April 2019]) includes structured abstracts of systematic reviews, by the Centre for Reviews and Dissemination in York.

The **Scottish Intercollegiate Guidelines Network** (SIGN) has published many clinical guidelines of relevance to AHPs. These can be accessed at www.sign.ac.uk (accessed 2 April 2019).

LEVELS OF EVIDENCE AND GRADES OF RECOMMENDATIONS

Previously, when examining and reporting on evidence, researchers and clinicians applied a grading system, for example the system proposed by Gray (2001):

- Level I: systematic review of multiple well-designed randomised controlled trials (RCTs). The term meta-analysis is used to describe quantitative approaches to synthesising evidence from multiple randomised controlled trials.
- Level II: one properly designed RCT of appropriate size.
- Level III: well-designed trials without randomisation single group pre–post cohort, time series or matched control studies.
- Level IV: well-designed non-experimental studies from more than one centre or research group.
- Level V: opinions of respected authorities, based on clinical evidence, descriptive studies, or reports of expert committees.

This system has been used in a number of therapy guidelines.

In 2004, the Grading of Recommendations Assessment, Development and Evaluation (GRADE), Working Group (http://www.gradeworkinggroup.org) proposed a system for grading the quality of evidence and the strength of recommendations that can be applied across a wide range of interventions and contexts. The GRADE system offers four levels of evidence quality: high, moderate, low, and very low (Guyatt, Cook, and Haynes 2004; Guyatt et al. 2008a), and classifies recommendations as strong or weak (Guyatt et al. 2008b).

Balshem et al. (2011) further the work of the GRADE working group and explain in detail what evidence is and is not (Table 1.1).

Table 1.2 summarises GRADE's (Balshem et al. 2011) approach to rating the quality of evidence, which begins with the study design (trials or observational studies) and addresses five reasons to possibly rate down the quality of evidence: risk of bias; inconsistency; indirectness; imprecision; publication bias. The table also suggests three reasons to possibly uprate the quality: large effect; dose response; and all plausible residual confounding (p. 404).

Signpost, see *Chapter 10: Selecting and Appraising Assessments and Outcome Measurements.*

The key to using the evidence is the ability to critically appraise it and make decisions as to whether the evidence is robust and whether it applies to your clinical situation and should be used to influence your practice. Critical appraisal has been defined as 'a method of assessing and interpreting the evidence by systematically considering its validity, results and relevance to the area of work considered' (Belsey and Snell 2003, p. 2). Criteria for examining the quality of research studies in order to assess the evidence are provided by Scottish Intercollegiate Guidelines Network (SIGN; www.sign.ac.uk [accessed 20 May 2019]):

- clear aim stated
- appropriate sampling strategy applied
- valid and reliable measurement tools used

TABLE 1.1   Significance of the four levels of evidence.

Quality level	Current definition (2011)	Previous definition (2004)
High	We are very confident that the true effect lies close to that of the estimate of the effect	Further research is very unlikely to change our confidence in the estimate of effect
Moderate	We are moderately confident in the effect estimate: The true effect is likely to be close to the estimate of the effect, but there is a possibility that it is substantially different	Further research is likely to have an important impact on our confidence in the estimate of effect and may change the estimate
Low	Our confidence in the effect estimate is limited: The true effect may be substantially different from the estimate of the effect	Further research is very likely to have an important impact on our confidence in the estimate of effect and is likely to change the estimate
Very low	We have very little confidence in the effect estimate: The true effect is likely to be substantially different from the estimate of effect	Any estimate of effect is very uncertain

Source: Balshem et al. (2011).

TABLE 1.2 GRADE approach to rating the quality of evidence.

Study design	Initial quality of a body of evidence	Lower if	Higher if	Quality of a body of evidence

Randomised trials	High ⟹	Risk of bias
		  −1 Serious
		  −2 Very serious
		Inconsistency
		  −1 Serious
		  −2 Very serious
		Indirectness
		  −1 Serious
		  −2 Very serious
		Imprecision
		  −1 Serious
		  −2 Very serious
		Publication bias
		  −1 Likely
		  −2 Very likely
			Large effect
			  +1 Large
			  +2 Very large
			Dose response
			  +1 Evidence of a gradient
			All plausible residual confounding
			  +1 Would reduce a demonstrated effect
			  +1 Would suggest a spurious effect if no effect was observed
				High (four plus: ⊕⊕⊕⊕)

				Moderate (three plus: ⊕⊕⊕O)
Observational studies	Low ⟹			Low (two plus: ⊕⊕OO)
				Very low (one plus: ⊕OOO)

Source: Balshem et al. (2011).

- adequate literature review provided
- all participants accounted for adequately
- statistical methods described fully and were appropriate
- statistical significance assessed
- outcomes clearly stated
- population similar to the clinical group of interest
- bias addressed.

Assessment is complex and the therapist needs to take many inter-relating factors into consideration. Therefore, assessment requires careful planning and conscious decision making in order to select the optimum assessment strategy for a particular client's needs. It is unlikely that one assessment will be suitable for all people with a particular diagnosis, so the AHP needs to combine the best evidence with a client-centred approach.

REFLECTION POINT

Now we have explored what evidence-based practice is, you can reflect upon your own assessment practice, or the assessment approaches that you have observed whilst on clinical placement if you are a student.

To assist you with reflecting on how much your practice is based on evidence, please turn to 'Worksheet 1.1', which you will find at the end of this chapter.

THE APPLICATION OF STANDARDISED ASSESSMENTS

A standardised assessment 'has a set, unchanging procedure' that the AHP must follow precisely when administering it; standardised assessments also require 'a consistent system for scoring' (RCOT 2020). The use of standardised assessments helps to 'ensure minimal variation in the way [tests are] carried out at different times and by different testers'. Reducing the amount of variation in test administration helps to make a test more reliable when it is applied over time or used by different AHPs. Test scores need to be stable over time and across testers if the results are to be used to measure clinical change in order to evaluate outcomes.

Signpost: For more details about standardisation, see *Chapter 7: Standardisation* and *Chapter 14: Test Development*.

Historically, AHPs have favoured the use of non-standardised assessments, particularly informal interview and unstructured observation (for example of movements, posture, and the observation of activities of daily living). AHPs have adapted existing standardised tests to suit their clinical environment (for example, see Shanahan 1992), with a trend towards the development of assessments on an individual department or service basis. This has the advantage that the assessment process can be tailored to the particular client group and to the practice environment. However, a major limitation is that majority assessments 'home grown' in individual departments are not rigorously standardised, nor are they backed by research that examines their reliability and validity (see Chapters 7 and 8).

Standardisation is defined as: 'made standard or uniform; to be used without variation; suggests an invariable way in which a test is to be used, as well as denoting the extent to which the results of the test may be considered to be both valid and reliable' (Hopkins and Smith 1993, p. 914).

Standardised test/measure/assessment/instrument has been defined as a: 'published measurement tool, designed for a specific purpose in a given population, with detailed instructions provided as to when and how it is to be administered and scored, interpretation of the scores, and results of investigations or reliability and validity' (Cole et al. 1995, p. 22).

In the environment of evidence-based practice, AHPs are being encouraged to utilise more standardised assessments in their practice in order to ensure that their assessments are as valid and reliable as possible and to enable the measurement of outcomes. Previously, many of the standardised tests that AHPs adopted were not developed by AHPs and were 'borrowed' from other fields, such as experimental and clinical psychology (see McFadyen and Pratt 1997). A disadvantage of this practice of 'borrowing' tests from other disciplines was that the tests did not always fit well with AHPs' philosophy and practice and the use of standardised tests was often rejected because they lacked good clinical utility and face validity (see *Chapter 8: Validity and Clinical Utility*). As a result, there was a need for AHPs to develop valid, reliable, sensitive, and clinically useful assessments of people's functional performance (Fisher and Short-DeGraff 1993). The last 20 years have seen developments in AHP research that have led to an increase in the number of standardised assessments that have been developed by AHPs. Clinicians now have a much wider choice of suitable standardised assessments from which to select appropriate measures for their client group.

AHPs have tended to undertake a formal assessment on referral and then informally monitor the person's progress during treatment. With the emphasis on evidence-based practice, it is no longer sufficient for AHPs to undertake one assessment to provide a baseline from which to plan treatment; ongoing evaluative assessment is also required to monitor the effectiveness of intervention in a reliable and sensitive manner.

THE USE OF STANDARDISED VERSUS NON-STANDARDISED ASSESSMENTS

Previously AHPs' assessment tasks and protocols were subjective and decentralised and 'the norms against which the patient's performance was judged was based upon the AHP's testing and treatment experiences with previous patients' (Borg and Bruce 1991, p. 541). As the allied health professions developed and strived to build a more scientific foundation for practice, there was an identified need for assessment processes to become standardised, evidence-based, and more centralised. However, even today a significant proportion of AHPs continue to adopt predominantly non-standardised forms of assessment. *NB: @OTalk data May 2019.*

Historically, several authors (e.g. Eakin 1989; McAvoy 1991) have discussed the trend for AHPs to continually reinvent the wheel in terms of the assessment tools they use. This was and is exemplified by the number of 'home-grown checklists' that clutter our practice, and the tendency to alter standardised assessments rather than identify appropriate AHP measures. There are a number of reasons why AHPs continue to use non-standardised assessments. For example, AHPs have reported the following reasons (Hong 1996; Hatfield and Ogles 2007; Laver 1994; @OTalk, May 2019):

- a lack of suitable standardised assessments;
- poor resources limit their ability to purchase standardised measures;
- limited access to training on the specifics of the assessment leading to difficulty in interpreting scores;
- standardised assessments can be lengthy to administer and AHPs report that they do not have the time or the length of the test makes it too tiring for patients;
- non-standardised assessments are flexible in terms of procedures, settings, and the manner in which the assessment is administered and are, therefore, perceived as being more client-centred;
- non-standardised assessments are seen as useful for observing functional ability in the person's home environment, for addressing the qualitative aspects of performance, and for exploring the dynamics between the client and caregiver.

Neale (2004) described the difficulty with standardised assessments and outcome measures. She reported that, in her work setting comprising a rehabilitation ward and stroke unit, her team 'use the Barthel ADL Index (Mahoney and Barthel 1965) which is completed at the weekly multi-disciplinary meeting . . . but it is not sensitive to the changes we see in patients during rehabilitation . . . the person can have the same score but still be showing marked improvement. We bemoan the Barthel, but the same difficulty arises with the other ADL assessments' (pp. 25–26). She commented on the issue of time: 'using a test takes up at least one treatment session to administer and more time to evaluate' (p. 25).

However, Neale (2004) also provided an example of how the use of a standardised assessment helped to identify a previously undiagnosed deficit:

I have acquired various standardised assessments for the department over the years. I do not use any with every patient. I learnt early that this may mean I miss things – when I first had the Balloons Test (Edgeworth et al. 1998), I practiced on one 'well recovering' stroke patient. Neither she nor I had noticed any indication of inattention in hospital. The test showed she missed the bottom left quadrant – and she subsequently reported the effects when serving food/covering a pie when at home. (p. 25)

Another common practice has been to take different parts of standardised tests or individual test items and integrate these into a 'therapist-constructed' tailored assessment battery for a specific client group or service (Hong 1996). However, once the standard procedure for test administration and scoring has been changed, even in a small way, the reliability and validity of that part of the test or test item can no longer be guaranteed (see Chapters 7 and 8). Therefore, although the test items might have been generated from a standardised test the ensuing 'therapist-made' assessment cannot be viewed as standardised. A further limitation of this practice, of using test items/parts drawn from standardised tests, is that the original source of, or reference for, the test item is rarely recorded on the tailored assessment and forms. This means that, once the AHPs involved in developing the tailored assessment leave the service, the AHPs who replace them are unaware of the original sources and the rationale for the development of the tailored 'therapist-constructed' assessment battery. Consequently, AHPs using inherited 'therapist-constructed' assessments can find it difficult to justify the reasons for carrying out these non-standardised assessments (Hong 1996).

If AHPs are using non-standardised assessments, it is critical that they are fully aware of their limitations. The findings from a non-standardised assessment are open to interpretation and are, therefore, much more subjective than the findings gained from a standardised measure. Furthermore, because detailed procedures for administering and scoring the test are rarely available for non-standardised assessments, it is not possible for the AHP to reliably repeat the assessment with the client in order to evaluate the effects of treatment. It is even more unreliable if another AHP tries to repeat the assessment with the same client at a later time.

AHPs should not underestimate the consequences of continuing to use non-standardised assessments where standardised measures of the same construct or area of function exist. This was demonstrated in a study by Stewart (1999). Stewart compared the results of a non-standardised assessment with a standardised measure of severity of disability in a group of elderly people. The purpose of her study was to examine if there were differences in outcomes and explore the consequences for service entitlement. The results of the study indicated that the non-standardised measure had 'restricted ability to identify and measure accurately the degree of disability of older people' and 'that because of the limited psychometric rigour of the [non-standardized measure] one consequence for service provision may be that a vulnerable group, elderly frail people, are denied services unnecessarily' (p. 422). Stewart concluded that 'when clinical judgement is based on objective assessment arising from the use of standardized instruments rather than intuitive guesswork, occupational therapists' decision making can be seen to be more rational and consequently defensible' (p. 422).

BENEFITS OF APPLYING STANDARDISED MEASURES

The use of improved, appropriate, sensitive, and standardised measures within occupational therapy and physiotherapy research and clinical practice would aid these professions at several different levels (Duncan and Murray 2012; Jette et al. 2009):

- **Health care policy level:** in a wide sense the principles of current health care (clinical governance, evidence-based practice, demonstrable effectiveness) demand accountability and quality of service; funding for services is becoming increasingly linked to evidence of effectiveness and efficiency.

- **Perception of the AHPs:** it is essential that AHPs present their assessment data, interventions, and outcome data in a format that educates other professionals, service users, and lay persons about the unique roles that AHPs have in the inter-disciplinary team.

- **Research/theory – practice gap within the professions:** AHPs continue to experience a gap between theory and related research and what is actually occurring in clinical practice.

- **Dissemination of findings:** the use of standardised assessments and outcome measures in research and results disseminated in professional literature, may be incorporated into clinical practice more easily if similar scales are already in use in practice and AHPs are comfortable with implementing different standardised tools.

- **Clinical research endeavours:** a vast majority of therapy research involves small sample sizes and research undertaken at a single site or in non-practice settings (e.g. simulated environments within university programmes); if outcomes measures were a routine aspect of therapy, then clinically based research and multi-centre trials would be much easier to undertake.

- **AHP level:** the use of standardised measures can improve communication among practitioners, foster consistency, and reaffirm knowledge and skill (Lewis and Bottomley 1994).

- **Client level:** the client receives an improved service in which assessment and outcome data is based on reliable, valid, and sensitive measures.

In conclusion, many non-standardised 'therapist-constructed' assessments continue to be used in practice and have both strengths and limitations. AHPs should be clear as to the theoretical foundations of all their assessment procedures, including both standardised and non-standardised tests. Where components of standardised tests are used in a 'therapist-constructed' assessment battery, AHPs should be able to quote the original source and the rationale for the test item's use in the ensuing non-standardised assessment. In cases where non-standardised assessments are used without such theoretical underpinning or rationale, professional credibility and client welfare can be at risk. Inadequate, and even inaccurate, decisions may be made from non-standardised assessments that can have negative consequences for both individual client care and, where the effectiveness of physiotherapy and occupational therapy intervention cannot be reliably demonstrated, for the service provision as a whole.

THE REQUIREMENT TO DEMONSTRATE EFFECTIVENESS

So what do we mean by the term 'effectiveness'? An effect is the power to produce an outcome or achieve a result. Effectiveness, in a clinical setting, relates to whether or not the anticipated therapeutic outcome is achieved during the therapeutic process. So the effect of therapy is the identifiable outcome that can be recorded at an agreed point (often the end) of the therapeutic process. Clinical effectiveness (also referred to as effective practice) is achieved when an action, intervention or system does what it is intended to do (RCOT 2020).

Two related, but significantly different terms, are efficacy and efficiency. These are also important for AHPs to consider and are defined briefly, along with some other terms related to effectiveness and outcome measurement, in Table 1.3.

TABLE 1.3   Definition of terms related to effectiveness and outcome measurement.

Term	Definition
Effectiveness	Whether treatments do more good than harm in those to whom they are offered under the usual conditions of care, which may differ from those in the experimental situation. Effectiveness is the measure of the ability of a programme, project or work task to produce a specific desired effect or result that can be measured. Relates to outcomes, not the efficiency of performance (Center to Advance Palliative Care n.d.).
Clinical effectiveness	'The degree to which a therapeutic outcome is achieved in real-world patient populations under actual or average condition of treatment provision' (Maniadakis and Gray 2004, p. 27).
Cost-effectiveness analysis	An analysis that 'compares the costs and health effects of an intervention to assess whether it is worth doing from the economic perspective' (Phillips and Thompson 2003, p. 1). Costs are categorised as: direct costs for the service and patient, service costs (staff time, equipment, drugs), patient costs (transport, out-of-pocket expenses), indirect costs (production losses, other uses of time), intangibles (e.g. pain, suffering, adverse effects) (p. 2).
Efficiency	Measure of production or productivity relative to input resources. Efficiency refers to operating a programme or project, or performing work tasks economically. Relates to resources expended or saved, not the effectiveness of performance.
Efficacy	This involves assessing whether a treatment actually works for those who receive it under ideal conditions and is the province of research. It has been defined as 'the degree to which a therapeutic outcome is achieved in a patient population under rigorously controlled and monitored circumstances, such as controlled clinical trials' (Maniadakis and Gray 2004, p. 27).
Outcome measure	A standardised instrument used by AHPs to establish whether their desired outcomes have been achieved.
Performance measure	Generic term used to describe a particular value or characteristic designated to measure input, output, outcome, efficiency or effectiveness. Performance measures are composed of a number and a unit of measure. The number provides the magnitude (how much) and the unit is what gives the number its meaning (what) (Center to Advance Palliative Care n.d.).
Performance measurement	A management tool for enhancing decision making and accountability. Performance measurement as a strategic process is used to assess accomplishment of organisational strategic goals and objectives (Center to Advance Palliative Care n.d.).

Why do we need to demonstrate effectiveness? 'All professions that hope to advance their practices must take three giant leaps forward to achieve their goals. They must first **document the status and process of practice**, then **develop valid standards of practice** and always they must **test the outcome** of their actions on behalf of their clients' (Cole et al. 1995, p. 2). As Cole et al. pointed out 'not everything we do in the name of therapy is successful or the final word' (p. 5). We may use practices that have been handed down from generation to generation of AHPs because they appear beneficial and we feel they make a difference, but nowadays 'clients should be ensured some appropriate level of outcome measurement' (p. 4) and 'individual therapists must determine what procedures are truly beneficial and directly related to outcomes' (p. 5).

So how do we demonstrate effectiveness? Standardised outcome measures are used to demonstrate whether or not your interventions are effective. Outcome data collected routinely will allow you to form a clearer idea over time about what aspects of your practice are effective and what aspects need to be changed, so you can base future treatment on the results of your findings with similar clients. Outcome measurement is undertaken by administering an outcome measure on at least two occasions. This is done to document change over time in the agreed focus of therapy in order to establish whether it has been influenced by the intervention to the anticipated degree and has achieved the desired outcome.

Cole et al. (1995) identified three basic standards for users of outcome measures:

- 'selecting the appropriate measure for a given population based on scientific evidence;
- administering the measure according to the developer's procedure;
- interpreting the results consistent with evidence of reliability and validity, and comparison to empirically derived norms of comparison group' (p. 171).

Signpost: For more information, see *Chapter 3: Purposes of Assessment and Measurement* and *Chapter 5: Test Administration Reporting and Recording.*

A FOCUS ON CLIENT-CENTRED PRACTICE

The World Health Organization (WHO 2001) emphasised that all health professionals should pay attention to insider perspectives of people with disability. In recent years, policy in the UK has had a greater focus on the service user being given adequate information to make an informed choice about his or her health and/or social care. Health and social care professionals are mandated to listen to the needs of the service user and respond to these identified needs as an integral part of any care package or therapeutic process (Clouston 2003; Edwards and Elwyn 2009). A series of National Service Frameworks (NSFs) have put an emphasis on placing the service user and his/her family at the centre of the health care process, not just as a service recipient.

Applying these principles means that the therapeutic intervention, whilst it may be influenced by guidelines, protocols, or standards, is not the same for each client with the same diagnosis. AHPs now have to consistently use self-report and proxy assessment methods to seek information about the wishes, needs, priorities, problems, and goals of the service user (and where appropriate the carer). AHPs have to analyse traditional observational assessment data in the light of self-report and proxy data and then negotiate the desired outcomes and therapeutic approach with the service user. AHPs have needed to develop client-centred outcome measures to capture self-report data reliably and provide robust evaluative measures of the client's and carer's perceptions and experience of the therapeutic outcome.

Signpost: For more information, see *Chapter 2: Methods of Assessment and Sources of Assessment Data.*

THE DEMAND FOR GOVERNANCE

'Clinical governance is a system for improving the standard of clinical practice' (Starey 2003, p. 1). The Department of Health (DoH) has defined clinical governance as a framework 'through which NHS organisations are accountable for continuously improving the quality of their services and safeguarding high standards of care, by creating an environment in which clinical excellence will flourish' (2004, p. 29). Clinical governance emphasises the responsibility that health organisations and their staff have to monitor the quality of their services and to continually work towards modernisation and improvement. Social care organisations and their staff, as outlined in *Modernising Social Services* (DoH 1998), hold similar responsibilities. This document outlined three main priorities: promoting independence; improving protection; and raising standards. An aspect of this is *Best Value*, which means that staff have to provide their services based on clear standards related to both the quality and the cost of the service and that services have to be delivered in the most effective, economic, and efficient way. For more information, see the UK government website: https://www.gov.uk/government/news/clinical-governance-guidance (accessed 21 May 2019). The Health and Social Care Information Centre was a special health authority that became a statutory body on 1 April 2005; this changed its name to NHS Digital on 20 April 2016. The NHS Long Term Plan (2019) highlights the importance of 'strong governance and accountability mechanisms in place for systems to ensure that the NHS as a whole can secure the best value from its combined resources' (p. 111).

Clinical audit: Clinical audit has been defined as

> *a quality improvement process that seeks to improve patient care and outcomes through systematic review of care against explicit criteria and the implementation of change. Aspects of the structure, processes, and outcomes of care are selected and systematically evaluated against specific criteria. Where indicated, changes are implemented at an individual, team, or service level and further monitoring is used to confirm improvement in health-care delivery.*
>
> (DoH 2004, p. 29)

Audit is the systematic and critical analysis of the quality of clinical care including diagnostic and treatment procedures, associated use of resources, outcomes and quality of life for clients (Johnston et al. 2000). Audit is a quality process that compares actual performance in a specific setting against agreed standards of practice.

THE USE OF STANDARDS, PROTOCOLS, GUIDELINES AND CARE PATHWAYS

What is the difference between a standard, a guideline, and a protocol? These three terms are defined briefly, along with some other relevant terms, in Table 1.4.

Practice guidelines: practice guidelines form part of the evidence base from which AHPs should work (see www.nice.org.uk/guidance). The National Institute for Health and Care Excellence (NICE) provides reviews of the evidence across broad health and social care topics. They are written on a clearly defined topic and require a systematic search in order to be based on the best available evidence. The development of practice guidelines involves the collection and review of:

- scientific evidence (literature reviews, meta-analyses, literature synthesis)
- professional opinions (experts)
- practice experience
- cost concerns.

TABLE 1.4   Definitions related to standards, protocols, and guidelines.

Term	Definition
Care pathway	'[A] pathway for a specific user group which determines locally agreed, multidisciplinary health practice and is based on the available guidelines and evidence' (DoH 2004, p. 29).
Standards	A basis for measurement. They provide a definite level of excellence. The Center to Advance Palliative Care (n.d.) defines a standard as an established measurable condition or state used as a basis for comparison for quality and quantity. The term 'standard' refers to a high level of quality, skill, ability, or achievement by which someone is judged. The Collins English Dictionary defines a standard as 'an accepted example of something against which others are judged or measured' or 'a level of quality'.
Protocols	Plans of care for clients presenting with similar conditions, diagnoses, or problems. The DoH (2001) defines a protocol as 'a plan detailing the steps that will be taken in the care or treatment of an individual' (p. 158).
Guidelines	Clinical guidelines are systematically developed statements that assist clinicians and clients in making decisions about appropriate treatments for specific conditions (NHS Executive 1996). Preferred practice guidelines provide the recommended approach to guide the provision of care related to a particular issue. They must be flexible to take into account the exceptions/variations needed to meet the wide range of client/family expectations and needs. Guidelines may be consensus- or evidence-based (Center to Advance Palliative Care n.d.).
Care management	The DoH (2001) defines this as 'a process whereby an individual's needs are assessed and evaluated, eligibility for service is determined, care plans are drafted and implemented, and needs are monitored and reassessed' (p. 152).
Care planning	'[A] process based on an assessment of an individual's assessed need that involves determining the level and type of support to meet those needs, and the objectives and potential outcomes that can be achieved' (DoH 2001, p. 152).
Care package	'[A] combination of services designed to meet a person's assessed needs' (DoH 2001, p. 152).

Once this information has been collected, draft guidelines are drawn up and a consensus and refining process is undertaken, which may involve:

- the input of experts;
- consensus conferences (usually involving representatives of the full range of stakeholders);
- methods for obtaining official commitment and sign-up from stakeholder organisations to the proposed guidelines;
- seeking any additional evidence and adding value judgements.

The output from this process would usually comprise:

- the clinical guidelines being formatted as a written document;
- publication and distribution of the guideline to all relevant staff/organisations;
- an implementation strategy to ensure that the guidelines lead to changes in practice where required.

Criteria for acceptable guidelines: Reinauer (1998) cites the work of Lohr (1997) who gives the following criteria for judging the quality of guidelines:

- Reliability and reproducibility
- Scientific validity
- Clinical applicability
- Clinical flexibility
- Clarity
- Multidisciplinary approach
- Scheduled review
- Documentation of procedures, evidence, etc.

Many clinical guidelines and statements of good practice highlight the importance of assessment.

For example, the *National Clinical Guidelines for Stroke*, which were developed by the Royal College of Physicians Intercollegiate Stroke Working Party (RCP 2016 [5th edition]), state that:

- Organisations and teams regularly involved in caring for people with stroke should use a common, agreed terminology and set of data collection measures, assessments, and documentation (Section 2.6.1).
- Measurement of function is central to the rehabilitation process.
- Many valid tools exist and it is important when considering the use of an assessment measure to understand which domain of the WHO ICF framework the instrument is measuring, and to ensure that the instrument is appropriate to the intervention in question (Wade 1992).
- Clinicians should be trained in the use of measurement scales to ensure consistent use within the team and to provide an understanding of their properties and limitations (Section 2.9).
- Routine screening should be undertaken to identify the person's level of functioning, using standardised measures (RCP 2016).

The Complexity of Assessment

Assessment involves highly complex skills that combine knowledge, experience, creativity, and original thought. From an outsider's viewpoint AHP assessment may look easy; an observer may think that it does not require a person to hold a degree in order to watch someone get dressed and to say whether s/he could do it or not, or to watch someone walk across a room and say whether s/he has problems with balance. Creek (1996) discusses the complexity of simple everyday activities, such as making a cup of tea, and explains how the therapeutic use of such activities requires training at an honours degree level. AHP assessment is actually very multifaceted and intricate.

The AHP needs to observe *how* the person performs and specify *where* and *when* s/he struggles. The AHP then hypothesises the *underlying causes* for the problems observed and records *how* the person responds to different prompts and cues. It is not enough to know that a person cannot manage a task, the AHP must also understand *why* in order to plan the appropriate treatment. For example, treatment will be very different for a person following a stroke who cannot dress owing to spasticity and reduced sensation in one arm compared to a person unable to dress because of visual neglect and body scheme deficits, although at first glance both the diagnosis and the functional problem may appear similar. The AHP has to use all available information and observations to estimate the person's *underlying capacity*, s/he then considers those observations and proxy report data about the person's *current function* and forms hypotheses for any *discrepancy* between likely capacity and actual functional performance. Then the AHP plans an intervention to support the person to maximise his/her capacity and reach his/her *full potential*. When developing an intervention the AHP has to *predict future outcomes* and plan *how* and *when* these outcomes will be measured in order to *evaluate the effectiveness* of the intervention.

There are several key reasons why physiotherapy and occupational therapy assessment is complex and needs to be multifaceted. These relate to the:

- nature of therapeutic practice;
- nature of human occupation and occupational performance;
- the complexity of measuring human function;
- influence of the demands of the assessment task;
- impact of the familiarity of the task;
- effect of the environment in which the assessment is undertaken;
- and the constraints of the practice setting.

These issues will now be explored briefly.

The Nature of Practice

The evolution of medicine and rehabilitation has been a mixture of science, philosophy, sociology, and intuition. Some of the finest practitioners may be some of the worst scientists. However, they may have an extraordinary intuitive science. Because of this fine mixture, it is difficult to quantify assessments, treatments, and outcomes. Nevertheless, this needs to be done.

(Lewis and Bottomley 1994, p. 139)

AHPs are engaged in practice that is focused upon recovery, rehabilitation, and remediation. They tend to use both quantitative and qualitative approaches to assessment. Consequently, some aspects of assessment are standardised, specific, and meticulous whilst other aspects are intuitive, fluid, and creative. AHPs have to balance, reconcile, and incorporate information from both approaches into the overall assessment process and resulting documentation. The proportion of art and science varies from AHP to AHP and is influenced by: the emphasis of their pre-registration education and training; the influence of supervisors, mentors, and peers; the nature of their continuing professional development (CPD); the clinical setting in which they work; and the type of client group they serve.

AHPs are trying to consider the whole person during the assessment process. Therefore, the domain of concern for an assessment is very broad and covers different levels of function from pathophysiology to societal limitation (see *Chapter 11: Applying Models to Assessment and Outcome Measurement*). An AHP considers macro issues such as the person's environment, family support, roles, and values in addition to undertaking micro-level assessment of very specific areas such as range of motion and muscle tone.

The therapeutic process is person-centred. This means that each assessment should be individually tailored to the person and should lead to an individualised intervention programme. More frequently services are developing protocols for people with similar diagnoses or problems and AHPs will use such protocols to guide their choice of assessment tools and interventions for a client group. The AHP needs to gain a clear picture of the individual, which includes his/her past life, present situation and hopes for the future, and his/her roles, motivation, locus of control, attitudes towards his/her condition and towards therapy. The AHP uses this information to understand how the medical diagnosis and prognosis may impact upon that person's quality of life. As the assessment progresses, and the unique aspects of the person's presentation emerge, the AHP refines the assessment in order to target the specific therapeutic needs and goals of the person.

AHPs work in a wide variety of practice settings so they need to be able to conduct assessments in a range of environments. This may involve undertaking an assessment in a person's home or workplace, a hospital ward or outpatient clinic, a therapy department, a GP practice, a school classroom, or a nursing home. AHPs do not always have easy access to all the environments of relevance to a client and will use simulated environments for assessment. The accuracy of the simulated environment will have a significant impact on the usefulness of the assessment scores for the prediction of the person's likely functioning in his/her natural environment (Austin and Clark 1993). For example, a mobility assessment undertaken on an expanse of level lino flooring in a physiotherapy department may not produce a good predictor of the person's safety when mobilising on different types of flooring in the cluttered environment of his/her home.

Therapy is provided frequently within a multidisciplinary context. AHPs need to liaise with other professionals and share the assessment process and results obtained for each service user and for the client group as a whole. When working in a team it is important not to have too much overlap, such that several members of the team ask the person the same questions, nor should there be any gaps in the assessment, where members of the team assume that another professional has assessed that area. This means that good communication and a clear understanding of the role of each member of the team is critical for an efficient, effective, and thorough multidisciplinary assessment.

Another factor that complicates assessment in a multidisciplinary setting is that of attempting to evaluate outcomes.

How can you be sure that your intervention has led to the observed changes in function, rather than the intervention performed by another team member or combination of interventions working in conjunction?

This can create an issue for AHPs. We are being encouraged to measure outcomes and demonstrate the effectiveness of our intervention. However, in many instances, we believe that our clients benefit from a multidisciplinary approach and that it would be unethical to withhold another intervention in order to limit potential confounding variables when measuring outcomes. The client's perspective in this has been well described by Bonnie Sherr Klein in her book *Slow Dance,* in which she describes her experience of having a stroke:

> After my exalted [physiotherapist] told me I should stop my acupuncture sessions with Bernard, I didn't have much faith in him either. 'If you do so many therapies at once, how can we tell which one is working?' he asked. 'I don't give a damn which one works,' I muttered to myself. 'I just want to get better.' It seemed like typical professional chauvinism. Bernard said no one thing was responsible for my progress; we were a team, all of us, including me.
>
> (Sherr Klein 1997, p. 220)

The Nature of Human Performance

Human behaviour is organised by roles. A **role** is a part played or a position held in a social context that fulfils an expected and/or chosen function and these roles are fulfilled through the performance of tasks, activities, and occupations. The individual sees **occupations** as part of his/her identity, and they can be categorised in terms of self-care, productivity and/or leisure occupations (RCOT 2020). An **activity** is a task or sequence of tasks, performed by an individual or a group that may contribute to an occupation or occupations (RCOT 2020). Whilst a **task** is defined as: 'a self-contained stage in an activity; a definable piece of performance with a completed purpose or product; a constituent part of an activity' (COT 2003, p. 60).

For AHPs **environment** means much more than the commonplace understanding of 'environment' as our physical surroundings; rather environment is defined as the set of circumstances and conditions (e.g. physical, social, cultural) in which a person lives, works and develops, that can shape and be shaped by occupational performance (RCOT 2020).

The performance of tasks, activities, and occupations can form everyday routines, which are habitual chains of behaviour with a fixed sequence, such as getting up, washed, dressed, and eating breakfast. Tasks, activities, and occupations also contribute to less frequent life events, such as giving birth to a child, planning a marriage ceremony, or achieving a qualification. Human behaviour is also organised in this way to enable some people to achieve exceptional things, such as a mountaineer climbing Everest, an athlete winning a race and becoming an Olympic medallist, or a person fighting for their life in a war zone. The ordinary or extraordinary things that people engage in each day are central to the manner in which each person lives his or her life. There are many factors that influence the occupations, activities, and tasks that people choose or feel compelled to do and which support or restrict their performance. These factors include wider environmental factors such as culture, norms, and values, and the person's social and physical environment and personal factors such as age, gender, personal capacity, and the impact of illness and adversity (Watson 2004). So not only must the AHP decide whether they will assess the person's ability through consideration of occupations and/or activities and/or tasks. They also have to assess the person's environment and evaluate the impact (whether supporting or limiting) of that environment on the person's ability to perform desired and necessary tasks, activities, and occupations.

Who we are, what we are, who we become, and how we achieve our dreams and aspirations are shaped by the tasks and activities we perform. However, these can also limit our potential and prevent us from achieving our goals and fulfilling our potential. Sometimes this is our choice, but for many people this results from a lack of opportunity. The constraints of their physical and sociocultural environment limit the variety and choice of their occupations (Watson 2004). As AHPs, we need to consider how this affects our clients, but we should also consider how this impacts the way in which we achieve our roles as AHPs.

For example:

Are we doing tasks and activities that could be delegated to other members of the team?

Is there an expectation to discharge patients in a set time frame that limits a full and personalised assessment process for each client?

Are the financial constraints of our organisation preventing us from purchasing a well-evidenced standardised assessment that we have identified as a valid and reliable outcome measure?

Each person has a unique set of experiences, values, norms, and expectations and these factors contribute to the nature of the therapeutic relationship formed between the client and AHP (Austin and Clark 1993, p. 22). People come to therapy with a unique set of roles, occupations, activities, and tasks. Although there are activities that everyone needs to do in some form or another, such as eating, sleeping, washing, toileting, and finding a way to move around, a large percentage of our activities are culturally and personally determined (see Abraham Maslow's 1943 work *Hierarchy of Needs*; and for use of Maslow's hierarchy by therapists, see Lewis and Bottomley 1994, pp. 70–71). This means that AHPs need to tailor their assessments for individual clients and cannot develop a standard process for assessment that can be applied in its entirety to every single client.

The Nature of Human Function and the Complexity of Measuring Outcomes

For AHPs, **function** is defined as the ability to perform tasks, activities and/or occupations to expected levels of competency. Dysfunction occurs when a person cannot perform tasks, activities and/or occupations to these normal standards of proficiency. Function is achieved through the interaction of performance components. These are subsystems within the individual, such as the motor system, the sensory system, or the cognitive and perceptual systems. As the interaction between the motor, sensory, perceptual, and cognitive systems is complex the definition of each system implicitly refers to the functioning of other systems. For example, Allport (1955) has defined perception as relating to our awareness of the objects or conditions about us and the impression objects make upon our senses.

Perception relates to the way things look, or the way they sound, feel, taste, or smell. Perception involves, to some degree, an understanding awareness, a 'meaning' or a 'recognition' of objects and the awareness of complex environmental situations as well as single objects. This definition implicitly refers to both the sensory and cognitive systems. For example, before an awareness of objects and conditions is registered sensory stimuli have been received from the environment, transmitted by the visual, auditory, gustatory, olfactory, and/or somatosensory systems to the brain, and the cognitive system is involved with accessing information, stored in the memory, required to recognise stimuli in the context of experience. It appears that tightly defined experimental conditions are required in order to attempt to evaluate the discrete functioning of any one system. In practice settings, where the aim is to assess the individual in their everyday context, the imposition of such experimental conditions impinges on the ecological validity of assessment. Therefore, during clinical evaluation it is preferable to evaluate the motor, sensory, perceptual, and cognitive systems together.

Function is dynamic, not static, and this can make it challenging to obtain a 'true' baseline of function at the start of the therapy process. Health professionals are being encouraged to embrace EBP. This means that AHPs need to evaluate the effects of their intervention using outcome measures. When undertaking assessment to evaluate the effects of an intervention the AHP needs to be aware that the person's scores on an outcome measure are open to a degree of 'error' and s/he will need to take any confounding variables into consideration when interpreting the person's performance on the outcome measure. A person's functioning can be influenced by several factors, for example:

- changing levels of pain
- concentration
- anxiety
- fatigue
- response to a drug regime
- level of stiffness.

Therefore, a single assessment might not present a true and complete picture of the person's ability. Variability in a person's function can be more extreme for certain diagnoses. People with Parkinson's disease, for example, may have very different levels of ability depending on the timing and effects of their medication. An AHP should try to undertake different parts of the assessment on different occasions, varying the time of day and the assessment environment. Test anxiety can impact performance, and clients' performance often improves as their AHP becomes familiar and good rapport is established.

When evaluating the outcome of intervention the AHP must be aware that a person's function may change for many reasons. For example, improvements may be observed as a result of a specific intervention or the success of a combination of interventions. This is important because therapy is rarely the sole intervention and often is provided in a multidisciplinary context. Other factors, that may result in observed improvements in function include:

- a belief/hope that change in function is possible
- a placebo effect
- a strong sense of locus of control
- good copying strategies
- high motivation
- good rapport with the AHP
- and feelings of acceptance and support.

When undertaking assessment to provide an accurate baseline and/or evaluate the effects of an intervention the AHP needs to define the specific area to be measured and will need to consider any confounding variables when interpreting the person's performance on the outcome measure.

Another factor that can complicate the measurement of outcomes is the person's level of insight. The AHP needs to assess whether the person has insight into the nature and severity of his/her condition because the need for insight is fundamental to the success of the therapeutic process. A lack of insight can impact on the accuracy of any self-report data collected from the service user and can hinder the negotiation of treatment goals and the formulation of an agreed plan for intervention. Insight may improve during the intervention and this can enable a more realistic treatment plan to be renegotiated. However, when goals are renegotiated mid intervention, the baseline assessment, which founded the original treatment goals, may no longer be accurate or appropriate to the renegotiated treatment goals and this can lead to serious complications in the interpretation of any measures of outcome (Austin and Clark 1993).

Interventions sometimes span several weeks, months, or even years. AHPs should, therefore, be aware that habituation effects may impact self-report and proxy data when measuring outcomes over a long time period. Some people progress through the intervention period constantly adapting to the changes in their ability or symptoms; because of these adaptations in response to treatment the service user and carer may lose sight of his/her original level of function and not notice the degree of change that has occurred since the baseline assessment (Austin and Clark 1993).

Timing the evaluation is an important consideration. For example, if AHPs are concerned with long-term benefits of intervention for their clients then a final assessment at discharge does not provide the whole picture when measuring outcomes. One must not assume that function will always plateau post discharge. Sometimes some of the progress achieved during treatment can be lost post discharge when the service user no longer has the AHP for support and encouragement or fails to keep up with an exercise programme once therapy is terminated. For other people the skills, abilities, and attitudes they acquired during the intervention period can inspire progress and function continues improve over time (Austin and Clark 1993). When measuring outcomes it is important to consider the intervention period or number of therapy sessions that are anticipated in order to obtain the desired change. The timings of measurements are critical and the AHP needs to judge the spacing of measurement and not undertake the final measurement too early before the service user has had the opportunity to gain the maximum change possible.

The Influence of the Level of Task Demand

Performance is affected by how demanding or difficult a task is and by the person's capacity, motivation, experience, and knowledge. AHPs need to take these factors into account during assessment. Experience, knowledge, and capacity are interrelated. This relationship is complex and subject to individual variation, so these factors are difficult to separate and assess in isolation. How an AHP structures the assessment and their reasoning and interpretation of assessment data is critical to their ability to untangle these complex influences upon performance. Task demand has been defined as 'the amount of cognitive and physical skill required to perform the task' (Culler 1993, p. 218). When a person goes to perform a task they firstly obtain factual information about the demands of a task. From this information they develop ideas, insights, and beliefs related to the task, and then create strategies to complete the task more efficiently.

A person's capacity, defined in terms of the amount of information that the central nervous system can handle and process, is limited. The brain has limits for the quantity of sensory information (experienced through the visual, tactile, auditory, olfactory, gustatory, and proprioceptive systems) that it can process at a time. For example, the auditory system can only process a certain amount of auditory stimulation at a time, which is why it is hard to concentrate on two people speaking simultaneously. All tasks place demands on the capacity of at least some of the body's sensory systems and, consequently, on the brain's ability to process sensory stimulation. The level and quality of a person's performance will be determined by the demands of a task if the demands of that task are within a person's capacity. For example, a person may have the capacity to perform two different tasks, such as eating cereal from a bowl with a spoon and eating a meal using a knife and fork. Although the person can do both tasks, they are likely to eat cereal with greater ease because it is a less demanding, easier, task. If the person reaches the maximum level of his/her capacity then performance will be limited by his/her capacity, not by the task demands.

Capacity alters in relation to both the normal developmental processes and to pathology. In terms of normal development, infants learn to use spoons before they learn to use knives and forks. Although organically based capacities decrease with age, many everyday tasks are considered to make relatively few demands, and on these tasks it is expected that performance will not vary with age (Welford 1993). However, some more complex tasks do load one or more capacities and performance can be a function of age. The onset of any limitation depends on the nature of the task demands, the individual's capacity, and on the rate at which capacities decline; i.e. the greater the capacity and the slower the rate of decline, the later will performance begin to decrease as a function of age (Craik 1977; Welford 1993). Capacity can be reduced as the result of an injury or illness. For example, a person who has experienced a stroke and who has associated motor and sensory deficits and a resultant limited capacity in the motor and sensory systems, may be unable to eat either using a spoon or using a knife and fork. The difference in task demand is not the issue, in this example, because the problems in task performance are related to the person's reduced motor and sensory capacity.

Performance at all ages is affected by the task demand, and the individual's capacity, experience, and knowledge. In addition, factors related to volition and societal expectations will also have an impact. Although all these factors (task demand, capacity, experience, knowledge, volition, and societal expectations) are acknowledged as important, it can be very difficult to distinguish between them and to identify the point at which a change in performance is related to pathology. This is why normative data provided in standardised normative assessments (see *Chapter 7: Standardisation*) is useful when an AHP needs to conduct a discriminative assessment (see *Chapter 3: Purposes of Assessment and Measurement*).

Some criterion-referenced assessments (see *Chapter 7: Standardisation*) take task demand into account and may present assessment items as a hierarchy from the simplest to the most complex task. For example, the Assessment of Motor Process Skills (AMPS; Fisher 1995) provides descriptions for a choice of Instrumental Activities of Daily Living (IADL) that have been calibrated through research to create a hierarchy from easiest to hardest task. Using hierarchies of task demand can save unnecessary testing time for both the AHP and client. For example, the Rivermead ADL Assessment (Whiting and Lincoln 1980) is structured in terms of a hierarchy of items comprising increasingly demanding personal and household tasks. The AHP decides where on the hierarchy to begin testing, based on their hypothesis about which tasks the person may not be able to manage. If the person can perform the selected task then the AHP ensures s/he can perform the three preceding tasks and then progresses testing up the hierarchy until s/he fails to perform three consecutive tasks. Other assessments may be graded so that the person can be presented with progressively more demanding tasks as his/her ability increases, for example an assessment of meal preparation could be graded from using a pre-packaged cold meal to preparing a hot, three-course meal using raw ingredients (Culler 1993).

The Impact of Familiarity on Performance

Familiarity and practice influence performance. When a person practices a task over time the demands of the task are learned and the person becomes more efficient in the use of his/her capabilities related to performing that task; the task becomes perceived as easier. A good example is learning to drive a car. Two adults may have the same capacities but the person who is familiar with driving a car will be better at driving than the person with no driving experience. Another example is that of cooking, 'it is less demanding for a person to cook a familiar recipe from memory than to follow a new recipe from a cookbook' (Culler 1993, p. 218). Therefore, AHPs need to be aware of how familiar or novel assessment tasks are to their clients. In addition, following a reduction in capacity, AHPs can use practice and repetition to increase a person's task performance and use ongoing reassessment of the task to monitor progress. When repeating an assessment in this way, the AHP must be able to differentiate between changes that result because the assessment is now familiar and changes that have resulted in the person's capacity. Improvements in motor function are an example of this. Therefore, parallel forms of an assessment (see *Chapter 9: Reliability*) could be used, where an unfamiliar task of the same demand and assessing the same capacity is given in place of the familiar assessment task.

The Influence of Environment upon Performance

The environment in which an assessment is undertaken may also impact upon performance and can have an enabling or constraining effect on a person's function (Law et al. 1996). The term environment usually makes people think about the physical elements (including accessibility, architectural barriers, and structural adaptations) of a person's setting. However, AHPs need to think about the environment in a broader context. In the *International Classification of Functioning, Disability and Health* (ICF), the World Health Organization (WHO 2001) describes disability and functioning as outcomes of interactions between health conditions (diseases, disorders, and injuries) and contextual factors. Contextual factors include external environmental factors, which are defined as 'the physical, social and attitudinal environment in which people live and conduct their lives' (p. 10, section 4) and are subdivided into social attitudes, architectural characteristics, legal and social structures, as well as climate and terrain.

The terms external environment and non-human environment have been used interchangeably in the therapy literature. Interaction with our environment facilitates the initial development, as well as maintenance of, all performance components (Mosey 1981). Cultural and social factors need to be taken into account when selecting appropriate occupations for assessment and treatment. The non-human environment, in the form of setting and tools, needs to be carefully selected and structured during assessment in order to ensure meaning for the patient and fulfil the therapeutic purpose. An individual must interact with the non-human environment to engage in occupations. An activity (such as washing) occurs in a physical and social environment (washing may take place in a bathroom or by a river and the activity will be influenced by social and cultural norms). The performance of an activity may also involve the use of objects (washing may require the use of a washing bowl or basin, soap, and towel). When an AHP uses the performance of daily living activities as a method of assessment s/he consciously structures an environment for this performance and selects specific tools for the patient to interact with. An intervention that increases the enabling aspect of the environment for an individual and thereby creates a compatible person–environment–occupation fit will increase, or with a progressive condition perhaps maintain, function. AHPs are involved with assessing and where necessary adapting a person's environment or teaching the person compensation techniques to help them to cope with the challenges placed by negotiating the environment with a particular impairment. For example, if an AHP modifies a kitchen to increase accessibility for a person in a wheelchair then the fit between the person's capacities, the kitchen environment and the activities of meal preparation, washing up, and laundry will improve leading to increased independence.

Familiarity with an environment may influence assessment results; the impact of familiarity does not just apply to the activity or task to be assessed but also to the familiarity of the environment in which the assessment is to be undertaken. For example, 'a familiar environment (e.g. kitchen at home) is less demanding than a new environment (e.g. clinic kitchen)' (Culler 1993, p. 219) and an AHP could expect a client to be more independent within his/her own kitchen than in unfamiliar kitchen areas. Even if the familiarity of an environment does not impact the final outcome of an assessment it may affect the speed at which the task is completed. It is quicker, as we know, to make a cup of tea in your own kitchen because you know where everything is kept. You will still be independent making a cup of tea in a friend's kitchen but probably it will take you more time because you will be searching in the unfamiliar environment for the items and ingredients you need. The home environment does not always facilitate function, for example, people may be able to mobilise better on the hard, flat surface of a physiotherapy department or hospital ward than on the different carpet textures (e.g. carpet, floorboards, rugs, lino, tiles) in their own homes.

The World Health Organization (WHO 2001) recommends that 'to assess the full ability of the individual, one would need to have a "standardized environment" to neutralize the varying impact of different environments on the ability of the individual' (p. 15). WHO suggests that there are a number of environments that can be used for this purpose:

a. an actual environment commonly used for capacity assessment in test settings;
b. an assumed environment thought to have an uniform impact;
c. an environment with precisely defined parameters based on extensive scientific research.

AHPs are often involved in conducting assessments in people's own home and work environments, as they need to evaluate both environmental barriers and environmental supports to performance. Assessment at home is considered useful because people are more likely to behave and communicate in their normal way in familiar surroundings. The AHP can build a more accurate picture of the person's needs during a home assessment. A home assessment can also facilitate access to the views and the needs of any carer. The environment selected for assessment is especially important for people with certain conditions. For example, the influence of context and environment on the function of a person with dementia is critical to assess (Tullis and Nicol 1999).

Where safety is of concern, it is critical to assess the person in the environment where s/he will be functioning to examine the relationship between potential environmental hazards and the person's ability. Once potential hazards have been identified, changes to the environment can be made to reduce the risks, for example a risk of falls. Some therapy assessments have been designed for use in the home environment. For example, the Safety Assessment of Function and the Environment for Rehabilitation (SAFER Tool; Letts et al. 1998) was developed to assess people's abilities to manage functional activities safely within their homes and the Home Falls and Accidents Screening Tool (Home Fast; Mackenzie, Byles, and Higginbotham 2000) was developed to identify hazards associated with falls in the home.

The Constraints of the Practice Setting

The practice setting will influence the AHP's choice of assessment and may serve to enhance or constrain the assessment practice. For example, if an AHP moves to a service that encourages standardised assessment and has a range of published tests available then knowledge of different tests and skills in standardised assessment may increase. Conversely, an AHP may be experienced with a particular standardised test but find that it is not available in a new practice setting or that with the demand of their new caseload there is not enough time to administer the test in full. It may not be possible in some settings to assess the client at several different times in varying test environments and cover all the areas of interest within the assessment. Therefore, the AHP needs to use clinical judgement to select the most effective assessment strategy within the physical and political boundaries of the practice environment. They may only be able to conduct a brief assessment and will need to make decisions about the person's overall ability and prognosis from limited data projections (see section on 'Predictive Validity' in *Chapter 8: Validity and Clinical Utility*). The quality of the AHP's clinical reasoning can be critical.

CONCLUSION

In conclusion, the AHP needs to be like an experienced chef: not following rigidly a set recipe but combining knowledge of different techniques and knowing which ingredients and flavours can be combined in a creative way for each particular situation.

> *Evidence based medicine is not 'cookbook' medicine. Because it requires a bottom up approach that integrates the best external evidence with individual clinical expertise and patients' choice, it cannot result in slavish, cookbook approaches to individual patient care. External clinical evidence can inform, but can never replace, individual clinical expertise, and it is this expertise that decides whether the external evidence applies to the individual patient at all and, if so, how it should be integrated into a clinical decision. Similarly, any external guideline must be integrated with individual clinical expertise in deciding whether and how it matches the patient's clinical state, predicament, and preferences, and thus whether it should be applied.*
>
> (Sackett et al. 1996, p. 71)

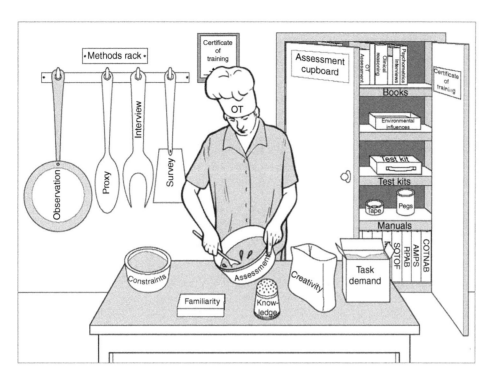

FIGURE 1.2   The AHP as a creative and expert chef. *Source*: Reprinted from Laver Fawcett (2002). © (2002), with permission from Elsevier.

AHPs need to adopt outcome measures that document the efficacy of their interventions, and guide clinical decisions and treatment planning. These measures need to be clinically appropriate, functionally relevant, valid, reliable, and responsive to change (Duncan and Murray 2012; Jette et al. 2009; Wright, Cross, and Lamb 1998). Not only should AHPs critique and implement valid and reliable assessments in their practice, they should also be prepared to add to the growing body of research into therapy measures. This may be by collaborating with a test developer to add to data on inter-rater reliability or by contributing your views to studies of clinical utility and aspects of validity.

Richards (2002) challenged AHPs to contribute to the national political agenda: 'it behoves . . . AHPs to contribute expert assessments which stand up to scrutiny, form a sound foundation for their intervention and link with valid outcome measures that clearly demonstrate the value of their contribution to efficient and effective service provision' (p. xviii).

We should not underestimate the responsibility we have to make sound judgements about our service users' abilities and dysfunction. The distance between theory and practice can sometimes feel like a wide chasm. We 'know' that we should be using valid, reliable, standardised measures in our practice. Assessment processes without a strong evidence or theoretical base are still occurring more often than we feel comfortable to admit. As, the demands of the everyday practice settings in which AHPs work, with limited time to review potential assessments and try them out, and few resources to purchase a new test, even when there is strong evidence for its application. No matter how competent an AHP is at providing treatment, this will be inadequate if it is based on faulty evaluation and decision making regarding the patient's deficits and the resulting intervention plan.

AHPs need to embrace EBP as an opportunity rather than a threat. It is about doing the very best we can for our clients. It also helps to further the development and standing of our professions, which assists in ensuring ongoing and ideally increased funding for providing occupational therapy and physiotherapy to those people who would benefit from these services. Achieving EBP is a step-by-step process. This book aims to assist AHPs to move towards a greater evidence base in their assessment and measurement practice. The first step is to raise a question or series of questions. Worksheets have been developed for each chapter to enable you to raise and answer questions related to different aspects of your assessment and measurement practice.

REFLECTION POINT

Let us begin with a global question:

How should I organise my assessment process in order to collect the right information, at the best time and in the most effective and efficient way to provide reliable, valid, and responsive measurement in a manner that is acceptable to my clients?

Once you have formulated a question as a focus for EBP, the second step is to search for evidence. Within the book we have reviewed literature and research that will provide foundational knowledge for helping you to start the journey towards answering this question. As it is such a big question, it is helpful to break it down into a series of more specific questions. We have noted the main chapter(s) that have been written to help you to answer each of these questions:

The following table provides signposting to other chapters in the book.

Why am I collecting assessment and measurement data?	See Chapter 3 on Purposes of Assessment and Measurement
Who is the best source for this information?	See Chapter 2 on Methods of Assessment and Sources of Assessment Data
What is the best method for collecting this information?	See Chapter 2 on Methods of Assessment and Sources of Assessment Data
What level of measurement is required?	See Chapter 4 on What is Measurement?
How can I ensure my measurements are valid?	See Chapter 8 on Validity and Clinical Utility
How do I evaluate whether my assessment process and the specific measures used are acceptable to my clients?	See sections on 'Face Validity' and 'Clinical Utility' in Chapter 8 and section on 'Test Critique' in Chapter 10
How can I ensure my measurements are reliable?	See Chapter 9 on Reliability
How can I ensure my outcome measures are responsive to a clinically relevant degree of change?	See Chapter 9 on Reliability
How do I prepare for an efficient and effective test administration?	See Chapter 5 on Test Administration, Reporting and Recording
How do I build rapport with my client?	See Chapter 5 on Test Administration, Reporting and Recording

How do I ensure that my test administration remains standardised?	See Chapter 5 on Test Administration, Reporting and Recording
How do I communicate the results of my assessment?	See Chapter 5 on Test Administration, Reporting and Recording
How do I combine the best available evidence with my clinical experience and my knowledge of my client's preferences?	See Chapter 6 on The Importance of Clinical Reasoning and Reflective Practice in Effective Assessment
How do I categorize the myriad of information and observational data collected about a person into a meaningful and organised assessment?	See Chapter 11 on Applying Models to Assessment and Outcome Measurement
How do I fit my assessment practice into the wider context of a multidisciplinary team and/or inter-agency approach?	See Chapter 11 on Applying Models to Assessment and Outcome Measurement
How do I set about identifying appropriate standardised tests for my service?	See Chapter 7 on Standardisation and Chapter 12 on Implementing the Optimum Assessment and Measurement Approach
How do I combine the best available evidence with my clinical experience and my knowledge of my client's preferences in order to implement the optimum assessment and measurement approach?	See Chapter 12 on Implementing the Optimum Assessment and Measurement Approach and Chapter 14 for a case study example

We have included a number of worksheets in this book, which can be used to focus your learning. If you are a pre-registration student you might use the worksheets on clinical placement to explore the assessment processes being used by your supervisor and his/her colleagues. If you are a practicing AHP you could use the worksheets, alone or with colleagues, as a focus for your own CPD – remember to put a copy of any completed worksheets in your CPD portfolio as evidence of your work – or for your team or department's service development activities.

WORKSHEET 1.1 Evidence-based Practice

Question	Comments
Do you currently base your assessment practice on evidence?	Yes, all assessments evidence based Partly, some assessments are evidence based No, none of the assessments used are evidence based
What else, apart from evidence, do you use to guide your assessment decisions/practice?	
Think of an instance where you changed your assessment practice based on evidence (e.g. acquired from journal article, conference presentation, or course)	What was your previous practice? What was the evidence that convinced you to change? What changes did you make? What have been the outcomes of the change?
What other areas of your assessment could benefit from being changed?	Do you need to seek more evidence related to these areas of assessment?

REFERENCES

@OTalk data, May 2019. See 'Introduction' chapter for full details.

Allport, F.H. (1955). *Theories of Perception and the Concept of Structure: A Review and Critical Analysis with an Introduction to a Dynamic-Structural Theory of Behavior*. Wiley.

Austin, C. and Clark, C.R. (1993). Measures of outcome: for whom? *British Journal of Occupational Therapy* 56 (1): 21–24.

Balshem, H., Helfand, M., Schünemann, H.J. et al. (2011). GRADE guidelines: 3. Rating the quality of evidence. *Journal of Clinical Epidemiology* 64 (4): 401–406. https://doi.org/10.1016/j.jclinepi.2010.07.015.

Belsey, J. and Snell, T. (2003). *What is Evidence-based Medicine?* London: Hayward Medical Communications.

Borg, B. and Bruce, M. (1991). Assessing psychological performance factors. In: *Occupational Therapy: Overcoming Human Performance Deficits* (eds. C. Christiansen and C. Baum), 538–586. Thorofare, NJ: Slack, Inc.

Center to Advance Palliative Care (n.d.). Toolkits for Palliative Care Programs. Available at capc.org (accessed 30 November 2020).

Clouston, T. (2003). Narrative methods: talk, listening and representation. *British Journal of Occupational Therapy* 66 (4): 136–142. https://doi.org/10.1177/030802260306600402.

Cole, B., Finch, E., Gowland, C. et al. (1995). *Physical Rehabilitation Outcome Measures*, 24–78. Baltimore: Lippincott Williams & Wilkins.

Craik, F.I.M. (1977). Age differences in human memory. In: *Handbook of the Psychology of Aging* (eds. J.E. Birren and K.W. Schaie). New York: Van Nostrand Reinhold.

Creek, J. (1996). Making a cup of tea as an honours degree subject. *British Journal of Occupational Therapy* 59 (3): 128–130. https://doi.org/10.1177/030802269605900310.

Culler, K.H. (1993). Occupational therapy performance areas: home and family management. In: *Willard and Spackman's Occupational Therapy*, 8e (eds. H.L. Hopkins and H.D. Smith), 207–269. Philadelphia: Lippincott Williams & Wilkins.

Department of Health (DoH) (1998). *A First Class Service: Quality in the New NHS*. London: Department of Health.

Department of Health (DoH) (2001). *Reference Guide to Consent for Examination or Treatment*, 1e. London: Department of Health.

Department of Health (DoH) (2004). *Choosing Health: Making Healthy Choices Easier*, vol. 6374. London: The Stationery Office.

Driever, M.J. (2002). Are evidenced-based practice and best practice the same? *Western Journal of Nursing Research* 24 (5): 591–597.

Duncan, E.A. and Murray, J. (2012). The barriers and facilitators to routine outcome measurement by allied health professionals in practice: a systematic review. *BMC Health Services Research* 12 (1): 96. https://doi.org/10.1186/1472-6963-12-96.

Eakin, P. (1989). Assessments of activities of daily living: a critical review. *British Journal of Occupational Therapy* 52 (1): 11–15. https://doi.org/10.1177/030802268905200104.

Edwards, A. and Elwyn, G. (eds.) (2009). *Shared Decision-Making in Health Care: Achieving Evidence-Based Patient Choice*. Oxford University Press. 9780199546275.

Fisher, A.G. (1995). *Assessment of Motor and Process Skills (AMPS)*. User Manual, Vol. 2. Fort Collins, CO: Three Star Press.

Fisher, A.G. and Short-DeGraff, M. (1993). Improving functional assessment in occupational therapy: recommendations and philosophy for change. *American Journal of Occupational Therapy* 47 (3): 199–201.

GRADE Working Group (2004). Grading quality of evidence and strength of recommendations. *British Medical Journal* 328 (7454): 1490. https://doi.org/10.1136/bmj.328.7454.1490.

Gray, J.A.M. (2001). *Evidence-Based Healthcare*. Elsevier Health Sciences.

Greenhalgh, T., Howick, J., and Maskrey, N. (2014). Evidence based medicine: a movement in crisis? *BMJ* 348: g3725. https://doi.org/10.1136/bmj.g3725.

Gustafsson, L., Molineux, M., and Bennett, S. (2014). Contemporary occupational therapy practice: the challenges of being evidence based and philosophically congruent. *Australian Occupational Therapy Journal* 61 (2): 121–123. https://doi.org/10.1111/1440-1630.12110.

Guyatt, G., Cook, D., and Haynes, B. (2004). Evidence based medicine has come a long way. *BMJ* 329: 990. https://doi.org/10.1136/bmj.329.7473.990.

Guyatt, G.H., Oxman, A.D., Kunz, R. et al. (2008a). What is "quality of evidence" and why is it important to clinicians? *BMJ* 336 (7651): 995–998. https://doi.org/10.1136/bmj.39490.551019.BE.

Guyatt, G.H., Oxman, A.D., Kunz, R. et al. (2008b). Going from evidence to recommendations. *BMJ* 336 (7652): 1049–1051. https://doi.org/10.1136/bmj.39493.646875.AE.

Hatfield, D.R. and Ogles, B.M. (2007). Why some clinicians use outcome measures and others do not. *Administration and Policy in Mental Health and Mental Health Services Research* 34 (3): 283–291. https://doi.org/10.1007/s10488-006-0110-y.

Hong, C.S. (1996). The use of non-standardised assessments in Occupational Therapy with children who have disabilities: a perspective. *British Journal of Occupational Therapy* 59 (8): 363–364. https://doi.org/10.1177/030802269605900804.

Hopkins, H.L. and Smith, H.D. (1993). *Willard and Spackman's Occupational Therapy*, 8e. Philadelphia: Lippincott Williams & Wilkins.

Jette, D.U., Halbert, J., Iverson, C. et al. (2009). Use of standardized outcome measures in physical therapist practice: perceptions and applications. *Physical Therapy* 89 (2): 125–135. https://doi.org/10.2522/ptj.20080234.

Johnston, G., Crombie, I.K., Alder, E.M. et al. (2000). Reviewing audit: barriers and facilitating factors for effective clinical audit. *BMJ Quality & Safety* 9 (1): 23–36.

Sherr Klein, B. (1997). *Slow Dance: A Story of Stroke, Love and Disability*. Toronto: Vintage.

Laver, A.J. (1994). The Development of the Structured Observational Test of Function (SOTOF). Doctoral dissertation. University of Surrey.

Laver Fawcett, A.J. (2002). Assessment. In: *Occupational Therapy and Physical Dysfunction: Principles, Skills and Practice* (eds. A. Turner, M. Foster and S. Johnson), 107–144. London: Churchill Livingstone. Chapter 5.

Law, M., Cooper, B., Strong, S. et al. (1996). The person-environment-occupation model: a transactive approach to occupational performance. *Canadian Journal of Occupational Therapy* 63 (1): 9–23. https://doi.org/10.1177/000841749606300103.

Law, M.C. and MacDermid, J. (eds.) (2014). *Evidence-Based Rehabilitation: A Guide to Practice*, 3e. Slack Incorporated. 10 1-61711-021-3.

Letts, L., Scott, S., Burtney, J. et al. (1998). The reliability and validity of the safety assessment of function and the environment for rehabilitation (SAFER tool). *British Journal of Occupational Therapy* 61 (3): 127–132. https://doi.org/10.1177/030802269806100309.

Lewis, C.B. and Bottomley, J.M. (1994). Assessment instruments. In: *Geriatric Physical Therapy: A Clinical Approach*. Norwalk, CT: Appleton & Lange.

Lohr, K.N. (1997). The quality of practice guidelines and the quality of health care. In: *Guidelines in Health Care Practice*. Report on a WHO Meeting, Schloss Velen, Borken, Germany, 26–28 January 1997. Copenhagen: WHO Regional Office for Europe.

Mackenzie, L., Byles, J., and Higginbotham, N. (2000). Designing the home falls and accidents screening tool (HOME FAST): selecting the items. *British Journal of Occupational Therapy* 63 (6): 260–269. https://doi.org/10.1177/030802260006300604.

Mahoney, F.I. and Barthel, D.W. (1965). Functional evaluation: the Barthel Index: a simple index of independence useful in scoring improvement in the rehabilitation of the chronically ill. *Maryland State Medical Journal* 14: 61–65.

Maniadakis, N. and Gray, A. (2004). Economic evaluation. In: *Outcome Measures in Orthopaedics and Orthopaedic Trauma*, 2e, 34–46. London: CRC Press.

McAvoy, E. (1991). The use of ADL indices by occupational therapists. *British Journal of Occupational Therapy* 54 (10): 383–385. https://doi.org/10.1177/030802269105401009.

McFadyen, A.K. and Pratt, J. (1997). Understanding the statistical concepts of measures of work performance. *British Journal of Occupational Therapy* 60 (6): 279–284. https://doi.org/10.1177/030802269706000614.

Mickan, S., Hilder, J., Wenke, R., and Thomas, R. (2019). The impact of a small-group educational intervention for allied health professionals to enhance evidence-based practice: mixed methods evaluation. *BMC Medical Education* 19 (1): 131. https://doi.org/10.1186/s12909-019-1567-1.

Mosey, A.C. (1981). *Occupational Therapy: Configuration of a Profession*, 67–69. New York: Raven Press.

Neale, M. (2004). Why I have difficulty with standardised assessments and outcome measures. *NANOT News: Journal of the National Association of Neurological Occupational Therapists* 24 (Winter): 25–26.

NHS Executive (1996). *Clinical Guidelines: Using Clinical Guidelines to Improve Patient Care within the NHS*. NHS Management Executive.

NHS (2019). The NHS Long Term Plan. https://www.longtermplan.nhs.uk (accessed 21 May 2019).

NHS Digital (n.d.). Patient Reported Outcome Measures (PROMs). https://digital.nhs.uk/data-and-information/data-tools-and-services/data-services/patient-reported-outcome-measures-proms (accessed 20 May 2019).

Phillips, C. and Thompson, G. (2003). *What is Cost-effectiveness?* London: Hayward Medical Communications.

Reinauer, Prof. Dr H. (1998). AWMF and Clinical Guideline Program in Germany. Presentation at the *International Conference on Clinical Practice Guidelines, 4* September 1998, Frankfurt/Main, Germany. Available at: https://www.awmf.org/service/gesamtarchiv/awmf-konferenz/frankfurtmain-4-sept-1998.html (accessed 8 December 2020).

Richards, S. (2002). Foreword. In: *Occupational Therapy and Physical Dysfunction: Principles, Skills and Practice* (eds. A. Turner, M. Foster and S.E. Johnson), 633. Edinburgh: Churchill Livingstone.

Royal College of Occupational Therapists (RCOT) (2020). Assessments and Outcome Measures Resource, 2020. Available to members at: https://www.rcot.co.uk/practice-resources/occupational-therapy-topics/assessments-and-outcome-measures.

Rycroft-Malone, J. (2004). The PARIHS framework—a framework for guiding the implementation of evidence-based practice. *Journal of Nursing Care Quality* 19 (4): 297–304. https://journals.lww.com/jncqjournal/Citation/2004/10000/The_PARIHS_Framework_A_Framework_for_Guiding_the.2.aspx.

Rycroft-Malone, J., Seers, K., Titchen, A. et al. (2004). What counts as evidence in evidence-based practice? *Journal of Advanced Nursing* 47 (1): 81–90. https://doi.org/10.1111/j.1365-2648.2004.03068.x.

Sackett, D.L., Rosenberg, W.M., Gray, J.M., et al. (1996). Evidence based medicine: what it is and what it isn't. *BMJ* 312: 71–72. https://doi.org/10.1136/bmj.312.7023.71.

Shanahan, M. (1992). Objective and holistic? Is this occupational therapy assessment in Ireland. *Irish Journal of Occupational Therapy* 22 (2): 8–10.

Starey, N. (2003). *What is Clinical Governance?* London: Hayward Medical Communications.

Stewart, S. (1999). The use of standardised and non-standardised assessments in a social services setting: implications for practice. *British Journal of Occupational Therapy* 62 (9): 417–423. https://doi.org/10.1177/030802269906200907.

Tullis, A. and Nicol, M. (1999). A systematic review of the evidence for the value of functional assessment of older people with dementia. *British Journal of Occupational Therapy* 62 (12): 554–563. https://doi.org/10.1177/030802269906201206.

Unsworth, C. (2000). Measuring the outcome of occupational therapy: tools and resources. *Australian Occupational Therapy Journal* 47 (4): 147–158. https://doi.org/10.1046/j.1440-1630.2000.00239.x.

Upton, D. and Upton, P. (2006). Knowledge and use of evidence-based practice by allied health and health science professionals in the United Kingdom. *Journal of Allied Health* 35 (3): 127–133.

Upton, P., Scurlock-Evans, L., Stephens, D., and Upton, D. (2012). The adoption and implementation of evidence-based practice (EBP) among allied health professions. *International Journal of Therapy and Rehabilitation* 19 (9): 497–503. https://doi.org/10.12968/ijtr.2012.19.9.497.

Veenstra, G.L., Ahaus, K., Welker, G.A. et al. (2017). Rethinking clinical governance: healthcare professionals' views: a Delphi study. *BMJ Open* 7 (1): e012591. https://doi.org/10.1136/bmjopen-2016-012591.

Wade, D.T. (1992). Measurement in neurological rehabilitation. *Current Opinion in Neurology* 5 (5): 682–686.

Watson, R. (2004). New horizons in occupational therapy. In: *Transformation through Occupation* (eds. R. Watson and L. Swartz). Wiley.

Welford, A.T. (1993). The gerontological balance sheet. In: *Adult Information Processing: Limits on Loss* (eds. J. Cerella et al.), 3–10. New York: Academic Press.

Whiting, S. and Lincoln, N. (1980). An ADL assessment for stroke patients. *British Journal of Occupational Therapy* 43 (2): 44–46. https://doi.org/10.1177/030802268004300207.

World Health Organization (2001). *International Classification of Functioning, Disability and Health (ICF)*. Geneva: World Health Organization.

Wright, J., Cross, J., and Lamb, S. (1998). Physiotherapy outcome measures for rehabilitation of elderly people: responsiveness to change of the Rivermead Mobility Index and Barthel Index. *Physiotherapy* 84 (5): 216–221. https://doi.org/10.1016/S0031-9406(05)65552-6.

RESOURCES

BMJ Best Practice (n.d.). What is the best evidence and how to find it. https://bestpractice.bmj.com/info/toolkit/discuss-ebm/what-is-the-best-evidence-and-how-to-find-it (accessed 2 April 2019).

Centre for Evidence-Based Medicine, University of Oxford (n.d.). Develops, promotes and disseminates better evidence for health care. https://www.cebm.ox.ac.uk/ (accessed 2 April 2019).

National Institute for Health and Care Excellence (NICE) (n.d.). Search 'evidence based practice'. https://www.evidence.nhs.uk/search?q=evidence+based+practice.

CHAPTER 2

Methods of Assessment and Sources of Assessment Data

OVERVIEW

In order to assess a new client, the allied health professional (AHP) must undertake a well-planned assessment process. This process might consist of the following steps:

1. Determine information required to make thorough clinical decisions and clarify what information is to be collected.
2. Identify relevant sources for this information.
3. Determine assessment methods to be used to collect this information from these sources.
4. Choose appropriate standardised tests to support informal assessment methods.
5. Undertake data collection procedures such as record/referral review, interviews, observations, and the administration of standardised measures.
6. Score any standardised test data (this might involve converting raw scores or plotting scores on a normative graph).
7. Analyse data.
8. Interpret data.
9. Report results (orally and in writing, may be required to record summaries on to a computer database).

This chapter is going to focus on steps 2 and 3 of this assessment process because AHPs need to be able to identify good sources of information and select appropriate methods for obtaining assessment data from these sources.

We discuss the merits of different methods of data collection. Methods used by AHPs include interview; observation; survey; referral information; medical notes; letters; telephone calls; and use of standardised tests. Sources of assessment data are described, including client self-report; proxy sources, such as family members, friends, neighbours, home care workers, voluntary workers, and other professionals involved with the client; and AHP observations and data collected by the AHP both formally, through standardised testing, and informally, e.g. by following a department checklist. Issues of culture, client age, technology, ethics, and confidentiality are discussed. Examples of published assessments for different methods and sources are provided. The chapter concludes with a detailed case study that illustrates how these different methods and sources can be combined to provide a thorough assessment.

QUESTIONS TO CONSIDER

What information needs to be collected?

What is the best method for collecting required assessment and measurement data?

Who will be the best source(s) for this information?

How do you determine if you have the information required to make thorough clinical decisions?

METHODS OF ASSESSMENT

A thorough assessment should involve a process that uses multiple methods for gathering and organising information required for making specific clinical decisions (Hayley et al. 1991). There are many different methods, both qualitative and quantitative, that can be used to help you collect, structure, and analyse assessment data.

The [Royal] College of Occupational AHPs (COT) outline the assessment methods used by AHPs in their position paper 'Occupational Therapy Defined as a Complex Intervention' (Creek 2003, 2009). COT states that 'the [AHP] uses assessment methods which are appropriate to their own abilities and to the client's needs and situation. These include:

- Interacting informally with the client
- Observing activity in the client's own living, working or social environments or in the clinical setting
- Setting the client specific tasks
- Carrying out standardised tests
- Interviewing clients and carers
- Asking questions and discussing the situation informally' (p. 21).

The Chartered Society of Physiotherapy extends this by listing a range of methods that are used in assessment, including:

- patient-reported outcome measures (PROMs)
- patient-reported experience measures (PREMs)
- clinician-completed observation scales
- task-specific activities/tests, e.g. sit to stand
- impairment tests, e.g. range of motion
- physiological tests.

(https://www.csp.org.uk/professional-clinical/research-evaluation/outcome-experience-measures).

It is useful to combine qualitative and quantitative methods to achieve a thorough assessment, because these have different functions and are designed to answer different questions (Eva and Paley 2004). Qualitative data collection methods include:

- informal observations (e.g. to note the person's facial expression, quality of movement, or social interactions with others)
- casual conversations with the client and their carers using open-ended questioning techniques
- the use of semi-structured interviews or questionnaires.

Qualitative information usually focuses on things like feelings, values, and perceptions of what has taken place or the significance of a problem.

The application of quantitative methods involves the administration of standardised or structured measurement, observational tests, and interview schedules. Data collected focuses on information and is expressed in the form of numerical scores. For example, quantitative data might comprise:

- raw or converted scores obtained by administering a standardised outcome measure
- data collected from observation testing methods, such as the range of movement of a joint
- structured self-report or proxy-report data, such as the number of times a particular daily living problem occurs over a set time period.

In addition to categorising methods in terms of whether the method yields qualitative or quantitative data, methods can be grouped in terms of whether they obtain direct or indirect data; examples of direct and indirect methods of data collection are provided in Table 2.1.

TABLE 2.1   Examples of direct and indirect methods of data collection used by AHPs.

Direct methods	Indirect methods
AHP Observations	Referral information (written, online letter or referral form, telephone)
Client self-report given direct to the AHP	Patient/client's previous records, such as medical, therapy, or social care records. These may be online through a shared data point.
Administration of a standardised test to the client by the AHP	Proxy reports from formal sources, such as the patient's GP, doctor, other members of a multidisciplinary team, workers from other statutory services, or teacher.
Administration of a standardised test to the carer by the AHP to assess the carer himself/herself (e.g. to examine the level of caregiver burden or parental stress)	Proxy reports from informal sources, such as the patient's parent, spouse, children, neighbour, friend, voluntary worker, or religious leader (e.g. priest).

SOURCES OF ASSESSMENT INFORMATION

In this section, we will describe the three main sources of information used by AHPs for assessment. These are client self-report (direct method), proxy report (indirect method), and AHPs' observational/collected data (direct method). We will describe the assessment methods used to collect data using each type of source and will provide examples of published assessments used by AHPs to collect data from each of these sources.

SELF-REPORT

The World Health Organization (WHO 2002, https://www.who.int/classifications/icf/en) emphasised that all health professionals should pay attention to insider perspectives of people with disability. WHO stated, in the International Classification of Functioning, Disability and Health (ICF), that 'disability and functioning are viewed as outcomes of interactions between health conditions (diseases, disorders and injuries) and contextual factors' (p. 10, https://www.who.int/classifications/icf/icfbeginnersguide.pdf?ua=1). Contextual factors are divided in the ICF into external environmental factors and internal personal factors. Internal personal factors 'include gender, age, coping styles, social background, education, profession, past and current experiences, overall behaviour pattern, character and other factors that influence how disability is experienced by the individual' (p. 10).

Clouston (2003) noted that 'involvement of the user in decisions about his or her own health and social care has become a key element of the changes encapsulated in the [British] Government's legislation. Listening to the service user and responding to his or her needs is an integral part of that change' (p. 136). As AHPs we need to engage the person in an assessment method that elicits information about these internal personal factors and the person themselves, as this is usually the most reliable source for this information.

Self-report assessment has been defined as 'a type of assessment approach where the patient reports on his or her level of function or performance' (Christiansen and Baum 1991, p. 858). Self-report is valuable in providing the AHP with a wide range of information, including:

- the person's description of his roles, occupations, routines, and values
- his living situation (including the physical environment and sociocultural influences)
- his goals for the future
- the presenting condition and his experience of illness or disability and the symptoms associated with any current problems
- his opinion about his current and previous level of function and occupational performance
- identification of available resources (financial, social, and emotional) that might be used to support the client (Hilko Culler 1993).

In addition to questioning about level of function, it can be helpful to consider individuals' perceptions of how important different activities are in their lives and also how satisfied they are with their current level of performance (Law et al. 1994).

This information helps AHPs to prioritise areas for further assessment and treatment. An example of this type of assessment is the *Canadian Occupational Performance Measure* (COPM 5th edition; Law et al. 2015; http://www.thecopm.ca), which is applied in the case study at the end of this chapter.

Self-report can be very useful as it enables the AHP to access information that only the client knows. 'Self-report assesses what the client says about what he or she is thinking, feeling or doing. Self-report is important because it is our only measure of cognitive activity (such as obsessions or negative self-statements) or of subjective experience (such as pain ...)' (Barlow et al. 1984, p. 124).

Previously, particularly within a medical model, the use of objective (quantitative) data has been favoured over subjective (qualitative) data and there was a 'belief that the patient's view was of no value in measurement' (Pynsent et al. 2004, p. 3). AHPs now have a more explicit interest in client-centred practice (Edvardsson 2015); it is very relevant for them to collect assessment data from the person they seek to treat (Law et al. 1994). We have come to the conclusion that although self-reports do not always coincide with observational or direct measures, 'it is not that self-report is an *inferior* measure, but rather that it is a *different* measure' (Barlow et al. 1984, p. 124). Carswell, et al. (2004) stated that 'without some measure of the client's perspective, it is difficult to imagine how one might engage in client-centred therapy' (p. 219). Hammell (2003), who believed that 'we cannot claim allegiance to client-centred philosophy when we are not paying attention to what disabled people are saying', echoes this (p. 48). Clouston (2003) emphasised the importance of 'listening to and valuing the voice of the user' and states that 'now, more than ever, ... [AHP]s have to show that this an integral part of their everyday practice' (p. 136).

An understanding of the client's perspective enables the AHP to find common ground from which to negotiate mutually agreed desired outcomes and treatment approaches, which are often referred to as 'treatment goals'. Jette (1995) noted that healthcare professionals working in a physical setting appear to have advocated and respected patient-level goals. Partridge and Johnston (1989), in a study that examined perceived control of recovery and predicted recovery from a physical disability, found that a person was more likely to recover faster if he perceived himself to be in control of his rehabilitation. Using self-report as a significant component of the assessment processes engages the client and facilitates his involvement and sense of control in his rehabilitation process. Therefore, self-report is a critical source of assessment data as it engages the person actively in the assessment process and elicits the client's own experiences, wishes, aspirations, and beliefs.

Self-report assessment provides subjective data, which helps the AHP to obtain a picture of the person and how he views his life, illness or disability, problems, and functioning. It is useful to try engage a client in some form of self-report assessment whenever possible; even a client who is considered to have little insight (for example, a person with severe dementia) will still have his perspective about what is problematic and may have ideas about what might help remedy the problem (Carswell et al. 2004). Even if these ideas are incongruent with the AHP's knowledge and experience of what is safe and possible, it is very helpful to know the belief system and expectations that the client is bringing into the therapeutic relationship.

Another group of clients who may have reduced levels of insight to engage in self-report are children. In the past, paediatric assessment focussed on the collection of observational data and information from proxy sources, such as parents and teachers. More recently, AHPs have come to understand the benefits of collecting self-report data from children. Sturgess et al. (2002) cite three reasons for using self-report with young children:

The first reason for using self-report with young children is that there is evidence that children hold a view about themselves which is unique, valid, and stable over time.

Secondly, increasingly sophisticated methods are being developed which provide ways for children to present this view reliably.

Lastly, children have a right to be intimately involved in the decisions being made about them. These arguments for using self-report are being substantiated by research and emerging clinical frames of reference (pp. 108–109).

Self-report data is critical when examining constructs such as pain. Pain is a very personal experience and is difficult to define and measure. In addition, research has indicated that carers overestimate pain relief following interventions compared with patients' reports. For example, see the study by Rundshagen et al. (1999), which examined patients' versus nurses' assessments of pain.

Self-report data can be collected using a range of methods including:

- structured, semi-structured or informal interview, given either face to face or via telephone
- a written format provided by standardised and un-standardised questionnaires, checklists, and surveys, which can be given to the person or sent via Web platforms, mail, or email for completion
- self-ratings, for example, on a Visual Analogue Scale (*VAS*) to rate pain
- self-monitoring through client journals, for example, to record symptoms, feelings, or activities undertaken
- card sorts (Barlow et al. 1984), for example, the Activity Card Sort (*ACS*; Baum and Edwards 2008; Laver-Fawcett 2019)
- narratives (for example, see Clouston 2003)
- play activities and the use of toys (e.g. dolls, dolls houses) for imaginary play and role play; joining children and participating actively in their play activities, particularly when the child is encouraged to direct the AHP and lead the play activity, can be very effective for opening up channels of communication (Swain 2004)
- the arts, such as drawings, paintings, sculpture, music to movement, and improvised drama (for example, see Dalton 1994).

Many methods for collecting self-report data are cost-effective in terms of time and resources. Self-report is very flexible, and as only a few materials are required – a pen and paper or a test form if a standardised test is being applied – the data can be collected easily in various environments including the person's own home, day care provider, outpatient clinic, ward, day hospital, workplace, school, etc. The critical question is how best to elicit what the person knows and feels and to distinguish between what they know and do not know and what they may or may not be prepared to share with you (Baldwin 1999, as cited in Sturgess et al. 2002).

An example of a structured interview self-report schedule is the Functional Life Scale (Sarno et al. 1973). An example of a self-report questionnaire is provided by the Satisfaction with Performance Scaled Questionnaire (Yerxa et al. 1988).

Self-report data is crucial for developing intervention goals that will have relevance and meaning for the person and, provided the person is able to communicate in some manner, should be a key component of all assessments no matter how brief. It can be used when the AHP does not have access to an environment suitable for observational testing or when the client refuses to undertake an observational assessment. In addition to being used as a baseline descriptive form of assessment, self-report is being increasingly used in measures of outcome. Adams (2002) warns about the levels of reliability in some self-report measures and stresses that 'care should be taken to ensure that any self-report account can be integrated as a valid and reliable outcome measure' (p. 173).

INTERVIEWING AS A MEANS OF COLLECTING SELF-REPORT DATA

The interview is commonly chosen by AHPs as the initial method of data collection and is a very useful method for collecting self-report data. Borg and Bruce (1991) reviewed the literature on interviewing and concluded that (a) interviewing is a crucial component of any assessment used to plan treatment; and (b) there are multiple ways to conduct an interview and not any one method is correct (p. 572). Smith (1993) stated 'an initial interview serves several vital purposes. It provides for:

1. collection of information about the patient to help develop objectives and plans for treatment;
2. establishment of understanding on the part of the patient about the role of the AHP and the purposes of the therapy process;
3. an opportunity for the patient to discuss the particular situation and think about plans for change' (p. 171).

In addition to collecting information for a baseline assessment, an initial interview forms the foundation for building rapport and forming the beginnings of an effective therapeutic relationship. Building good rapport is essential to obtaining a full history from the person, and so the AHP should consciously try to put the client at ease. AHPs need to be aware of how differences or similarities between themselves and their clients (for example, age, gender, and sociocultural background) can serve to either facilitate or hamper the development of rapport and the establishment of an effective therapeutic relationship.

It is important for the AHP to provide introductory information to set the scene for the first contact, and for a potential therapeutic relationship, this information should include:

- introducing themselves to the client;
- outlining their role as an AHP;
- explaining the purpose of the interview;
- describing the type of service that can be provided in that practice setting; and
- discussing the degree of confidentiality that applies by letting the client know with whom the AHP might share interview information.

When conducting an interview, AHPs should check that the person is able to hear, comprehend, and attend to the conversation. The nature of the assessment environment can serve to facilitate or disrupt the assessment process, so it is important that

AHPs ensure a quiet, private interview environment that is free from interruptions and distractions.

We recommend you should consider the nature of the referral when judging what the most appropriate environment will be. For example, Sturgess et al. (2002) noted that for children who have experienced traumatic or stressful events, removal to a separate room might make them feel isolated or trapped, and an environment where they are reassured by the presence of other children may make the child more relaxed and responsive. The ambient temperature should also be comfortable for the nature of the assessment: neither too hot, which might make a client feel drowsy and could reduce concentration, nor cold and draughty, particularly if the person being asked to undress for a physical assessment. Where possible, the person's usual environment should be selected, as the person is more likely to feel at ease in a familiar place. In addition, the person is likely to feel more empowered in their own environment, whereas in a therapy department the AHP needs to consider consciously that they are in their familiar place and that this environment may feel alien to the client.

It is important for the AHP to consider non-verbal body language. We recommend you should choose carefully where you sit in relation to the person; for example, a formal set-up with the AHP sitting behind a desk might not be conducive to providing a relaxed atmosphere. Instead, set up two comfortable chairs at a 90° angle to each other; removing the barrier of the desk and the direct confrontation of sitting opposite the person can help facilitate the sharing of information. The chair selected needs to be of an appropriate height and style to facilitate safe transfers and ensure comfort, particularly during a long interview or test administration. A number of authors have categorised factors that can influence the client, the AHP, and/or client–AHP interaction during an interview and that may facilitate or impede successful data collection using the interview method.

In the next section, we shall outline two pieces of work that describe influential factors which AHPs need to be mindful of while preparing for, during, and reflecting upon an interview. Fidler (1976, as cited by Smith 1993, p. 170) described **four filters** that impact the interactions between people and can be significant in distorting the interview or observation process, these are:

1. 'Perceptual: how sensory stimuli (colour of clothing, perfume) affect the way the other person is perceived;
2. Conceptual: the knowledge base brought to the interaction;
3. Role: the way each person perceives the role he or she is to play in the interaction;
4. Self-esteem: the way each person feels about himself or herself'.

AHPs need to be aware of these four filters and how they may influence their objectivity during an assessment, and also how they may influence the response of the client to the AHP and impact the formation of an effective therapeutic relationship.

Borg and Bruce (1991) categorised factors that can influence an interview process in a slightly different way. They also identify four influences for the AHP to consider:

1. The environmental factors, including the institution the AHP works for and the specific environment selected as the interview setting. Environmental issues have already been discussed above; in addition Borg and Bruce (1991) recommended:
   (a) selecting an atmosphere that conveys a feeling of warmth;
   (b) ensuring a minimum of distractions by putting a sign on the door indicating that an interview is in progress and by switching mobile/office

phones to silent and letting the answer-phone pick up messages during the course of the interview; and

(c) pre-planning so that any questionnaire, task, or test materials that might be required during the interview are collected in advance and easily accessible during the interview.

2. The influence of the AHP, which includes 'the [AHP's] interview skills, personal values, beliefs and theoretical orientation' (p. 573), all of which can influence the interview outcome. Recommended interviewing skills involve the AHP being an active listener who is aware of the impact of verbal and non-verbal communication and understands how facial expression, or a movement such as nodding, can convey acceptance or criticism of the client's comments or behaviour. When an AHP is able to actively listen, respect, and identify with the client's viewpoint, while maintaining their own identity, they become empathetic. Clients who experience genuine empathy from their AHPs are more likely to develop rapport and form effective therapeutic relationships. The AHP's theoretical orientation will shape the topics covered and the manner in which questions are asked; it will also influence the way in which the AHP analyses the information obtained and the nature of any hypotheses generated from this analysis.

3. Client influences: as with the AHP, the client brings a unique set of values, beliefs, and experiences to the assessment. As the person is presenting for therapy, he is likely to also come with needs, expectations, and perhaps some anxiety. Borg and Bruce (1991) further describe clients' factors as follows: 'they may be fearful, wonder what is permissible to discuss, or may have a specific agenda they wish to share. Their previous therapy experiences may confirm their discomfort or support their investment in therapy' (p. 573). So it is important for the AHP to allow sufficient time for an initial interview to explore and understand any client-focussed influences.

4. Dynamic interactions between AHP and client: The fourth area identified by Borg and Bruce (1991) they labelled 'Patient Symptoms and Interviewer responses'. The dynamic interactions that occur while establishing the therapeutic relationship are affected by the nature of the client's presenting problem, AHP–patient responses, and time–pressure. The presenting problem can have a varying impact depending upon its nature. For example, an AHP needs to be particularly mindful of responses when interviewing clients with mental health problems. The client may misinterpret the AHP's verbal and non-verbal communication, particularly if the client is experiencing paranoid or psychotic symptoms.

When interviewing young children, AHPs are advised to ask questions in a clear, direct, and unambiguous manner and to use concrete stimuli (such as objects, pictures, or photographs) to support the self-report by clarifying both the AHP's question and the child's verbal response. Care must be taken when selecting stimuli to ensure they are not over-stimulating, distracting, or confusing (Sturgess et al. 2002).

Benjamin (1974, as cited by Smith 1993) 'delineated three parts to an interview: initiation, development and closing' (p. 171).

The **initiation phase of an interview** involves:

- the AHP explaining the purpose of the interview, including the parameters, how long it should take, the type of topics to be discussed, and how the AHP plans to use the information

- the AHP describing their role in relation to the client in the clinical setting
- the AHP endeavouring to establish mutual understanding, respect, and trust with the client in order to build rapport and set the foundations for an effective therapeutic relationship.

The **development phase of an interview** involves the following:

- The AHP, in the role of interviewer, poses a series of questions to elicit information and to explore issues with the client.
- This phase is facilitated by having a list of planned questions or an outline of topics to be covered to help focus the interview and ensure that important information vital to an accurate baseline assessment and identifying relevant treatment objectives is not omitted.
- During this phase it is helpful if the AHP asks open questions that elicit a descriptive response, as opposed to closed questions which produce a one-word (yes, no, may be) type answer.
- Lewis (2003) has detailed that during the development phase of an interview the AHP needs to be skilled in asking one question at a time, tolerating silence, listening carefully, observing both verbal and non-verbal responses, restating or clarifying questions when needed, and encouraging the patient to continue to stay on track.

The **closing phase of an interview** involves the following:

- The AHP identifies that either the list of questions/topics to be addressed have all be covered and she has obtained the necessary information for this stage of the assessment process or that the allotted time has expired.
- The AHP should indicate to the client that the interview is coming to a close.
- The AHP should make clear that the interview is finishing and that there is no further opportunity at this time to bring up new issues.
- If there is further relevant information to be discussed, another time should be identified for continuing with the interview.
- If time allows, the AHP should summarise the key points that have been discussed to double-check that she has correctly understood and interpreted the information gained.

Communication, Insight, and Capacity Issues

One disadvantage of self-report is that the information provided 'may not accurately reflect patient performance' and the person's report of his functioning 'may vary considerably from actual performance observed by the AHP' (Culler 1993, p. 212). When selecting self-report as an assessment method, the AHP should be aware that a number of conditions might make the interview difficult to conduct and could lead to reduced reliability of the data collected. Prior to an initial interview, the AHP should check referral data to see if there are any factors that might indicate difficulties using a self-report method. These could include communication problems arising from speech problems, such as aphasia or dysarthria, or from hearing impairment. Cognitive capacity to provide a reliable self-report also should be considered. When the referral indicates a diagnosis such as dementia, acute confusional state, stroke, or traumatic brain injury, the AHP should be alert to the possibility of a related cognitive deficit and should be prepared to explore the issue of cognitive capacity to self-report. Extremes in mood state, such as depression or mania, can also influence the person's ability to engage effectively in the interview process. This may be associated with skewed responses; for example, a person with depression might underestimate his opportunities, resources, and abilities, whereas a person who is feeling elated during a period of mania might overestimate his opportunities, resources, and abilities. Although it is very important to gain insight to the person's viewpoint whatever his condition, in cases where the person's level of insight is questionable, it is particularly useful to compare self-report data with AHP observations, standardised test results, and proxy report.

Cultural Issues and Self-Report Data Collection

When conducting any assessment, and in particular interviews, AHPs should take into account the person's cultural background. It can be more difficult to establish good rapport when dealing with language barriers and differences in accepted forms of verbal and non-verbal communication. When the AHP and client cannot communicate directly, then a bilingual interpreter, volunteer, or family member can be used as a translator. Where possible try to obtain an outside interpreter. Although family members can be very helpful, they might not always be the best interpreter 'since they may be uncomfortable interpreting intense personal feelings ... or may distort what has been said due to their own interpretations' (McCormack et al. 1991, p. 21). In addition, there might be some information that a person prefers to keep confidential, and he may not want to discuss some things in front of family members. AHPs should try to use interpreters of the same sex and age as the person where possible, because generational and gender differences can affect the interview, particularly when the person is a first-generation immigrant. In addition to language barriers, the AHP should be aware of other factors that could impede the assessment process. These can occur when individuals' backgrounds lead to a distrust of health and social care providers and the health/social care system, or when people have a strong sense that these do not fit with their cultural traditions (McCormack et al. 1991). The AHP's goals for assessment, rehabilitation, and empowerment may need to be adapted if the person comes from a culture where a reliance upon family for care and support following an accident or illness exists, as opposed to an expectation to work towards maximising remaining skills in order to return to a maximum level of independence.

Although AHPs use self-report in the initial stages of assessment to form a picture of the person and the problems to be addressed through therapy, self-report can also be a useful method for monitoring progress during intervention. Used formally, self-monitoring is 'a process whereby the patient records specific behaviours or thoughts as they occur' (Christiansen and Baum 1991, p. 858). Self-report is particularly useful for monitoring any side effects related to an intervention, for example, increased pain following a series of prescribed physiotherapy exercises. Some standardised self-report tools have been developed as outcome measures that can be used to evaluate progress over time; the COPM (originally published in 1991, http://www.thecopm.ca), for example, provides a useful change score when used for reassessment. In addition, self-report data is an essential component of any service evaluation. An increased emphasis on clinical governance and best value is linked to a requirement for involving service users, not just in decisions about their own service provision, but also in an evaluation of the strengths and weaknesses of that service and an involvement with the identification of changes that need to be made to modernise service provision.

Examples of Self-Report Assessments

The following standardised tests are examples of self-report measures that can be used by AHPs.

Communication Checklist – Self-Report (CC-SR)

This is an example of a self-report instrument for older children and adults with communication impairments, with a particular emphasis on pragmatic difficulties (Bishop et al. 2009). This 70-item questionnaire is suitable for older children, adolescents, or adults who speak in sentences and have a reading age of at least 10 years. Fifty behavioural statements focus on communicative weaknesses and 20 on communicative strengths. In order to circumvent lack of self-awareness, some items are rated on the feedback the informant has received from other people (e.g. 'People tell me that I talk too much'). Z-scores, scales scores, and percentiles are provided for three composites: Language Structure, Pragmatic Skills, and Social Engagement (https://www.pearsonclinical.co.uk/ForAlliedHealthProfessionals/allied-health--assessments.aspx?tab=2).

Canadian Occupational Performance Measure (COPM)

The COPM is a good example of a robust self-report measure that can be used with a wide range of clients ranging from school-aged children up to older adults and with people who have a wide range of diagnoses, including both physical and mental health problems. It was developed in 1991 as a measure of performance, including the importance of performance problems and the client's level of satisfaction with performance. The COPM is a well-established standardised assessment and outcome measure, which is now published in its 5th edition (http://www.thecopm.ca/casestudy/psychometric-properties-of-the-copm). The COPM 'has been officially translated into 35 languages' and is used 'by occupational AHPs in over 40 countries throughout the world' (http://www.thecopm.ca). In a review of the literature published on the COPM (Carswell et al. 2004), 88 papers were identified the COPM in the title or the abstract. These reported on its psychometric properties, or its contribution to research outcomes or its contribution to OT practice; this level of publications from a wide variety of authors indicates how widely the COPM has become accepted in both practice and research.

The COPM has a semi-structured interview format. It is usually first completed as an initial assessment so that therapy objectives can be based upon problems selected by the client. The assessment covers the domains of self-care, productivity, and leisure. The client rates identified occupational performance issues in terms of importance (10 = extremely important to 1 = not important at all) and then rates the most important issues in terms of performance (10 = able to do it well to 1 = not able to do it) and satisfaction with that performance (10 = extremely satisfied to 1 = not satisfied at all). Following an agreed period of intervention, the COPM is administered again, and the client rates the same problem activities for performance and satisfaction, and their scores are summed and averaged. The differences between the initial, baseline scores, and the follow-up scores are calculated to provide a change score, which indicates the outcome. Although the COPM was primarily developed as a self-report tool, it can also be used successfully as a proxy measure with a carer, such as a parent or spouse. (Note: For an example of the COPM applied in practice, see the case study 'Scott' at the end of this chapter.)

Life Experienced Checklist (LEC)

Ager (1990) developed the LEC as a quality of life measure designed to gauge 'the range and extent of life experiences enjoyed by an individual' (p. 5). It comprises a 50-item checklist, divided into five domains: home, leisure, relationships, freedom, and opportunities. The LEC can be used 'with a wide range of client groups, including individuals with learning difficulties, the elderly and both mental health in-patients and out-patients' (p. 5). The LEC can be used as a self-rating tool or as a proxy measure. For clients/carers who have sufficient reading comprehension, the LEC is administered as a self-report checklist, and some services post it to the client and/or carer for completion; it can also be administered as an interview. The LEC has a dichotomous scoring system, in which either an item applies to the client or not, so each question has be written to elicit a clear yes or no response, and the client (or AHP if administered as an interview) simply ticks the items that apply. For example, an item from the Leisure domain is 'I visit friends or relatives for a meal at least once per month' (p. 2 of the LEC form).

Visual Analogue Pain Scale

AHPs have used Visual Analogue Scales (VAS) since the late 1960s (Lasagna 1960). A VAS comprises either a 100 mm or 30 cm line, drawn either horizontally or vertically, and labelled with two verbal expressions at the extreme ends to indicate the maximum and minimum points on a continuum of a sensation or feeling. VAS is used for the assessment of intensity or magnitude of a subjective experience, such as pain, breathlessness, or fatigue. The Visual Analogue Pain Scale (*VAPS*; Strong et al. 1990), is used for obtaining a self-report from clients on the intensity of their pain. The scale uses a horizontal 100-mm-long line with ends labelled 'no pain' on the left and 'unbearable pain' on the right. The client is asked to mark or point to the position on the scale that represents the intensity of his pain, and the AHP then measures the distance from the left end to the client's mark (range 0 to 100). Therefore, a client must be able to conceptualise a sensory continuum and partition a closed range as an indication of their experience of pain on that continuum. AHPs find this simple to administer and easy to score (Pynsent et al. 2004).

Occupational Performance History Interview (OPHI)

Kielhofner and Henry (1988) developed the OPHI. It covers the domains of organisation of daily routines; life roles, interests, values, and goals; perceptions of ability and responsibility; and environmental influences. The OPHI comprises 39 questions and focuses on the past and present for each area. There is a Life History Narrative Form for summarising data. Scoring uses a 5-point ordinal scale (5 = adaptive to 1 = maladaptive). In 2004, a second version was published (https://www.moho.uic.edu/productDetails.aspx?aid=31).

PATIENT-REPORTED OUTCOME MEASURES (PROMs)

PROMs are questionnaires measuring the patients' views of their health status (NHS England, https://www.england.nhs.uk/statistics/statistical-work-areas/proms). PROMs have been a programme of evaluation of surgical outcomes based on questionnaires completed by patients before and after their surgery in England since 2009. Eligible patients are those treated by or on behalf of the English NHS for the following procedures: hip replacements, knee replacements, varicose vein surgery, and groyne hernia surgery. **PREMs** are questionnaires measuring the patients' perceptions of their experience while receiving healthcare services, such as timeliness of service delivery, the environment, and facilities (Bull et al. 2019).

PROMs are being used more widely across healthcare (Chan et al. 2019), though Calvert et al. (2019) raised a number of challenges for us to consider to maximise the impact of patient-reported outcome assessment for patients and society. They suggested that multiple questionnaires could be burdensome for the patient and that 'patients may be unsure why they are being asked to complete a PROM, who will access their responses, and how the data will be used' (p. 3). However, they go on to say that sharing of PROM data may offer huge benefits to society through better health outcomes and use of resources. We need to be mindful of the principles of patient-centred care that incorporate the patient voice and patient-reported outcomes into our practice, such as the timely explanation of information based on patient need and delivery of the information in a way that can help patients take effective actions to manage their own health and well-being (Nelson et al. 2015). Yorkston and Baylor (2019) suggest that the use of PROMs may allow us as AHPs to focus treatment on issues that patients view as valuable and to document the outcomes of these interventions.

The COSMIN initiative (https://www.cosmin.nl, Mokkink et al. 2016) was formed to improve the selection of outcome measurement instruments by developing methodological guidelines based on consensus reached in a broad international panel of experts, and is a useful resource for identifying the right measure for your patients to complete (https://www.cosmin.nl/finding-right-tool). The COSMIN focus started with PROMs. See Chapter 7 for further details.

Examples of Generic PROMs

EuroQoL (EQ-5D™ Index, https://euroqol.org/euroqol) collates responses given in five broad areas (mobility, self-care, usual activities, pain/discomfort, and anxiety/depression) and combines them into a single value. This questionnaire is an example of a generic PROM as it measures well-being regardless of a person's illness or disorder, and is used by AHPs (Kyte et al. 2015).

EuroQol Visual Analogue Scales (EQ-VAS) is a simple and easily understood 'thermometer'-style measure based on a patient's self-scored general health on the day that they completed their questionnaire. The scale provides an indication of their health that is not necessarily associated with the condition they have and which may have been influenced by factors other than healthcare. Feng et al. (2014) have suggested that 'in applications where the *patients'* view of their overall health is the measurement goal, the EQ-VAS is *prima facie* more appropriate than the use of EQ-5D profile data weighted by general public preferences' (p. 985).

Examples of Specific PROMs

Oxford Hip Score/Oxford Knee Score/Aberdeen Varicose Vein Questionnaires combine into a single score a patient's answers to a number of health questions of particular relevance to hips, knees, or varicose veins (Kwong et al. 2018).

PROXY REPORT

In addition to seeking information directly from a client, information can be obtained from a number of other (proxy) sources. A proxy is formally defined as 'a person or agency of substitute recognized by law to act for, and in the best interest of the patient' (Centre for Advanced Palliative Care 2005). However, in the context of therapy assessment, the term *proxy* is used more widely to refer to an informant (e.g. carer, professional) who has knowledge about the circumstances or condition of the client who is able to share that knowledge with the person's permission or without breaking laws of confidentiality.

A proxy report is sometimes referred to as an informant interview (Borg and Bruce 1991). A proxy or informant report can be particularly helpful when a client has communication difficulties or lacks insight into his problems and level of ability. To assist AHPs in prioritisation of referrals prior to assessment, or when the AHP wants to understand how a primary carergiver (such as a parent or spouse) is coping with their carer role, or when the AHP wishes to check whether the client's perspectives and priorities are consistent with those of his family/teacher/healthcare providers. Where the client has a condition that impacts his ability to provide an adequate self-report use of a proxy as translator to interpret sign language, symbol boards, facial expression, and body language or as someone who knows the person's pronunciation and use of language sufficiently well to translate is very helpful. In addition, where the client has communication difficulties, the relevance of the perceptions and views of the family/caregivers becomes even more critical (Tullis and Nicol 1999), such as when working with children, people with communication problems (such as following a stroke), and people with dementia. Swain (2004), for example, states that 'though a physiotherapist working, for instance, with a person with learning difficulties may have difficulties understanding him or her, it is often the case that others, including members of a young person's family, other professions or an advocate are "tuned in" to him or her' (p. 218).

Proxy sources may include:

- the person's primary caregiver (either an informal carer such as a family member, neighbour, or volunteer, or a formal caregiver, warden, nursing home staff, or home help);
- other members of the AHP's multidisciplinary team (for example, occupational therapists, physiotherapists, speech and language therapists, psychologist, social worker, nurse, doctor);
- other health professionals involved with the client's care (such as their general practitioner [*GP*], health visitor, or district nurse); and
- other professionals working with the client (such as a case manager, teacher, or lawyer).

A proxy report can be of value because, in the majority of cases, other people will spend much more time than the AHP with the client and will have opportunities to see how the client is managing over a longer time frame and in a different and/or wider range of settings. For example, in an inpatient setting, nurses on the ward will be in greater contact with the patient, and in an outpatient setting, the parent or partner will have seen how the person is managing in the home environment, while a colleague, employer, or teacher could share information about the person's abilities and problems in a work or school setting.

A proxy report may be obtained in person through interviewing the proxy face to face or over the telephone, through case conferences, ward rounds, and team meetings or via written data. Written information from family members and neighbours might involve letters or the use of standardised or un-standardised checklists and questionnaires. Written information from other professionals might comprise referrals, letters, medical notes, and assessment reports. Increasingly, much of this information is held in electronic formats and, depending on the clinical setting, might be accessible via a computer database, for example, in a secondary care setting via the hospital's intranet. Reports and information from colleagues from other organisations and settings might be sent via Web application platforms, post, or email.

Proxy reports are being increasingly used to assist AHPs screen referrals to help determine whether the referral is appropriate and/or to help prioritise referrals. Green et al. (2005) undertook a study that explored the value of parent and teacher reports using two standardised questionnaires in order to identify which referrals would require a full clinic-based observational assessment. They found that the parent report was quite reliable in the identification of appropriate referrals. Nevertheless, they had a poor response rate from the teacher proxies and found that the increased time required by the AHPs to chase schools to increase the return rate resulted in little cost benefit for their goal of better managing their waiting list.

The initial interaction with the person's family/caregiver (often referred to as the carer) can provide the foundation for building effective partnerships with carers. This can be critical to support the person and their carer to manage complex issues in the home/community environment and to integrate the intervention into the person's daily routines at home. An initial interview with a carer can serve several purposes, including the forming of a working relationship, the gathering of information about the client and his environment, and the provision of information to the carer about the AHP's role, strategies for supporting the client, available services, and carer support structures. In some practice settings (such as an acute, short-stay inpatient setting), the AHP may only have the opportunity to meet the carer on one or two occasions, for example, when the family come into a ward to visit or during an assessment home visit. In this case, the AHP may need to interweave both the obtaining of data for assessment and intervention in the form of instruction, advice, support, etc.

Clark et al. (1995) identified four main types of interaction categories that occur between AHPs and carers during assessment and treatment:

1. *Caring interactions* that focussed on friendliness and support
2. *Partnering interactions* that involved seeking and acknowledging input and reflective feedback to help caregivers make changes/modify behaviour or to affirm existing caregiver practices
3. *Informing interactions* that involved gathering information, explaining information, and clarifying information
4. *Directing interactions* that involved the provision of instruction and advice.

The type of information provided by a proxy will vary considerably depending upon the amount of contact the proxy has with the person, their relationship, and their degree of involvement. Discrepancies can decrease between proxy reports and self-reports if the assessed concept is one that concrete objective behaviours are able to be referred to (e.g. the ability to eat, bathe, etc.). However, discrepancies often arise when proxies are asked to evaluate more subjective and abstract experiences (e.g. pain and emotional well-being; Perkins 2007). The AHP needs to be aware of these factors in order to evaluate the value and reliability of the proxy's report.

In some instances, it can be useful to seek informal and/or standardised assessment data from more than one proxy, for example, both a child's parents, a parent and teacher, or all the children of a client. A mother and father might have different perceptions about a child's abilities and needs, as might children in relation to their parent's condition and problems. When interpreting discrepancies in viewpoints among multiple proxy reports, it is helpful to reflect on the amount of time a proxy spends with the client and also any cues that suggest the nature of the relationship between a proxy and client. For example, Abidin (1995), author of the Parenting Stress Index (PSI), states that when the PSI is administered to both a child's parents, 'spreads of up to 10 raw score points between mothers and fathers are to be expected' (p. 8). Abidin (1995) notes that where the mother is the primary caretaker of a child with a behaviour disorder, AHPs should expect the father's PSI scores to be lower. He explains that 'this does not indicate that fathers' perceptions are less clouded by their own situations, but [that] the mothers' greater involvement with child care leaves them open to greater stress associated with their children's behaviour' (p. 8).

Examples of Assessments That Use Information from a Proxy

Memory and Behaviour Problem Checklist (MBPC)

The MBPC is used with carers of people with dementia. Zarit et al. (1986) published the original version, and Teri et al. (1992) reported on a revised version. It can be administered by interview or using a self-completion survey format. The RMBPC covers items such as sleep disturbance, wandering, aggressive outbursts, and help needed with self-care. Items are scored on a five-point ordinal scale that measures the frequency and intensity of the observed problems (0 = problem has never been observed to 4 = indicates that problem occurs daily or more often).

Pediatric Evaluation of Disability Inventory (PEDI)

Hayley et al. (1992) developed the PEDI to assess the functioning of children aged 6 months to 7.5 years. It covers the domains of self-care, mobility, and social functioning. A proxy report can be gained from parents, or from teachers or rehabilitation professionals who are familiar with the child. The PEDI assesses capability using a Functional Skills Scale and performance of functional activities using a Caregiver Assistance Scale. A Modifications Scale records environmental modifications and equipment used by the child in routine activities of daily living (ADL).

The Health Utilities Index (HUI®)

HUI is a family of generic health profiles and preference-based systems for the purposes of measuring health status, reporting health-related quality of life, and producing utility scores (Horsman et al. 2003, http://www.healthutilities.com).

The 15-item questionnaire (15Q) is designed for self-completion, includes 15 multiple-choice HUI questions, and takes approximately 5–10 minutes to complete. The 40-item questionnaire (40Q), with a built-in skip-pattern based on item response, is designed for interviewer administration either face to face or by telephone. Each of the 15Q and 40Q formats of HUI questionnaires are available in two versions: a self-assessment version, to collect information from people about their own health; and a proxy-assessment version, to collect information about the health status of study subjects from people other than the subjects themselves.

Infant-Toddler Symptom Checklist

The Infant-Toddler Symptom Checklist (DeGangi 1995) is a proxy measure developed for use with parents of 7- to 30-month-old infants and toddlers. The Symptom checklist can be used stand alone as a screen to identify infants and toddlers 'who are at risk for sensory-integrative disorders, attentional deficits, and emotional and behavioural problems' (p. 1). It can also be used alongside other observational developmental measures to aid diagnosis. The measure covers nine test domains: self-regulation; attention; sleep; eating or feeding; dressing, bathing and touch; movement; listening and language; looking and sight; and attachment/emotional functioning. It comprises five age-banded checklists (for 7–9, 10–12, 13–18, 19–24, and 25–30 months) and a general screening version that can be used across a 7–30-month child population when it is not convenient to select an age-appropriate version, for example, handed to parents to complete in an outpatient clinic waiting room. The symptom checklist can be either given to parents to self-complete or can be filled in during an interview. For parent self-completion, the authors provide an example cover sheet that explains the scoring and asks parents to record demographic information and details about the child's birth, delivery, medical problems, etc. The manual states that it takes approximately 10 minutes. Most items are rated on a 3-point ordinal scale:

1. Never or sometimes, if the child has never had this difficulty, or has it infrequently or some of the time
2. Most times, if this a difficulty the child experiences frequently or most of the time at present
3. Past, if this was a problem in the past, but is no longer a problem.

Canadian Occupational Performance Measure (COPM)

Although the COPM (Law et al. 1991; see earlier summary in section titled 'Self-Report') was designed primarily as a self-report measure, it can also be used as a proxy-report measure with a carer (such as a parent or spouse). Carswell et al. (2004) found a number of studies in their literature review that 'showed how the COPM could be used to gather information from proxy respondents on behalf of clients who cannot report reliably on their own occupational performance' (p. 216). Wallen and Ziviani (2012) found that COPM can be used as a valid proxy assessment.

Measures That Assess the Proxy (e.g. Caregiver and Parent Burden Scales)

In some cases, where the proxy is an informal carer, such as a spouse, parent, sibling, or child, the carer may also be the focus of part of the assessment. Where carer burden is identified, and intervention, such as respite, education, and counselling, is called for, then the proxy also might become a service user in his/her own right.

Life Satisfaction Index – Parents (LSI-P)

The LSI-P (Renwick and Reid 1992) is a self-report tool used to assess parents' quality of life and experience of parenting a child with a disability. The LSI-P was developed as a research tool to explore the nature of quality of life for parents of a child with a disability. The LSI-P addresses five domains: (a) general well-being; (b) interpersonal relationships; (c) personal development; (d) personal fulfilment; and (e) leisure and recreation. The LSI-P is a 45-item index (9 items per domain) based on a series of statements that the parent rates on a Likert-type scale. Items are scored on a 6-point scale: 1 = strongly disagree; 2 = disagree; 3 neither agree nor disagree; 4 = agree; 5 = strongly agree; and 6 = not applicable. The LSI-P can be a self-administered questionnaire or administered in the context of an interview. The LSI-P is a useful assessment to use with parents at the first appointment; they can be asked to complete it at home, or it can be administered as an interview, which provides the AHP with the opportunity to discuss parents' responses to statements.

Caregiver Stress Index

The Caregiver Stress Index (Robinson 1983) comprises 13 items covering stressful aspects of caring, including demand on time; physical strain; emotional adjustment; changes in personal plans; work adjustment; sleep disturbance; inconvenience; and upset related to changes in the cared-for person. Construct and predictive validity were established by the developer on a sample of 85 family carers of older people admitted to hospital owing to physical conditions (Robinson 1983). The original version uses a dichotomous 2-point scale. Thornton and Travis (2003) found that the Modified CSI is easily administered and scored and can be a useful method for detecting strain levels among informal caregivers.

Parenting Stress Index (PSI)

The PSI (Abidin 1983, 1997) is a proxy measure developed for use with parents of children aged 1 month to 12 years. The PSI is a normative assessment, and original norms were based on 2633 mothers (age 16 to 61 years, mean age 30.9) of children aged 1 month to 12 years. References are provided for research using the PSI with a wide range of child populations including birth defects (e.g. spina bifida, congenital heart disease), communication disorders (e.g. hearing impairment, speech deficits), attention deficit hyperactivity disorder (*ADHD*), autism, developmental disability, learning disabled, premature infants, at risk/abused children, and other health problems (such as asthma, diabetes, and otitis media). Originally developed in the United States with norms mainly based on a white American population, the PSI has since been used in a number of cross-cultural studies and has been translated into Spanish, Chinese, Portuguese, Finnish, Japanese, Italian, Hebrew, Dutch, and French. The manual describes the PSI as a screening and diagnostic tool. The parent is given a seven-page reusable item booklet containing a front sheet with scoring instructions and 120 questions. The parent is given a separate answer sheet/profile form and is asked to circle his/her answer for each of the 101 PSI items and on the 19 item Life Stresses scale if required. For most items, an ordinal scale is used. The majority of items are scored on a 5-point Likert-type scale: strongly agree; agree; not sure; disagree; and strongly disagree. (Note: For more details on the PSI, see the detailed Test Critique provided in Chapter 10.)

OBSERVATIONAL ASSESSMENT METHODS

AHPs should not just rely upon self-report and the proxy report for the assessment because some research studies have found discrepancies between reported and observed function. Some authors state that the most reliable form of functional assessment is considered to be direct observation.

Although the term *observational methods* is used here, it refers more widely to methods in which the AHP directly uses their senses to assess some aspect of the client's problem or situation. Although visual observations and the use of verbal instructions/questions to elicit the client's response as a behaviour/reply will form the basis for a significant proportion of direct therapy assessment, the use of other senses can be very important. For example, some assessment methods use active listening (e.g. auscultation of lung sounds), smell (e.g. smells can help the AHP identify a problem with incontinence or the risk of the person consuming food that has gone off), or touch (where the AHP is assessing the degree of resistance in a muscle as an indication of stiffness or spasticity). AHPs are trained in direct observational skills, and many therapy assessments will involve some sort of observation.

This method of assessment provides data about the person's level of ability to perform specific tasks in specific environments and yields useful information from the process used to attempt the assessment task and from the quality of the person's performance. AHPs, particularly physiotherapists, also use direct observational/auditory assessment to measure physiological processes such as respiratory rate, blood pressure, and heart rate using methods such as percussion, palpation, and sphygmomanometers.

Occupational therapists are trained in activity analysis, and a particular area of their expertise is considered to be 'in assessing clients and drawing inferences based on their direct observation of the client's performance' (Law 1993, p. 234). Fisher and Bray Jones (2006) refers to this as a 'performance analysis', which she defines as 'the observational evaluation of the quality of a person's task performance to identify discrepancies between the demands of a task and the skill of the person' (p. 2). She recommends an assessment approach that involves the AHP observing and evaluating a client's skill as he 'engages in the course of actions that comprises the process of performing occupations' (p. 3).

There are several ways of observing clients, and AHPs create opportunities to observe clients in a variety of formal, structured activities and informal, unstructured situations. For example, you may:

- administer a standardised test that requires the performance of test items which are observed and recorded;
- set up an activity for the person to perform and then observe from the sidelines; or
- choose to be a participant-observer who will observe the client's performance while engaged in an activity or task together with the person.

If you can create opportunities to interact informally as a participant-observer in situations where role differentiation is less defined than in a formal testing situation, they can often obtain information (for example, on roles, interests, values, and ability) that might otherwise be difficult to assess accurately or might not come to light. Therefore, it is desirable to build opportunities for informal contact into the assessment if possible, particularly where an in-depth assessment is required and the therapeutic relationship is likely to last for some time – such as with a person with a long-term mental health condition who will have an AHP care coordinator from a community mental health team or a person with a stroke or head injury who will be treated in a rehabilitation unit over several weeks or months). Informal situations can be created even in more formal hospital environments, for example, by escorting a patient from the ward to the therapy department and seeing how they mobilise, manage the lift, or explore and purchase items in the hospital shop or restaurant. It can also be useful to allow few minutes before or after a treatment session to interact informally with the person and their family or carer, for example, in the waiting room or while family are visiting the person's bedside on the ward.

The ability of an individual to perform a set task to a specified standard is straightforward to observe. However, the underlying functions that impact task performance, such as the functioning of the sensory, perceptual, and cognitive systems, cannot be observed directly. Within the allied health professions, it is accepted that you will draw inferences from observed behaviours about underlying functional status. The accuracy and value of observational assessment is dependent on the expertise of the AHP undertaking the observation and the thoroughness and objectivity with which observations are recorded.

You should be aware that there is a risk when drawing inferences from observed behaviour that your own subjective feelings will influence the behaviours that you focus upon during the observation and the way in which these behaviours are interpreted. AHPs construct inferences in the form of hypotheses, and this is linked to a process called diagnostic reasoning, which is explored later in Chapter 6.

There are some areas of assessment where it is particularly useful to use a formal or standardised assessment method, rather than informal observation. For example, when measuring range of movement, informal observational assessment has been found to be unreliable and goniometric measurement has been found to be superior (Atkins 2004). Atkins also cites literature indicating 'that the visual inspection of gait is unsystematic, subjective and observer skill dependent' and states that 'even skilled observers miss subtle abnormalities and have difficult quantifying simple parameters such as cadence, stride length and velocity' (2004 p. 361). However, sometimes an AHP may be aware that a standardised measurement would be more reliable, but might not have access to the relevant equipment or test, or be unable to apply it in their clinical setting. For example, gait analysis is often undertaken as a subjective observation in the client's own home or in a ward setting. However, it can be measured more objectively when equipment is available in a physiotherapy department to undertake gait laboratory analysis, such as force and pressure measurements at the foot–ground interface and using electromyography to provide data on muscle action potentials.

A large proportion of therapy and rehabilitation assessments (both standardised and non-standardised) involve the observation of the performance of ADL. Examples include the following:

- Functional Independence Measure (*FIM*; Granger et al. 1993)
- Klein-Bell Activities of Daily Living Scale (Klein and Bell 1982)
- Rivermead ADL Assessment (Lincoln and Edmans 1990; Whiting and Lincoln 1980)
- Rivermead Mobility Index (Collen et al. 1991), which assesses a range of mobility tasks considered essential to basic ADL.

Another large group of assessments comprises batteries of observational tasks developed to assess functioning at an impairment level. Examples include the following:

- Alberta Infant Motor Scale (*AIMS*; Piper et al. 1992)
- Chedoke-McMaster Stroke Assessment (Gowland et al. 1993)
- Chessington OT Neurological Assessment Battery (COTNAB; Tyerman et al. 1986)
- Peabody Developmental Motor Scales (Folio and Fewell 1983)
- Rivermead Perceptual Assessment Battery (*RPAB*; Whiting et al. 1985).

A few observational assessments provide data across several levels of function. Examples of observational assessments that examine performance of ADL, at the disability level, and provide information about functional limitations and/or underlying impairment, such as motor and cognitive functioning, include the following:

- Arnadottir OT-ADL Neurobehavioural Evaluation (*A-ONE*; Arnadottir 1990)
- Assessment of Motor Process Skills (*AMPS*; Fisher 2003)

- Kitchen Task Assessment (*KTA*; Baum and Edwards 1993)
- Structured Observational Test of Function (*SOTOF*; Laver and Powell 1995).

COMBINING METHODS

The critical advice here is to obtain multiple measures to produce a complete assessment of the client's progress. It is especially important to use multiple measures, because the measures might produce different results.

(Barlow et al. 1984, p. 124)

The most comprehensive way in which to conduct an assessment is to collect data from several sources using a range of assessment methods and then compare the data looking for similarities and differences in the findings. You may choose to interview people about their ability rather than conduct an observational assessment due to the time required. It is usually not feasible to observe all areas of ability relevant to the person; the most reliable method is to interview individuals and their proxies about their performance in the full range of their activities and then select a few key activities/areas of functioning for direct observation/testing. Although self-reports and proxy reports can be a useful adjunct to observational data, they rarely replace observational assessment completely. Green et al. (2005) reported that a parent report was valuable, but that it did not replace the full clinical assessment undertaken by the AHP, as there were inadequate levels of specificity obtained from the proxy measure. Hammell (2004) warns that observational assessment cannot be a truly objective exercise because the client who is being assessed may not share judgements made by an AHP. Therefore, the most valid and reliable assessment will combine data collection methods and compare and contrast the findings from each of the sources. The more significant the decisions that are to be made from the assessment, such as deciding who is fit to return home and who might require long-term institutional care, the more critical it is that the assessment fully represents all viewpoints.

Sturgess et al. (2002) describe the benefits of combining observational methods, such as filming, with self-report and parent reports when assessing young children. They cited research that demonstrated that children's views are different from those of their parents. They noted that the parent could only provide an opinion about how they think a child feels and that this can be contaminated by the adult's view of how they think the child should feel or how they think they would have felt themselves in a similar situation.

Sometimes you might acquire different, and even conflicting, information from different sources. In this situation, it is helpful for you to develop a series of hypotheses about the client and their situation and then to examine these hypotheses using all the information available. When interpreting hypotheses using discrepant information from different sources, it is helpful to judge the data in the context of the motivations, fears, and viewpoints of the people who provided the conflicting opinions. Factors that influence performance, such as pain, fatigue, medication, and mood, can result in people forming different, yet valid, perceptions about a person's ability. What you might observe a person do in a hospital environment on one occasion may be very different from what the person's family observe them doing regularly at home.

Velozo (1993) described how we should combine methods to provide a thorough assessment of a person's ability to work. The suggested assessment process included the following:

1. Review of medical, educational, and vocational records
2. Interviews with the patient, family, employer, teachers, and other personnel

3. Observation
4. Inventories and checklists
5. Standardised and non-standardised evaluations.

An example of an assessment that combines methods is the **PEDI**. The PEDI (Hayley et al. 1992) is a good example of a therapy assessment that combines data collection methods within a standardised assessment. The PEDI requires the use of AHP observation and interview with the parent, and in this chapter we have explored how as AHPs we use a wide range of data collection methods and sources of information in order to undertake a thorough assessment. These methods and sources are summarised in Figure 2.1.

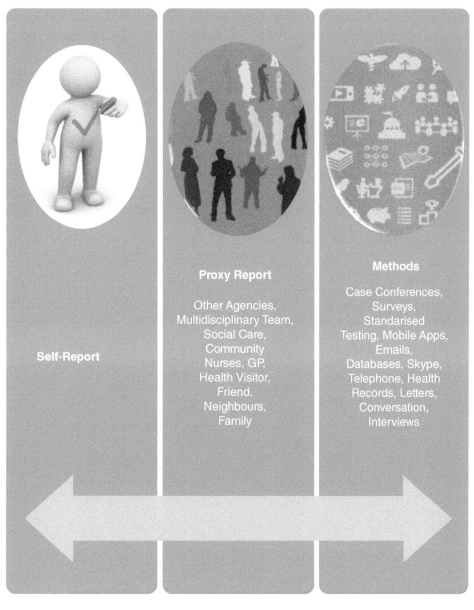

Self-Report

Proxy Report

Other Agencies,
Multidisciplinary Team,
Social Care,
Community
Nurses, GP,
Health Visitor,
Friend,
Neighbours,
Family

Methods

Case Conferences,
Surveys,
Standarised
Testing, Mobile Apps,
Emails,
Databases, Skype,
Telephone, Health
Records, Letters,
Conversation,
Interviews

FIGURE 2.1   The wide range of data collection methods and sources used by AHPs.
Source: From Laver-Fawcett (2002). © 2002, Elsevier.

DOCUMENTATION

You need to find logical ways to structure and document the myriad of information and observations that are obtained when combining data collection methods. One method commonly used is that of problem-orientated documentation, which is a structured system of documentation that has four basic components (Cameron and Turtle-Song 2002):

1. A summary of **subjective** data (gathered from the client and any proxy)
2. A summary of any **objective** data (gathered from structured observations or the administration of standardised tests)
3. An **assessment** and **analysis** which is generated from both sources of data
4. The **plan** for treatment.

These are sometimes referred to as SOAP notes, which stands for: subjective, objective, assessment (the analysis of data to formulate an understanding of the client's problems) and plan (for intervention/management/treatment; Gossman et al. 2019). Identified problems are numbers. Each subsequent entry in the notes can refer to one or more problems, with the related problem number written in the margin. Entries are only made when there is something of significance to report, such as new information or a change in functioning. Therefore, the last entry for a numbered problem should be the most up to date, regardless of when it was written. Not every SOAP heading has to be used for each entry; for example, you may record something said by the client and their assessment of what this meant, but have not undertaken any related direct measurement, nor need to take action at this point. In this case, entries will be made under the headings S and A only. For an example of a SOAP entry, see Box 2.1.

Electronic Records

As Electronic Health Records (*EHR*) became normal practice in health and social care settings (Hastings 2010), others have suggested we may need to record our notes as APSO rather than the traditional SOAP, so that the Assessment and Plan appear first when reviewing a person's health record (Gossman et al. 2019; Pearce et al. 2016).

AHPs need to be scrupulous about their documentation and record keeping to prevent being exposed to negligence claims or breaking of confidentiality laws. AHPs must make their records carefully, avoiding abbreviated or ambiguous notes and ensuring that any handwritten notes are legible. No document should be open to misinterpretation as AHPs may have to rely on them should their practice face a legal challenge, which could occur several years later. Therefore, notes should be accurate, contemporaneous, concise, legible, logical in sequence, and signed after each entry.

Ethical Practice, Data Protection, and Confidentiality

Engaging in ethical practice is one key competency for [AHPs] therapists (Van der Kaay et al. 2019, p. 210). Confidentiality of this information is critically important. AHPs are

---

Box 2.1   Example SOAP Notes

S = Subjective: This includes relevant comments, feelings, or opinions made by the patient/carer about a specific problem.

e.g. *Mr Brown says he does not know why he had to come today, refusing to join the reminiscence group. Spoke to wife on the telephone: Mrs Brown reports her husband was very agitated this morning and did not want to get on the ambulance to come to the day hospital.*

O = Objective: This is what the therapist does, observes, or measures, and should be repeatable had it been undertaken by another therapist. Treatment/interventions given can also be recorded here, in addition to assessment information.

e.g. *Reassessed Mr Brown on the 6-item Cognitive Impairment Test (6 CIT) to see if there was a further decline in mental state. Scored 21/28. Previous score from GP referral undertaken two months ago was 14/28, indicating an increased level of impairment.*

Used Reality Orientation techniques with Mr Brown in a one-to-one session for 30 minutes, orientating him to where he was, why his GP had referred him to the day hospital, day, date, time, and looked at the newspaper together.

A = Assessment/Analysis: This is a statement of the therapist's professional opinion based on the information recorded under S and O. Hypotheses with therapist's rationale can be written here.

e.g. *Mr Brown's 6 CIT scores indicate increased level of cognitive impairment, and Mr Brown appeared more disorientated and agitated today; this may be related to multi-infarct dementia, and Mr Brown may have suffered from another infarct. He might also have an infection that is causing the sudden deterioration in function.*

Mr Brown appeared to respond well to the one-to-one attention and Reality Orientation approach.

P = Plan: This is what the therapist plans to do about the problem, in the short or long term.

- *Ask duty psychiatrist to undertake a physical examination today and check for a chest infection, urinary tract infection, etc.*

- *Report to Consultant psychiatrist at the next multidisciplinary team (MDT) meeting the change in six CIT scores.*

- *Involve Mr Brown in a Reality Orientation Group each morning on arrival to the day hospital.*

- *Educate Mrs Brown in the Reality Orientation approach for her use with Mr Brown at home.*

---

ethically and legally obliged to safeguard confidential information relating to a client. Security of information and records are very important. AHPs are obliged to keep all information secure and only release records to people who have a legitimate right and need to access them. The Health Care Professions Council in the United Kingdom sets out a set of standards of performance, conduct, and ethics by which all registrants must work (HCPC, 2016; see https://www.hcpc-uk.org/standards/standards-of-conduct-performance-and-ethics). These include communicating appropriately, respecting confidentiality, managing risk, reporting concerns about safety, and keeping records of your work.

AHPs should be aware of local and national policies on electronic notes (which include emails, computerised records, letters) and should adhere to these policies. All AHPs should also be aware of other codes of practice, policies, and law related to confidentiality issues, such as the Data Protection Act 2018, the NHS Constitution for England (2015), and the Rights Act (1998).

THE USE OF CASE SCENARIOS TO SUPPORT METHODS OF ASSESSMENT IN PRACTICE

For students, the process of selecting and pulling together the results of a number of different methods of assessment may feel daunting. Case histories/studies/scenarios can be an excellent way of understanding how theory translates into practice and of illustrating an approach in a clinical setting. In addition to the detailed case study presented below, the following references may also be of interest:

- Baum et al. (2000) in their article 'Measuring Function in Alzheimer's Disease'. The paper describes a range of measures including self-report, proxy, and observational measures and illustrates how these can be applied to an assessment process through the case of a 62-year-old man with dementia and his wife.
- Unsworth's text (1999), *Cognitive and Perceptual Dysfunction: A Clinical Reasoning Approach to Evaluation and Intervention,* contains a number of detailed case studies. For example, Laver and Unsworth (1999) have written a case study about a 29-year-old man who experience cerebral bleeding leading to stroke, in which an assessment process using standardised self-report, proxy-report, and observational measures are applied.

Case Study: Scott

by Sally Payne, Claire Howell, and Alison Laver-Fawcett

This case study illustrates how an occupational therapy service assembled a toolkit of standardised assessments to gather information from a range of sources using a number of different methods. The first part of this study describes the service and the rationale for the measures that therapists selected to use. The second part shows how these assessments are applied in a clinical setting through the case of a teenage boy, whom we will refer to as 'Scott'.

About the Occupational Therapist

Sarah qualified as an occupational therapist 15 years ago and has spent much of this time working with children and young people in the NHS. She has worked as a member of two multidisciplinary preschool child development teams, and with a variety of agencies when working with school-aged children in the community. Sarah leads a small community paediatric occupational therapy service in an urban area on the edge of a large city with a population of 220 000.

The Setting

The community paediatric occupational therapy service uses the Person-Environment-Occupational (*PEO*) model of practice (Law et al. 1996) to guide the development, delivery, and evaluation of services to children, young people, and their families. The PEO model encourages a 'top-down' approach to occupational therapy referral, assessment, intervention, and evaluation with improved occupational performance being the aim of therapy. The PEO is a trans-active model of occupational behaviour in which occupational performance is considered to be the product of a dynamic relationship between people, occupations or roles, and their environment (Law et al. 1996). The occupational therapist facilitates change in the person, environment, and/or occupational dimensions to improve occupational performance.

Any adult who knows the child well and who has a concern about their occupational performance can refer children and young people to the occupational therapy service. Occupational therapy involves developing collaborative relationships with the child or young person and his or her parents/carers, teachers, and other professionals. Assessment and intervention plans are tailored to meet the needs of each individual.

The occupational therapy team use a combination of standardised and non-standardised assessments to gain both qualitative and quantitative information about a young person's strengths, needs, and priorities. Although quantitative data is useful for help with the diagnosis and for providing evidence when applying for additional resources for the child, qualitative data is most useful in helping to identify the young person's strengths, the impact of difficulties on their daily life, their priorities for intervention, and for guiding intervention planning.

Assessment Process

Assessment tools used by the team were selected to be congruent with the chosen model of practice. Selected assessments that are occupation-focussed include the:

- AMPS (Fisher and Bray Jones, 2006)
- School AMPS (Fisher et al. 2007)
- *COPM* (Law et al. 2015).

Component-based assessments are also used by the therapists as part of diagnostic process, including the:

- Movement ABC-2 (Henderson et al. 2007)
- Developmental Test of Visual Motor Integration (*VMI*; Beery and **Beery** 2010).

Occupational therapists also use the following to explore a young person's sensory processing patterns in the context of their home and/or school environment:

- Sensory Profile 2 (Dunn 2014).

These tools are used to support the information gained from informal interviews with the child/young person and parents/carers, and general observations made by the therapist. A thorough assessment usually starts with a telephone call to the parents/carers to clarify the assessment aims and parents' concerns.

Summary of the Strengths and Limitations of Selected Assessment Tools: Observational Assessments

The AMPS (Fisher and Bray Jones 2006) is a standardised observational assessment that allows the therapist to simultaneously assess a person's ability to perform ADL (domestic and personal) and the quality of their motor and process skills. Motor skills are the observed actions that the person uses to move himself or objects during the tasks performed, and include walking, reaching, manipulating and lifting. Process skills are how a person sensibly organises himself, his tools, and his actions over time, and reflects how effective he is at overcoming or compensating for any problems that he encounters.

The AMPS assessment is usually undertaken in the individual's home. Individuals (from three years of age) select two or more familiar activities that they are willing to demonstrate. Tasks frequently chosen by young people include preparing a bowl of cereal and a cold drink, making a jam sandwich, and dressing. The therapist observes the person performing his activities and rates his motor and process abilities. The results are computer-analysed. This test was selected for use in this community paediatric occupational therapy service for the following reasons:

- The AMPS has been standardised internationally and cross-culturally on more than 46 000 subjects (AMPS International).
- It is a standardised test of occupational performance that clearly demonstrates to parents and others the link between skills and occupational performance.
- It can be used with children, young people, and adults.
- It is very popular with the children and young people, who enjoy choosing their activities and carrying them out. Tasks chosen are meaningful to the individual, and are culturally appropriate.
- It is a sensitive tool that demonstrates why a person has difficulty performing daily tasks.
- The test is carried out in the young person's own environment, and so demonstrates the interaction of the person, the environment, and the activity.
- It helps with intervention planning and reflects an individual's own circumstances.
- It can be used to objectively measure therapy outcomes.

Disadvantages of the AMPS are that therapists have to attend a five-day training course to qualify to use the tool, and must use it regularly to maintain standardisation. Although AMPS is increasingly being used with paediatric populations, published evidence of its use with children is currently limited.

The School AMPS (Fisher et al. 2007) is a modified version of the AMPS and is a standardised assessment tool for measuring a young person's schoolwork task performance within their own classrooms and routines. The therapist observes the young person in class, and assesses the motor and process skills used to perform school activities as chosen by the class teacher. The therapist develops a collaborative relationship with the class teacher to understand the teacher's expectations of the individual and the class, the class routine, and the tools that the child is expected to at school. Assessment results are computer-analysed and can be used to demonstrate the young person's motor and process skills in comparison to other children of the same age. This test was chosen for use in the service for the following reasons:

- The School AMPS is a valid, reliable assessment tool.
- It is a sensitive measure of occupational performance and demonstrates the interaction between the young person, their environment, and their school-work activity.
- It clearly demonstrates to teachers the role of the occupational therapist and facilitates collaborative working between therapists and teachers.
- It takes account of the roles and role expectations of the young person within a particular class environment.
- Interventions arising from the assessment are relevant to the individual.
- It can be used as an objective measure of change following intervention.

Disadvantages: In order to use the School AMPS, therapists must attend a five-day course to qualify to use the tool and must use it regularly to maintain standardisation. It can sometimes be difficult to plan a school observation that includes appropriate tasks, so pre-planning and liaison with teachers is essential.

The Movement ABC-2 (Henderson et al. 2007) is a standardised norm-referenced assessment for children from 4 to 16 years old. It provides objective quantitative data on children's motor performance in the areas of manual dexterity, aiming and catching, and balance. Children's scores are compared to a norm sample to indicate whether the child is performing at or below the level expected for their age. Additional qualitative data is collected to indicate how the child performs each task.

This assessment was chosen for use in the community paediatric occupational therapy service for the following reasons:

- The Movement ABC-2 is a valid, reliable assessment of impairments of motor function.
- It has been standardised on over 1100 children in the United Kingdom (as stated in the Movement ABC Manual 2007).
- It has been used extensively for research and clinical purposes (Harris et al. 2015; Smits-Engelsman et al. 2013)
- With practice, it is fairly quick to administer (taking between 30 minutes to 1 hour).
- It is recommended as a valid and reliable tool to be used during the diagnosis of developmental coordination disorders (Blank et al. 2019).

Limitations: Although this assessment is extensively used by occupational therapists in the United Kingdom (Payne 2002), it is also used by educationalists and other health professionals. It can, therefore, be difficult to explain the unique contribution of occupational therapy if this is the only assessment used. It is a measure of component skills and does not take account of contextual factors: it cannot be assumed that the child who scores well on the Movement ABC does not have difficulty performing ADL in the classroom or at home. It can be difficult to use this test to monitor change over time as the test activities vary between age bands. This test seems to emphasise children's difficulties as it is often obvious to them when they have 'failed'. It also requires a certain amount of preparation and space to administer. It is only standardised for young people up to age 16 years, 11 months.

The Developmental Test of VMI (Beery and Beery 2010) is a standardised test of VMI for people aged three years and over. Individuals copy a series of increasingly complex geometric forms, and an individual's score is calculated as the number of patterns that have been successfully copied, prior to three consecutive failures. Two supplemental tests examine visual perception and motor coordination using the same stimulus patterns as the VMI. Raw scores are converted to standard scores and scaled scores to give an indication of how the person has performed in comparison to other people of the same age.

This assessment was chosen for use in this community paediatric service for the following reasons:

- The VMI has been standardised on 1737 individuals aged 2018 years and 1021 adults aged 19+ (as stated in the VMI 6th Edition manual, Beery and Beery 2010).
- It is useful for identifying children who may have difficulty integrating the visual and motor skills required for writing and drawing.
- It can suggest to the therapist that further assessment of motor or visual skills is required.
- It is quick to administer and can be used with individuals or groups.
- It can help parents and professionals understand a child's current level of development and suggest approaches for developing skills.
- This assessment can be used to evaluate change in VMI after intervention that has focussed on this area.

Limitations: This test was standardised on an American population, and the authors recommend that local norms be developed, but this impractical for a small therapy service. Although scoring criteria is given, scoring can still be quite subjective. The VMI is used by a range of professionals, particularly those in education, and so it can be difficult to demonstrate the unique role of the occupational therapist if this is the only test used. Children who perform well on the VMI may still have difficulty with visual perceptual or motor skills within a classroom context.

Assessments Using Reports from a Proxy (Parent, Teacher)

The Sensory Profile 2 (Dunn 2014) is a suite of judgement-based questionnaires completed by caregivers and teachers of children aged 0–14 years. Questionnaires evaluate a child's sensory processing patterns in the context of home, school, and community-based activities. Separate questionnaires are available for caregivers of children aged birth–3 months, 3–36 months, and 3–14 years. Teachers of children aged 3–14 years can complete the School Companion Sensory Profile 2.

This tool was chosen for use in this service for the following reasons:

- Increasing numbers of children are being referred to the service following concerns about the impact of their responses to sensory stimulation on their participation and performance of everyday activities.

- The Sensory Profile enables the therapist to systematically capture the child's responses to sensory input in their typical environment at home, school, and in the community.
- The Sensory Profile enables the therapist to identify environmental and task-specific sensory factors that support or hinder a child's occupational performance.
- The tool facilitates collaborative planning with the caregiver and/or teacher and is useful for identifying areas of need for intervention planning.
- The Sensory Profile can be administered and scored using a paper or digital version.

Limitations: Although no special training is required to administer the Sensory Profile, a sound understanding of sensory processing theory is necessary to interpret the findings.

Self-Report Assessments

The COPM (5th edition) developed by Law and colleagues has already been mentioned as a good example of a self-report assessment earlier in this chapter. The COPM individualised outcome measure is used for assessing and evaluating the child's self-perception in occupational performance, and covers the constructs of self-care, productivity, and leisure. The area of self-care includes personal care, functional mobility, and community management. The area of productivity includes paid or unpaid work, household management, and school or play. Leisure includes quiet recreation, active recreation, and socialisation. Function is rated in terms of importance, performance, and satisfaction on three 10-point scales. The COPM can be administered separately to the child and his/her parent or carer. It takes between 20 to 40 minutes to administer. This test has been selected for use in this service for the following reasons:

- The test has acceptable levels of test–retest reliability (Law et al. 1998).
- The test has good clinical utility (Law et al. 1994).
- It encompasses the occupational performance areas of self-care, productivity, and leisure.
- It incorporates the roles and role expectations of the child.
- It considers the importance of performance areas to the child and the parent.
- It considers the child and parent's satisfaction with present performance.
- It focuses on the child's own environment, thereby ensuring the relevance of the problems to the child.
- It allows for input from members of the child's social environment (e.g. parent, teacher) if the child is unable to answer on his or her own behalf.
- The test has been used for previous research in child populations, for example, studies with children with cerebral palsy (Law et al. 1997; Pollock and Stewart 1998; Wilcox 1994).
- The test is useful for measuring the outcomes of intervention from the client's perspective.

This test is easier to use with older children who are able to understand the concepts of performance and satisfaction. With younger children, it is helpful to use pictures and visual scales to help the children identify their priority areas, and satisfaction with these: at present, these have to be developed locally.

The *Perceived Efficacy and Goal Setting System 2* (*PEGS*; Missiuna et al. 2004) can be used to help children aged 5–9 years evaluate their performance of everyday activities and set goals for intervention. Using a set of cards that illustrate self-care, school, and leisure activities, children identify those that are challenging and those they are motivated to work on. Parents and teachers complete an additional questionnaire regarding the child's ability to perform daily tasks to identify their priorities. This assessment has been chosen for use by the service for the following reasons:

- The self-report format support child-centred practice, enabling children to identify their own strengths and difficulties and prioritise goals for intervention.
- Use of the caregiver and teacher questionnaires provides multiple perspectives on a child's performance of daily activities.
- PEGS-2 facilitates collaborative goal setting and the creating of intervention plans addressing occupations that matter to the young person.

Limitations: The age range for this assessment is limited (5–9 years), and the cards include pictures of activities that may be less familiar to children living in the United Kingdom. The assessment requires young people to have some insight (and the motivation) to identify tasks they do well and those they struggle with.

Case Study: Scott's Referral Information

Thirteen-year-old-Scott was referred for the advice of an occupational therapist by his mother. She indicated on the referral form (see Figure 2.2) that school activities were the main area of concern, closely followed by ADL and leisure activities. Specific difficulties were identified with using a knife and fork, tying shoelaces, managing buttons, and other fine motor tasks. At school, Scott's writing was very laboured and required great concentration, and his hand hurt after a period of writing. In Physical Education classes (PE), he found slow movements difficult, and appeared clumsy when moving quickly. Scott's mum felt he had general difficulties with perceptual tasks. Other information on the referral form indicated that Scott had a diagnosis of verbal dyspraxia, and that he attended a mainstream secondary school with support from a specialist language resource centre. He was receiving speech and language therapy at school. Scott had seen an occupational therapist previously (when he was seven years old), who, his mother reported, had provided useful advice and help with tying shoelaces.

Information Gathering: Proxy Report from Scott's Parent and Teacher

The referral included questionnaires completed Scott's parents (see Figure 2.3) and teachers. These have been developed by the occupational therapy service, and the school questionnaire is based on the Occupational Therapy Referral Form and Behaviour Checklist (Dunn 2000). Information provided through the questionnaires is used to help prioritise the referrals. Very occasionally, parents indicate that they do not wish the school to be contacted. This request is respected, and if the primary area of concern relates to self-care activities, then the occupational therapist focuses on this area for assessment and intervention. If, however, there are concerns relating to school issues, then this is discussed with the parents in person, and an appropriate plan is agreed with them.

Scott's Occupational Therapy Referral Form

Family Name: .... Jones ....   **Child's Name**: ...Scott ....
Address: ....   Tel No   ....
    ....   DOB   ....
    ....   Post code   ....

Parent/Carer's Names   **Relationship**
Mary Jones ....   Mother ....
Steve Jones ....   Father ....

GP Name   Dr Smith ....   **Consultant**   Dr Black ....
Address   ....   Base   ....
....

Other professionals involved   **Diagnosis**   Verbal Dyspraxia ....
Jane Sykes, SaLT ....

School/Nursery attended   **Teacher**   Mrs B ....
    ....   Tel: ....

○ Please indicate if you are making a referral for the following reasons:
    ○ The child has an acute/deteriorating/life-limiting condition
      (please circle)
    ○ Malfunction/breakdown of essential equipment putting
      child/carer at risk
● Please indicate the main performance area of concern:

Activities of daily living School Nursery Play/leisure

Reason for referral: Scott still has difficulty using a knife and fork. Tying shoelaces, doing up buttons, any fine motor control tasks. School – writing is very laboured, needs great concentration and his hand hurts after a few minutes. Sports/PE – finds slow movements hard but performs fast movements clumsily. Experiences general difficulties with perceptual skills.

Date of referral: 19.9.19

Parent/Carer: I agree for this referral to be made to occupational therapy

Signed: Mary Jones   Print: MARY JONES

Referrer: Mary Jones   Signed: Mary Jones

Designation: Parent   Contact no.

Please return this form to: Occupational Therapy, 41 Old Street, Anytown
    Tel:

FIGURE 2.2   Completed referral form for Scott.

Information provided by Scott's parents indicated concerns regarding dressing, following instructions, a poor sense of danger, and difficulty accessing mainstream leisure opportunities. Scott's mum was concerned that Scott had developed many avoidance strategies, and that his currently good level of self-esteem might suffer as he struggled to succeed at increasingly challenging activities.

The school questionnaire was completed and returned by his teacher (see Figure 2.4). It indicated that Scott had an Education, Health and Care Plan, and was supported by specialist teaching from the language resource centre.

**Scott's Occupational Therapy Referral
Parent/Carer Questionnaire**

Child's Name;	*Scott Jones*	DoB:
Date sent:		

Scott has been referred for an occupational therapy assessment. To help with the evaluation we would be grateful if you could complete the questionnaire and return it to the occupational therapy department by:.........

The information that you provide will remain confidential

Family
Mum's Name:.........*Mary Jones*..............   Dad's name: _Steve Jones_

Siblings: ....*Susie*.....................   ....

....

With whom does the child live?   _Family_..

Tel: ....

School/Nursery
School/Nursery   ....
Tel: ....
Address: ....

• *If you do not wish us to contact the school/nursery please tick here.*

Listed below are some of the areas in which an occupational therapist may be able to help a child. Please tick the areas that your child finds difficult and comment if appropriate

Activities of daily living

✓ Dressing – *buttons, zips, laces, doing a tie*

✓ Eating and drinking – *using a knife, opening tins, spreading any thing on bread*

✓ Toileting

○ Washing/bathing

○ Seating at home

School/Nursery

✓ Using a pencil/writing   *Writing very laborious, can only manage for short periods*

○ Using computer equipment

○ Concentration/attention

✓ Following instructions.   *If too much information is given*

○ Moving around the school

Organisation

FIGURE 2.3   Completed parent questionnaire for Scott.

Play/Leisure

- ✓ Avoids activities such as Lego. Jigsaws

   - ○ Dislikes playground equipment e.g. slide, round about *The opposite, does not see potential dangers and throws himself at every activity*

   - ○ Prefers sedentary (quiet) play

   - ○ Always seems very active

- ✓ Has difficulty accessing leisure opportunities *Attends leisure opportunities organised by local support group, but mainstream sports have not been successful due to competition, teasing, misunderstanding of coach.*

Please comment on any other concerns that you have about your child in the space below
Scott has learned various strategies to avoid certain activities. As he gets older his difficulties become more apparent to peer group. We are concerned that this will affect his self-esteem.
Thank you for your help!

Signature of person completing the form: *Mary Jones*

Date:　　　　　　　　　　　　　　Name (Print)

Relationship to the child: *Mother*

Please return this form to: Occupational Therapy
　　　　　　　　　　　　　41 Old Street
　　　　　　　　　　　　　Anytown
　　　　　　　　　　　　　Tel:

FIGURE 2.3　(Continued)

Difficulties identified by school indicated that Scott seemed weaker than other children and had problems running; he avoided drawing and had an awkward pencil grip; he found it difficult to manage tools such as a ruler and set of compasses; he found it generally difficult to produce written work and worked slowly; and he was easily distracted in class. No sensory processing issues were identified. Scott's teachers forwarded an example of his written work. The occupational therapist noted that this was difficult to read, letters were poorly formed and squashed together, and he seemed to have pressed hard.

Therapist's Reflections upon Initial Data

The referral information suggested that Scott's mother had a good understanding of occupational therapy and what it might have to offer her son. It gave clear indications of the functional areas of difficulty, and also demonstrated a concern for Scott's self-esteem. Sarah also recognised that Scott, at 13 years old, would have his own ideas about what was important to him, and that is was possible that Scott's priorities would be different from those of the parents. At 13, Scott would also have developed his own strategies and ways of managing.

The school questionnaire indicated that Scott was attending a mainstream school, which suggested that his cognitive levels were comparable to his age peers. However, he received extra professional support for language. Despite this, he continued to have difficulty demonstrating his potential in the written form.

Sarah was aware that people with verbal dyspraxia also have difficulties with coordination, and this was reflected in the information provided by parents and school. Previous experience and research evidence also suggests that people may

Scott's Occupational Therapy Referral
Teacher Questionnaire

Scott Jones (dob) has been referred for an occupational therapy assessment. To help with the evaluation we would be grateful if you could complete the questionnaire and return it to the occupational therapy department by

Thank you very much for your help!

Formal evaluations
  • **Cognitive tests**
Name of test   ....
Full score: ....
    Verbal: ....
    Performance: ....

  • **Academic levels**
Reading   *≤6.01*........................... Date of assessment: *July 2002*.........
Spelling   *≤6.00*........................... Date of assessment: *Sept 2001*.......
Maths   .... Date of assessment:...........

  • **Other pertinent evaluations**
....   Date of assessment...........
....   Date of assessment...........

When is the child due to change school?   *N/A –at secondary*...............

Does the child have an Education, Health and Care Plan? *Yes*..........

Please tick the statements that are pertinent to this child
Gross motor
  ✓ Seems weaker than other children his/her age
  ✓ Does not have the endurance other children his/her age have for an activity
  ✓ Difficulty with hopping, jumping, skipping or running compared to others his/her age
  ✓ Appears stiff and awkward in his/her movement
  ✓ Clumsy, does not appear to know how body works, bumps into others or objects, never quite sits in chair correctly
  ○ Does not seem to understand concepts such as right, left, front or back as it relates to his/her body
  ○ Shies away from playground equipment. May only play on one particular item
  ○ Poor posture (always seems to be learning against something, shoulders slump forward)
  ○ Has difficulty with transitions between activities and locations
  ✓ Requires adaptation of the physical environment to access educational opportunities (e.g. seating, positioning, modified PE equipment etc.)

Fine Motor
  ✓ Difficulty with drawing, colouring, tracing
  ✓ Performs these activities quickly and result is usually sloppy
  ✓ Avoids fine motor activities
  ✓ Problem holding pencil, grasp may be very loose or very tight
  ✓ Printing is too dark, too light, too large, too small
  ○ Does not seem to have a dominant hand
  ✓ Has difficulty manipulating school tools such as ruler, paintbrush, compass
  ✓ Has difficulty or is unable to produce hand-written work

Academic
  ✓ Distractible
  ○ Restless
  ✓ Slow worker
  ○ Disorganised, messy desk
  ○ Short attention span
  ○ Hyperactive
  ○ Can't follow directions
  ○ Never completes assignments

FIGURE 2.4   Completed teacher questionnaire for Scott.

Sensory processing
- ○ Withdraws from touch
- ○ Touches everything
- ○ Avoids being close to others
- ○ Fearful of being off the ground
- ○ Doesn't like playground equipment such as slide, swing
- ○ Can't seem to stop moving, craves swinging, rocking
- ○ Trouble discriminating shapes, letters of numbers
- ○ Cannot complete puzzles appropriate for age
- ○ Difficulty copying designs, letters of numbers
- ○ Difficulty tracking (e.g. reading or following teacher's arm movements)

Emotional and behavioural responses
- ○ Does not like to have routine changed
- ○ Is easily frustrated
- ○ Cannot get along with others
- ✓ Accident prone
- ○ Copes better 1:1 or in a small group

Personal care
- ○ Needs assistance with toileting
- ○ Needs assistance or extra supervision with meals/drinks/snacks

Please attach a typical example of the child's writing and their most recent IEP

Signature of person completing the form:

Date:

FIGURE 2.4   (Continued)

have perceptual and organisational difficulties (e.g. Schoemaker et al. 2001; Wilson and Mckenzie 1998). The therapist was aware that these areas would need to be considered when assessing Scott's performance problems.

Initial Assessment: Proxy Report from Scott's Mother

The assessment started with a telephone consultation with Scott's mother. This enabled the therapist and parent/carer to prioritise the young person's needs in order to focus the assessment appropriately.

Scott's mum explained that Scott spent some time each day in the language resource centre for small group work to develop reading and writing skills. He also had speech therapy input at school on a weekly basis. Scott was supported by a number of different learning support assistants in several mainstream classes where there was a large written component. Scott's mum was frustrated that Scott often did not note down his homework accurately, and she felt that with the level of support that Scott received his homework should be recorded precisely. She reported that she provided a lot of support for Scott at home by scribing and helping him to organise his work. The family had purchased a 'Read out loud' computer system and site licences to use the software at school and at home. Scott used this frequently at home, for example, to read back his work and when researching using the Internet, but his mum felt that more use could be made of this system at school.

Scott's mum explained that she was a member of the local Aphasic support group, and had been a member of the local Dyspraxia Support Group when it was active some years ago. She regularly acted as the parent contact for local authority consultations on educational issues for children with speech and language needs. Sarah recognised that this mother was very supportive and understanding of Scott's needs. Sarah hypothesised that Scott's mother would actively engage in the assessment and intervention process, and may have additional experience and insights that would help the therapist to develop a family-centred intervention.

Sarah asked Scott's mum if she could provide some information about Scott's performance of self-care activities. She then asked questions about dressing, eating, washing, and so on, using a prompt sheet based on the PEDI (Hayley et al. 1992). This has been adapted by the therapists to cover children over the age of seven years, and ensures that information is gathered on all aspects of self-care. It also helps to clarify areas of concern, and informs the therapist of any compensations that the young person and family are already using.

At the end of this conversation, Sarah reflected back to Scott's mother that the current areas of concern seemed to be

- difficulty producing legible, timely written work at school,
- a need to help Scott develop independence skills at home, and
- a need to maintain and promote self-esteem.

Sarah and Scott's mother agreed that it would be useful to meet with Scott at home to identify his concerns, strengths, and priorities, and to observe Scott as he participated in some activities to gain a clearer picture of any underlying difficulties. Sarah was particular about involving Scott in the assessment process to engage him in identifying and prioritising intervention areas. She felt that there was a greater likelihood of a positive outcome if this was the case.

The Home Assessment Visit: Self-Report and Observational Assessment

A visit was arranged for the therapist to meet Scott at home after school with his mother. Sarah was concerned that Scott should not be withdrawn from school as he was already experiencing difficulties keeping up with schoolwork. She also felt it was important to meet Scott in his own environment as this helps young people to feel more comfortable about sharing the challenges they face. Sarah explained to Scott that an occupational therapist is interested in finding out how a person manages their daily occupations and the aspects of these that are difficult or challenging. The therapist explained that she was interested in knowing whether there were any activities that Scott would like to participate in but felt unable to do so at present, and also what activities he enjoyed and what he considered to be his strengths. Scott told the therapist that he was good at swimming, riding a bike, and organising himself. Sarah was a bit surprised at the last comment, but on reflection, hypothesised that Scott was referring to the strategies he and his mother had put in place to accommodate his organisational difficulties. Scott said that he had difficulty with writing and spelling, and that his hand ached at times. He could not tie his shoelaces or his school tie (his mother had adapted his tie so that it fastened at the back with Velcro), and he did not enjoy ball games. Scott shared that he enjoyed being in the Scouts and had participated in many weekend activities with them. He was currently having individual swimming lessons. and had recently achieved an adult swimmer certificate. He attended the dance club at school, and was the only boy in his year to do so.

Scott showed Sarah some of his schoolbooks and explained that he was often provided with handouts to reduce the amount of writing. He felt his drawings were not as good as those of his peers. Sarah asked Scott about using a computer; Scott said he liked to use the computer at home but was not able to use it much at school.

Direct Observational Assessment Using a Standardised Tool

Sarah decided to use the Assessment of Motor and Process Skills (AMPS, Fisher and Bray Jones 2006). The therapist has found that young people enjoy choosing and participating in the assessment activities and, unlike with some of the component-based assessment tools, it is unusual for a person to feel that they have 'failed' the test because the activities they have chosen are familiar to them. The AMPS would provide good information about the effect of any motor and process difficulties on Scott's performance of self-care activities.

Sarah was able to identify several activities that Scott might like to perform from information he had provided. Scott decided to prepare a bowl of cereal and a cold drink, and to change the covers on his duvet. The therapist invited Scott's mother to watch Scott perform the tasks as long as she did not say anything!

After Scott had completed the activities, Sarah reflected back to Scott and his mother the areas that she thought he had found difficult. These included:

- positioning himself effectively in front of his workspace;
- managing tasks that require the use of both hands together;
- manipulating objects;
- maintaining smooth, fluent arm movements;
- holding objects securely;
- handling objects; and
- organising equipment.

Scott seemed to have difficulty accommodating for his difficulties, so that they persisted throughout the activities. Scott and his mother agreed this was a true reflection of the difficulties he experienced, at home and, at school, and in other ADL.

At the end of this visit, Sarah agreed to contact Scott's teachers to discuss school issues with them. A further home visit was arranged to discuss the assessment findings and to make a plan for future intervention.

The School Visit: Proxy Report and Direct Observational Assessment

Sarah arranged to meet with the head of the resource centre, Mrs B., and Scott's speech therapist at school, and to observe Scott in a science lesson. This lesson was chosen as it would have a written component, and Scott would be using some small equipment. Mrs B. described Scott as having a very positive attitude towards school. However, he had difficulty organising his ideas and writing these down. He had support to help him with reading and spelling. It was not always possible to read his work, but he was allowed to use a computer to write up his work 'in best'. Technology lessons were identified as challenging; Scott had various teachers who did not all understand his needs. Scott had in the past injured himself when using some equipment, and was felt to be at risk of harm. Support was provided in these lessons. The resource centre had provided all teaching staff with a student profile explaining Scott's difficulties and the accommodations they could make. This included the recommendation that Scott be provided with handouts enlarged to A3 size, and gapped worksheets where possible to reduce the amount of writing.

Scott was observed in a science lesson using a School AMPS format (Fisher et al. 2007). An assistant supported Scott during this lesson. The assistant sat to his left side and provided help to understand the task, to move on to the next stage, to sequence the activity, and to support the ruler when drawing lines. The assistant also glued Scott's worksheet into his book and helped him to pack his bag at the end of the lesson. Scott participated in the lesson by putting up his hand to answer questions. However, Sarah observed that he did not sit squarely in front of the desk, compromising the fluency of arm movements to control his pen. His workspace was cluttered, and Scott appeared to be distracted by objects around him, such as his eraser. He had difficulty drawing lines with the ruler, and organising his graph on the page so that it was not too squashed. The lesson ended with an activity that Scott completed on a worksheet rather than copy from the board.

At the end of the lesson, the teacher reported that Scott's behaviour had not been affected by Sarah's presence in the class. She informed the therapist that Scott enjoyed science, but it was difficult for him to record his work in a way that could be assessed to accurately reflect his ability. The therapist felt that that the assistant had provided too much help at times; for example, the occupational therapist believed that Scott could have managed to glue in his own worksheet. The therapist decided that she would suggest a session with the assistant, during which she could advise her about appropriate prompts and cues to help to improve Scott's independence skills in the classroom.

Needs Identification: Assessment Report

Sarah then wrote a detailed assessment report for Scott and his family that could be shared with his speech and language therapist and school staff. This included a summary of the assessment process and performance analysis, and the identification of the difficulties affecting Scott's performance of everyday activities at home and at school. Strengths and needs were organised under the person/environment/occupation headings.

Person-level issues

For Scott these could be divided into those that related to motor or to process aspects. Motor difficulties included balance and the ability to position himself appropriately in relation to his workspace. Scott used increased effort to perform activities, and had difficulty with activities that required the use of two hands together or the manipulation of small objects. He tired quickly. Process difficulties included difficulty organising his work and materials so that he sometimes knocked them over, organising his work on the page, and sequencing activities. He had difficulty moving on to the next part of the activity, and sometimes stopped too soon or during an action to do something else. This interrupted the flow of his work. However, despite these difficulties Scott appeared to be very determined, and at school was willing to participate in class discussions. He had taken on board many strategies that he and his mother had developed and seemed pleased to be in control of implementing these strategies to help himself. He had a wide range of after-school activities and achieved success in these pursuits.

Environmental level issues

These were different for home and school. At home, Scott could be quite focussed. Scott and his family had accommodated many of his needs and structured their routines and physical environment to help promote Scott's independence and self-esteem. They made good use of timetables and colour coding. Scott was accepted for himself and his interests were encouraged. At home, Scott was seen as a person first, and as someone with a disability second.

At school, Scott received good support from the resource centre, and the therapist was encouraged to see the accommodations that the science teacher had made by providing a worksheet. In lessons, Scott was encouraged to speak out, despite his language difficulties. The use of support assistants enabled Scott to participate in the learning experience and to demonstrate his learning on paper. Despite this support, Scott still found it difficult to remain focussed, particularly towards the end of the lesson when he typically did not record his homework.

Occupational level issues

(i.e. the tasks or activities that a person performs during his daily life): For Scott, these included the following:

- Production of written work at school: This difficulty was a consequence of the interaction between language difficulties, physical and process difficulties, and the school environment.
- Dressing: Scott was not independent in the more complex activities of tying shoelaces and a school tie.
- Snack preparation: Scott had difficulty with the organisation of the activity, and the handling of tools and equipment.

Goal Setting, Action Planning, and Setting a Baseline for Outcome Measurement

Sarah shared the assessment report with Scott and his parents, who agreed that this painted a good picture of Scott, his strengths and difficulties. Scott and his mother agreed that a referral could be made to the community physiotherapy department for advice with regard to balance and stability. The physiotherapists accepted the referral and following a physiotherapy assessment, shoe inserts were provided to correct his foot position.

Sarah explained that she could offer some time-limited intervention to work on some specific skills. Sarah used the COPM (Law et al. 2015) as a self-report assessment to help her prioritise and measure some relevant, client-centred treatment goals for Scott. Using the COPM, Scott identified handwriting, tying shoelaces, and tying a tie as being his priorities for intervention. His baseline performance and satisfaction ratings are provided in Table 2.2.

TABLE 2.2   Scott's COPM identified problems and baseline scores.

Performance problems	Performance (out of 10)	Satisfaction (out of 10)
Tying shoelaces	2	3
Tying a tie	2	1
Handwriting	2	2

TABLE 2.3   Scott's COPM baseline total scores.

Scott's Total Performance Score	2
Scott's Total Satisfaction Score	2

Sarah then calculated a total performance score (sum of the scores divided by number of areas scored, i.e. 6/3) and a total satisfaction score; these are provided in Table 2.3.

A series of after-school visits were arranged to work on these areas with Scott at home. A further school visit was arranged to discuss the assessment findings and their implications with Scott's teachers.

Interventions

Scott had identified developing neater writing as a priority for intervention. However, Sarah felt that the time was right for considering alternative methods of written communication at school. She raised this issue with Scott and his parents, who were very keen to explore this idea further. Sarah forwarded to Scott's parents some information about an initiative for helping children with communication difficulties through the provision of assistive technology. Sarah also discussed this possibility with Scott's teachers. The necessary paperwork was completed by school staff, with encouragement from Scott's parents, and an assessment requested to identify and supply the appropriate equipment.

While at the school, Sarah also suggested that Scott might benefit from using a sloping work surface when working on literacy skills in the resource centre. The resource centre staff were keen on this idea, and Sarah provided a wooden slope for Scott to try. The head of the centre decided to ask the technology department to produce some similar slopes for several of the children to use while in the centre. Meanwhile Sarah and Scott worked on tying shoelaces and his school tie during five home visits. A cognitive, task-specific approach was adopted in which Sarah encouraged Scott to develop the skills to complete the tasks independently. Strategies used included the therapist breaking down the task into each component and modelling these, and Scott developing his own verbal prompts to remind himself of the actions to be taken. Each week the strategies were modified and amended. After eight weeks, Scott was able to complete both activities independently.

Measuring the Outcome

At the first home visit during the intervention stage, Sarah videoed Scott attempting to tie his laces and tie. Consent was given by Scott and his parents for the video to be used for therapeutic and professional training purposes. During the last home visit, another video was taken of Scott successfully performing the tasks. Scott also repeated the COPM and re-rated his performance and satisfaction (see Tables 2.4 and 2.5). Scott was not asked to re-rate his performance and

TABLE 2.4   Scott's COPM identified problems and follow-up scores.

Performance problems	Performance (out of 10)	Satisfaction (out of 10)
Tying shoe laces	8	8
Tying a tie	7	8

TABLE 2.5   Scott's COPM follow-up total scores.

Total Performance Score	7.5
Total Satisfaction Score	8

satisfaction with the third activity, handwriting, as this area was not targeted for intervention while alternatives were being explored.

Sarah calculated COPM change scores to evaluate overall improvement. Scott scores gave an overall performance score of 7.5 at follow-up, Sarah deducted the baseline score of 2, and this gave a change in performance score of 5.5. Scott scores gave an overall satisfaction score of 8 at follow-up, which minus the baseline score of 2 gave a change in satisfaction score of 6 points. Validity studies conducted on the COPM have indicated that a change score of 2 or more represents an outcome that is considered clinically important by the client, family, and therapist (Carswell et al. 2004; Law et al. 1998) Scott's change scores were above 2 for both performance and satisfaction, indicating clinically important change following intervention.

Discharge

At the last home visit, Scott's parents indicated how pleased they were with the progress that he had made. Sarah explained that although she was not going to offer a formal review or further intervention at this stage, she would be happy to see Scott again in future if other issues arose. Scott's mother regularly attends the new local support group for parents of children with coordination disorders. Sarah has also invited Scott's mother to share her experiences as the parent of a young person with a coordination disorder at secondary school at meetings for parents of children who are due to transfer to secondary school. This inside information has been well received by both therapists and parents.

Reflecting on the Data Collection Methods You Use in Your Practice

At the end of each chapter, you will find templates for worksheets designed to assist you in applying principles of assessment and outcome measurement to your own practice.

Please go to Worksheet 2.1 found on p. *92*.

REVIEW QUESTIONS

Reflecting on the questions below will help you to check you have understood the content of this chapter. If you are unsure, go back and re-read the relevant section or follow up on any of the publications referenced to explore an area in further depth:

2.1   What is meant by direct and indirect assessment methods?

2.2   What are the three categories of sources for gathering assessment data?

2.3   What methods could you use for collecting self-report data?

2.4   List the types of informants/proxies an AHP might use.

2.5   What methods could you use for collecting proxy/informant report data?

2.6   What are the three main phases of an interview?

2.7   What factors might influence the outcome of an interview?

2.8   Give an advantage and a disadvantage for using self-report data.

You will find brief answers to these questions at the back of this book on p. 445.

WORKSHEET 2.1   Reflecting on Data Collection Methods

Data Collection method	What data do you currently collect using this method?	What decisions do you need to make from this data?	What assessments (standardised or un-standardised) do you currently employ to collect data using this method?	Is this assessment method adequate? YES or NO	List potential assessments that you could employ to collect data using this method
Observation					
Self-report from service user/ client/patient					
Proxy report (other professional, next of kin, other carer)					

REFERENCES

Abidin, R. R. (1983). Parenting Stress Index: Manual, Administration Booklet,[and] Research Update.

Abidin, R. R (1995). PSI: Parenting stress index. *Professional Manual (3rd Ed)* Psychological Assessment Resources.

Abidin, R.R. (1997). Parenting stress index: a measure of the parent–child system. In: *Evaluating Stress: A Book of Resources* (eds. C.P. Zalaquett and R.J. Wood), 277–291. Lanham, MD, US: Scarecrow Education.

Adams, J. (2002). The purpose of outcome measurement in rheumatology. *British Journal of Occupational Therapy* 65 (4): 172–174. https://doi.org/10.1177/030802260206500404.

Ager, A. (1990). *The Life Experiences Checklist (LEC)*. Windsor: NFER-Nelson.

Árnadóttir, G. (1990). *The Brain and Behavior: Assessing Cortical Dysfunction Through Activities of Daily Living (ADL)*. Mosby Incorporated.

Atkins, R.M. (2004). The foot. In: *Outcome Measures in Orthopaedics and Orthopaedic Trauma* (eds. P. Pynsent, J. Fairbank and A. Carr), 357–368. CRC Press.

Baldwin, W. (1999). Information no one else knows: The value of self-report. In: *The Science of Self-Report: Implications for Research and Practice* (eds. A.A. Stone, C.A. Bachrach, J.B. Jobe, et al.). Psychology Press.

Barlow, D.H., Hayes, S.C., and Nelson-Gray, R.O. (1984). *The Scientist Practitioner: Research and Accountability in Clinical and Educational Settings (No. 128)*. Pergamon.

Baum, C. and Edwards, D.F. (1993). Cognitive performance in senile dementia of the Alzheimer's type: The Kitchen Task Assessment. *American Journal of Occupational Therapy* 47 (5): 431–436.

Baum, C.M. and Edwards, D. (2008). *ACS: Activity Card Sort*. AOTA Press, American Occupational Therapy Association.

Baum, C.M., Perlmutter, M., and Edwards, D.F. (2000). Measuring function in Alzheimer's disease. *Alzheimer's Care Today* 1 (3): 44–61.

Beery, K. E., & Beery, N. A. (2010). The Beery-Buktenica Developmental Test of Visual-motor Integration (Beery VMI): With Supplemental Developmental Tests of Visual Perception and Motor Coordination and Stepping Stones Age Norms from Birth to Age Six: Administration, Scoring, and Teaching Manual. Pearson.

Benjamin, L.S. (1974). Structural analysis of social behavior. *Psychological Review* 81 (5): 392.

Bishop, D.V.M., Whitehouse, A.J.O., and Sharp, M. (2009). *Communication Checklist-Self Report (CC-SR)*. San Antonio, TX: The Psychological Corporation.

Blank, R., Barnett, A.L., Cairney, J. et al. (2019). International clinical practice recommendations on the definition, diagnosis, assessment, intervention, and psychosocial aspects of developmental coordination disorder. *Developmental Medicine & Child Neurology* 61 (3): 242–285.

Borg, B. and Bruce, M.A. (1991). Assessing psychological performance factors. In: *Occupational Therapy: Overcoming Human Performance Deficits* (eds. C. Christiansen and C.M. Baum), 538–586. Thorofare, NJ: Slack.

Bull, C., Byrnes, J., Hettiarachchi, R., & Downes, M. (2019). Reliability and validity of patient-reported experiences measures: A systematic review. Delivered at Emerging Health Policy Research Conference (Annual). Sidney, Australia. http://hdl.handle.net/2123/20562

Calvert, M., Kyte, D., Price, G. et al. (2019). Maximising the impact of patient reported outcome assessment for patients and society. *BMJ* 364: k5267. https://doi.org/10.1136/bmj.k5267.

Cameron, S. and Turtle-Song, I. (2002). Learning to write case notes using the SOAP format. *Journal of Counseling & Development* 80 (3): 286–292. https://doi.org/10.1002/j.1556-6678.2002.tb00193.x.

Carswell, A., McColl, M.A., Baptiste, S. et al. (2004). The Canadian occupational performance measure: a research and clinical literature review. *Canadian Journal of Occupational Therapy* 71 (4): 210–222. https://doi.org/10.1177/000841740407100406.

Centre for Advanced Palliative Care (2005) Lexicon on the CAPC Manual.

Chan, E.K., Edwards, T.C., Haywood, K. et al. (2019). Implementing patient-reported outcome measures in clinical practice: a companion guide to the ISOQOL user's guide. *Quality of Life Research* 28 (3): 621–627. https://doi.org/10.1007/s11136-018-2048-4.

Christiansen, C. and Baum, C.M. (1991). *Occupational Therapy: Overcoming Human Performance Deficits*. Slack.

Clark, C.A., Corcoran, M., and Gitlin, L.N. (1995). An exploratory study of how occupational therapists develop therapeutic relationships with family caregivers. *American Journal of Occupational Therapy* 49 (7): 587–594. https://doi.org/10.5014/ajot.49.7.587.

Clouston, T. (2003). Narrative methods: talk, listening and representation. *British Journal of Occupational Therapy* 66 (4): 136–142. https://doi.org/10.1177/030802260306600402.

Collen, F.M., Wade, D.T., Robb, G.F., and Bradshaw, C.M. (1991). The Rivermead mobility index: a further development of the Rivermead motor assessment. *International Disability Studies* 13 (2): 50–54.

Creek, J. (2003). *Occupational Therapy Defined as a Complex Intervention*, 1. London: College of Occupational Therapists.

Creek, J. (2009). Occupational therapy defined as a complex intervention: a 5-year review. *British Journal of Occupational Therapy* 72 (3): 105–115. https://doi.org/10.1177/030802260907200304.

Culler, K.H. (1993). Occupational therapy performance areas: home and family management. In: *Willard and Spackman's Occupational Therapy*, 8e, 207–269. Philadelphia: Lippincott Williams & Wilkins.

Dalton, M.P. (1994). *Counselling People with Communication Problems*, vol. 11. Sage.

DeGangi, G.A. (1995). *Infant/Toddler Symptom Checklist: A Screening Tool for Parents*. Psychological Corp.

Dunn, W. (2000). Best practice occupational therapy: In community service with children and families. Slack Incorporated.

Dunn, W. (2014). *Sensory Profile 2 Manual*. The Psychological Corporation.

Edvardsson, D. (2015). Notes on person-centred care: what it is and what it is not. *Nordic Journal Of Nursing Research*. 35 (2): 65–66.

England, N.H.S. (2015). *The NHS Constitution for England*. London: Department of Health.

Eva, G. and Paley, J. (2004). Numbers in evidence. *British Journal of Occupational Therapy* 67 (1): 47–48. https://doi.org/10.1177/030802260406700107.

Feng, Y., Parkin, D., and Devlin, N.J. (2014). Assessing the performance of the EQ-VAS in the NHS PROMs programme. *Quality of Life Research* 23 (3): 977–989. https://doi.org/10.1007/s11136-013-0537-z.

Fidler (1976) In, Smith, H. D. (1993)). Assessment and evaluation – an overview. In: *Willard and Spackman's Occupational Therapy*, 8e, 169–172. Philadelphia: JB Lippincott.

Fisher, A.G. (2003). *Assessment of motor and process skills. Administration and Scoring Manual.* Fort Collins, CO: Three Star Press.

Fisher, A. G., & Bray Jones, K. (2006). Assessment of motor and process skills: Vol. 1. *Development, standardization, and administration manual.*

Fisher, A., Bryze, K., Hume, V., and Griswold, L. (2007). *School AMPS: School Version of the Assessment of Motor and Process Skills.* Fort Collins, CO: Three Star Press.

Folio, M. R., & Fewell, R. R. (1983). Peabody developmental motor scales and activity cards. DLM Teaching Resources.

Gossman, W., Lew, V., & Ghassemzadeh, S. (2019). SOAP Notes. In *StatPearls [Internet].* StatPearls Publishing. https://www.ncbi.nlm.nih.gov/books/NBK482263 accessed 28.08.19

Gowland, C., Stratford, P., Ward, M. et al. (1993). Measuring physical impairment and disability with the Chedoke-McMaster Stroke Assessment. *Stroke* 24 (1): 58–63.

Granger, C.V., Hamilton, B.B., Linacre, J.M. et al. (1993). Performance profiles of the functional independence measure. *American Journal of Physical Medicine & Rehabilitation* 72 (2): 84–89.

Green, D., Bishop, T., Wilson, B.N. et al. (2005). Is questionnaire-based screening part of the solution to waiting lists for children with developmental coordination disorder? *British Journal of Occupational Therapy* 68 (1): 2–10. https://doi.org/10.1177/030802260506800102.

Hayley, S.M., Coster, W.J., and Ludlow, L.H. (1991). Pediatric functional outcome measures. *Physical Medicine and Rehabilitation Clinics of North America* 2 (4): 689–723. https://doi.org/10.1016/S1047-9651(18)30678-8.

Hayley, S.M., Coster, W.J., Ludlow, L.H. et al. (1992). *Pediatric Evaluation of Disability Inventory (PEDI) Manual.* Boston: New England Medical Center.

Hammell, K.W. (2003). Changing institutional environments to enable occupation among people with severe physical impairments. In: *Using Environments to Enable Occupational Performance* (eds. L. Letts, P. Rigby and D. Stewart), 35–53. Thorofare, NJ: Slack.

Hammell, K.W. (2004). Deviating from the norm: a sceptical interrogation of the classificatory practices of the ICF. *British Journal of Occupational Therapy* 67 (9): 408–411. https://doi.org/10.1177/030802260406700906.

Harris, S.R., Mickelson, E.C., and Zwicker, J.G. (2015). Diagnosis and management of developmental coordination disorder. *CMAJ: Canadian Medical Association journal = journal de l'Association medicale canadienne* 187 (9): 659–665. https://doi.org/10.1503/cmaj.140994.

Hasting, M., Jones, R., Jenkins, F., & Middleton, K. (2010). Allied health records in the electronic age. In *Managing Money, Measurement and Marketing in the Allied Health Professions* (p. 96). Oxford: Radcliffe Publishing.

Henderson, S.E., Sugden, D.A., and Barnett, A.L. (2007). *Movement Assessment Battery for Children*, 2e. London, UK: Harcourt Assessment.

Horsman, J., Furlong, W., Feeny, D., and Torrance, G. (2003). The health utilities index (HUI®): concepts, measurement properties and applications. *Health and Quality of Life Outcomes* 1 (1): 54. https://hqlo.biomedcentral.com/articles/10.1186/1477-7525-1-54.

Human Rights Act (1998) UK Public General Acts Human Rights Act 1998 (legislation. gov.uk) (accessed 14/01/2021)

Jette, A.M. (1995). Outcomes research: shifting the dominant research paradigm in physical therapy. *Physical Therapy* 75 (11): 965–970. https://doi.org/10.1093/ptj/ 75.11.965.

Klein, R.M. and Bell, B. (1982). Self-care skills: behavioral measurement with Klein-Bell ADL scale. *Archives of Physical Medicine and Rehabilitation* 63 (7): 335–338.

Kielhofner, G. and Henry, A.D. (1988). Development and investigation of the occupational performance history interview. *American Journal of Occupational Therapy* 42 (8): 489–498. https://doi.org/10.5014/ajot.42.8.489.

Kwong, E., Neuburger, J., and Black, N. (2018). Agreement between retrospectively and contemporaneously collected patient-reported outcome measures (PROMs) in hip and knee replacement patients. *Quality of Life Research* 27 (7): 1845–1854. https:// doi.org/10.1007/s11136-018-1823-6.

Kyte, D.G., Calvert, M., Van der Wees, P.J. et al. (2015). An introduction to patient-reported outcome measures (PROMs) in physiotherapy. *Physiotherapy* 101 (2): 119–125. https://doi.org/10.1016/j.physio.2014.11.003.

Lasagna, L. (1960). The clinical measurement of pain. *Annals of the New York Academy of Sciences* 86 (1): 28–37. https://doi.org/10.1111/j.1749-6632.1960.tb42788.x.

Laver Fawcett, A.J. (2002). Assessment. In: *Occupational Therapy and Physical Dysfunction: Principles, Skills and Practice* (eds. A. Turner, M. Foster and S. Johnson), 107–144. London: Churchill Livingstone. Chp. 5.

Laver-Fawcett, A.J. (2019). *The Activity Card Sort – United Kingdom Version (ACS-UK): Test Manual.* York: York St John University.

Laver, A.J. and Powell, G.E. (1995). *The Structured Observational Test of Function (SOTOF).* NFER Nelson.

Laver, A.J. and Unsworth, C. (1999). *Cognitive and Perceptual Dysfunction: A Clinical Reasoning Approach to Evaluation and Intervention* (ed. C. Unsworth). FA Davis.

Law, M. (1993). Evaluating activities of daily living: directions for the future. *American Journal of Occupational Therapy* 47 (3): 233–237. https://doi.org/10.5014/ajot.47.3.233.

Law, M., Baptiste, S., Carswell-Opzoomer, A. et al. (1991). *Canadian Occupational Performance Measure.* Toronto: CAOT.

Law, M.C., Baptiste, S., Carswell, A. et al. (1998). *Canadian occupational performance measure: COPM.* CAOT Publ. ACE.

Law, M., Baptiste, S., Carswell, A. et al. (2015). *Canadian Occupational Performance Measure (COPM)*, 5e. COPM | Canadian Occupational Performance Measure (thecopm.ca).

Law, M., Cooper, B., Strong, S. et al. (1996). The person-environment-occupation model: a transactive approach to occupational performance. *Canadian Journal of Occupational Therapy* 63 (1): 9–23.

Law, M., Polatajko, H., Pollock, N. et al. (1994). Pilot testing of the Canadian occupational performance measure: clinical and measurement issues. *Canadian Journal of Occupational Therapy* 61 (4): 191–197. https://doi. org/10.1177/000841749406100403.

Law, M., Russell, D., Pollock, N. et al. (1997). A comparison of intensive neurodevelopmental therapy plus casting and a regular occupational therapy program for children with cerebral palsy. *Developmental Medicine & Child Neurology* 39 (10): 664–670.

Lewis, S.C. (2003). *Elder Care in Occupational Therapy.* Slack Incorporated.

Lincoln, N.B. and Edmans, J.A. (1990). A re-validation of the Rivermead ADL scale for elderly patients with stroke. *Age and Ageing* 19 (1): 19–24.

McCormack, G.L., Llorens, L.A., and Glogoski, C. (1991). Culturally diverse elders. In: *Occupational Therapy and the Older Adult* (ed. J.M. Kiernat), 11–25. Gaithersburg, MD: Aspen Publishing Co.

Missiuna, C., Pollock, N., and Law, M.C. (2004). *The Perceived Efficacy and Goal Setting System*. PsychCorp.

Mokkink, L.B., Prinsen, C.A., Bouter, L.M. et al. (2016). The COnsensus-based Standards for the selection of health Measurement INstruments (COSMIN) and how to select an outcome measurement instrument. *Brazilian Journal of Physical Therapy* 20 (2): 105–113. https://doi.org/10.1590/bjpt-rbf.2014.0143.

Nelson, E.C., Eftimovska, E., Lind, C. et al. (2015). Patient reported outcome measures in practice. *BMJ* 350: g7818. https://doi.org/10.1136/bmj.g7818.

Partridge, C. and Johnston, M. (1989). Perceived control of recovery from physical disability: measurement and prediction. *British Journal of Clinical Psychology* 28 (1): 53–59. https://doi.org/10.1111/j.2044-8260.1989.tb00811.x.

Payne, S. (2002). Standardised tests: An appropriate way to measure the outcome of paediatric occupational therapy? *British Journal of Occupational Therapy* 65 (3): 117–122.

Pearce, P.F., Ferguson, L.A., George, G.S., and Langford, C.A. (2016). The essential SOAP note in an EHR age. *The Nurse Practitioner* 41 (2): 29–36. https://doi.org/10.1097/01.NPR.0000476377.35114.d7.

Perkins, E.A. (2007). Self-and proxy reports across three populations: older adults, persons with Alzheimer's disease, and persons with intellectual disabilities. *Journal of Policy and Practice in Intellectual Disabilities* 4 (1): 1–10. https://doi.org/10.1111/j.1741-1130.2006.00092.x.

Piper, M.C., Pinnell, L.E., Darrah, J. et al. (1992). Construction and validation of the Alberta Infant Motor Scale (AIMS). *Canadian Journal of Public Health= Revue canadienne de sante publique* 83: S46–S50.

Pollock, N. and Stewart, D. (1998). Occupational performance needs of school-aged children with physical disabilities in the community. *Physical & Occupational Therapy in Pediatrics* 18 (1): 55–68.

Pynsent, P., Fairbank, J., and Carr, A. (2004). *Outcome Measures in Orthopaedics and Orthopaedic Trauma*. CRC Press.

Renwick, R.M. and Reid, D.T. (1992). Life satisfaction of parents of adolescents with Duchenne muscular dystrophy: validation of a new instrument. *The Occupational Therapy Journal of Research* 12 (5): 296–312. https://doi.org/10.1177/153944929201200503.

Robinson, B.C. (1983). Validation of a caregiver strain index. *Journal of Gerontology* 38 (3): 344–348. https://doi.org/10.1093/geronj/38.3.344.

Rundshagen, I., Schnabel, K., Standl, T., and Am Esch, J.S. (1999). Patients' vs nurses' assessments of postoperative pain and anxiety during patient-or nurse-controlled analgesia. *British Journal of Anaesthesia* 82 (3): 374–378. https://doi.org/10.1093/bja/82.3.374.

Sarno, J.E., Sarno, M.T., and Levita, E. (1973). The functional life scale. *Archives of Physical Medicine and Rehabilitation* 54 (5): 214. https://www.ncbi.nlm.nih.gov/pubmed/4701402.

Schoemaker, M.M., van der Wees, M., Flapper, B. et al. (2001). Perceptual skills of children with developmental coordination disorder. *Human Movement Science* 20 (1-2): 111–133.

Smith, H.D. (1993). Assessment and evaluation – an overview. In: *Willard and Spackman's Occupational Therapy*, 8e, 169–172. Philadelphia: JB Lippincott.

Smits-Engelsman, B.C., Blank, R., van der Kaay, A.C. et al. (2013). Efficacy of interventions to improve motor performance in children with developmental coordination disorder: a combined systematic review and meta-analysis. *Developmental Medicine & Child Neurology* 55 (3): 229–237. https://doi.org/10.1111/dmcn.12008.

Strong, J., Ashton, R., Cramond, T., and Chant, D. (1990). Pain intensity, attitude and function in back pain patients. *Australian Occupational Therapy Journal* 37 (4): 179–183. https://doi.org/10.1111/j.1440-1630.1990.tb01265.x.

Sturgess, J., Rodger, S., and Ozanne, A. (2002). A review of the use of self-report assessment with young children. *British Journal of Occupational Therapy* 65 (3): 108–116. https://doi.org/10.1177/030802260206500302.

Swain, J. (2004). Interpersonal communication. In: *Physiotherapy: A Psychosocial Approach. Researching Together: A Participatory Approach* (eds. S. French and J. Sim), 317–331. Oxford: Butterworth Heinemann.

Teri, L., Truax, P., Logsdon, R. et al. (1992). Assessment of behavioral problems in dementia: the revised memory and behavior problems checklist. *Psychology and Aging* 7 (4): 622. https://doi.org/10.1037/0882-7974.7.4.622.

Thornton, M. and Travis, S.S. (2003). Analysis of the reliability of the modified caregiver strain index. *The Journals of Gerontology Series B: Psychological Sciences and Social Sciences* 58 (2): S127–S132. https://doi.org/10.1093/geronb/58.2.S127.

Tullis, A. and Nicol, M. (1999). A systematic review of the evidence for the value of functional assessment of older people with dementia. *British Journal of Occupational Therapy* 62 (12): 554–563. https://doi.org/10.1177/030802269906201206.

Tyerman, R., Tyerman, A., Howard, P., & Hadfield, C. (1986). The Chessington OT neurological assessment battery. In *International Journal of Rehabilitation Research* (Vol. 9, No. 4, pp. 423-423). 2-6 Boundary Row, London, England SE1 8HN: Chapman Hall LTD.

Van der Kaay, S., Jung, B., Letts, L., and Moll, S.E. (2019). Continuing competency in ethical decision making: an interpretive description of occupational therapists' perspectives. *Canadian Journal of Occupational Therapy* 86 (3): 209–219.

Velozo, C.A. (1993). Work evaluations: critique of the state of the art of functional assessment of work. *American Journal of Occupational Therapy* 47 (3): 203–209. https://doi.org/10.5014/ajot.47.3.203.

Wallen, M.A. and Ziviani, J.M. (2012). Canadian occupational performance measure: impact of blinded parent-proxy ratings on outcome. *Canadian Journal of Occupational Therapy* 79 (1): 7–14. https://doi.org/10.2182/cjot.2012.79.1.2.

Whiting, S. and Lincoln, N. (1980). An ADL assessment for stroke patients. *British Journal of Occupational Therapy* 43 (2): 44–46.

Whiting, S., Lincoln, N.B., Bhavnani, G., and Cockburn, J.E. (1985). *Rivermead Perceptual Assessment Battery*, 61. Windsor: NFER-NELSON.

Wilcox, A. L. (1994). Verbal Self-guidance: An Exploratory Study with Children with Developmental Coordinationa Disorders. Unpublished thesis. University of Western Ontario.

Wilson, P.H. and McKenzie, B.E. (1998). Information processing deficits associated with developmental coordination disorder: a meta-analysis of research findings. *Journal of Child Psychology and Psychiatry* 39 (6): 829–840.

World Health Organisation (WHO) (2002). *Towards a Common Language for Functioning, Disability and Health - ICF*. WHO/EIP/GPE/CAS/01.3 Original: English Distr.: General. WHO: Geneva. https://www.who.int/classifications/icf/icfbeginnersguide.pdf?ua=1

Yerxa, E.J., Burnett-Beaulieu, S., Stocking, S., and Azen, S.P. (1988). Development of the satisfaction with performance scaled questionnaire (SPSQ). *American Journal of Occupational Therapy* 42 (4): 215–221. https://doi.org/10.5014/ajot.42.4.215.

Yorkston, K. and Baylor, C. (2019). Patient-reported outcomes measures: an introduction for clinicians. *Perspectives of the ASHA Special Interest Groups* 4: 1–8. https://doi.org/10.1044/2018_PERS-ST-2018-0001.

Zarit, S.H., Todd, P.A., and Zarit, J.M. (1986). Subjective burden of husbands and wives as caregivers: a longitudinal study. *The Gerontologist* 26 (3): 260–266. https://doi.org/10.1093/geront/26.3.260.

RESOURCES

The COnsensus-based Standards for the selection of health Measurement INstruments (COSMIN) https://www.cosmin.nl/finding-right-tool

EuroQoL – https://euroqol.org/euroqol

NHSDigitalhttps://digital.nhs.uk/data-and-information/data-tools-and-services/data-services/patient-reported-outcome-measures-proms

NHS England – https://www.england.nhs.uk/statistics/statistical-work-areas/proms

CHAPTER 3

Purposes of Assessment and Measurement

OVERVIEW

This chapter focuses on the reasons why allied health professionals (*AHPs*) need or are required to assess clients and categorise these reasons in terms of the different timings of assessment throughout an intervention process. In this chapter, we will explore four distinct purposes of assessment:

1. descriptive
2. discriminative
3. predictive
4. evaluative assessment.

Examples of published assessments that address these different purposes will be provided, and a case scenario will be used to demonstrate how these different assessments can be used. Table 3.1 (P. 113) later in the chapter gives a brief overview of each assessment type. The chapters ends with a case study.

QUESTIONS TO CONSIDER

The purpose of conducting an assessment needs to be conscious and articulated. Before you start an assessment process, you need to be able to answer some basic questions:

- *Why am I doing this assessment?*
- *What information do I need to collect?*
- *What decisions will I need to make from this information?*
- *What will be the benefit to the client (and where relevant, the carer) from undertaking this assessment?*

Articulating the answers to these questions enables the AHP to select an effective and efficient assessment approach. An AHP must not only understand the purpose of the assessment but must also be able to educate the service user, and where appropriate the carer, about the purposes and procedures involved in the assessment process. We must be able to explain the specific rationale for using any standardised measures as part of this assessment process. The requirement to explain the purpose of an assessment to the service user has been identified as a standard for practice (England NHS 2016). So, being able to answer the questions stated at the start of this chapter helps the AHP to provide a clear explanation to the client and carer about why the assessment is necessary and why the assessment approach has been selected.

PURPOSES OF ASSESSMENT

Purposes for assessment may be categorised in several ways, the most frequent of which are categorisation in terms of the timing of an assessment and categorisation based on the reason for the assessment and the related use of the data collected. When selecting a specific assessment or an overall assessment strategy for a person, it is essential that the AHP considers the purpose for which the assessment information is gathered and how the results or the assessment might be interpreted and used. When undertaking a critique of potential assessments, it is vital to consider the intended purpose of the assessments under review because the content, methods, psychometric properties, and clinical utility of an assessment should be evaluated against its intended purpose. In terms of client assessment, assessments can be grouped in terms of four main purposes: **Descriptive, Discriminative, Predictive, and Evaluative** (Kirshner and Guyatt 1985; Law 1987). Some assessments are developed to address just one of these four purposes. However, there are many assessments that can be used for a combination of purposes. Later in this chapter, we will also consider these further in the section titled 'Definition of a Comprehensive Assessment'.

PLANNING AN ASSESSMENT APPROACH

It is useful to think about the process when planning an assessment approach and to consider carefully the optimum timing for the assessment(s) within the intervention process. This process has been described as 11 major steps (Creek 2003):

1. referral or reason for contact
2. information gathering
3. initial assessment
4. reason for intervention/needs identification/problem formulation
5. goal setting
6. action planning
7. action
8. ongoing assessment and revision of action
9. outcome and outcome measurement
10. end of intervention or discharge
11. review.

Steps 2, 3, 4, 8, and 9 explicitly relate to assessment, and steps may be taken more than once.

1. **Referral:**

   Referral is the *process* through which an AHP encounters a potential client. Referrals are made in a variety of ways depending on the service specification and policy and may be received as a self-referral (Holdsworth et al. 2018), an e-referral through electronic records, and a letter or email communication. Other referrals may be made verbally, either via telephone (such as to a Fast Response service) or in a ward round or multidisciplinary team meeting. The amount of information provided in a referral can also vary greatly, both in terms of what the service specifies as minimum information required for a referral to be accepted and because referrers vary greatly in the level of information they provide (Volkmer et al. 2018). At the end of the intervention process, the AHP may also make a referral to put the client and/or carer in contact with another required agency or professional.

2. **Information Gathering:**

   The *information* provided in a referral is not always enough. AHPs, therefore, chose to gather more information about the person, the reason for the referral, and the presenting problem prior to conducting the initial assessment. At this stage, the AHP often engages in a screening process; this is a review of referral and other available information to determine if the referral is appropriate and services are relevant and necessary. Where a service operates a waiting list, the referral might also be prioritised in terms of urgency in order to categorise the referral and place the person the appropriate waiting list. For example, some services use three categories for sorting referrals:

   a. crisis: contact to be made within four hours and the client to be see within one working day, e.g. to prevent an admission to hospital

   b. urgent: client to be seen within seven working days

   c. non-urgent: client to be seen when the service has capacity.

3. **Initial Assessment:**

   On *referral*, the AHP will need to conduct an initial assessment or **screening assessment**. The purpose of this level of assessment is to identify potential problems areas for further in-depth assessment. Initial assessment has been defined as:

Definition of Initial Assessment

The first step in the ... process following referral; the art of gathering relevant information in order to define the problem to be tackled, or identify the goal to be attained, and to establish a baseline for treatment planning. (Creek 2003, p. 54)

Some services triage referrals at this stage to either prioritise referrals for a waiting list system or to signpost the client to the most relevant service or team member. Screening is an investigative process used by AHPs to determine the need for a comprehensive assessment and potential intervention. The initial assessment is used to provide a baseline for treatment planning. An initial or screening assessment may be short and take only one session (for example, the assessment of an inpatient being referred for a total hip replacement or in an intermediate care team). In some settings, the initial assessment may require several sessions, perhaps comprising an initial interview, an informal observation of aspects of function, and the administration of a standardised assessment battery, for example when deciding the appropriateness of a referral to a community mental health team or a referral for a period of intensive rehabilitation in a Stroke Unit.

4. **Needs Identification and Problem Formulation:**
   Problem *formulation* can be seen as both an event and process, the process being suggestion, discussion, reflection, feedback, and revision (Johnstone and Dallos 2013). If we reconsider Figure 2.1 (in Chapter 2), we see that as an AHP as an AHP you will gather data and information from many sources, and therefore the identification of the key problems for the client may change over the assessment period. Using an assessment tool such as *Canadian Occupational Performance Measure (COPM)* can support improvement in practice, including knowledge of client perspective, and clinical decision making through collaborative identification of need and problem formulation (Colquhoun et al. 2012).

5. **Goal Setting:**
   Following the determination of the need for an intervention, a plan for an intervention is required, including measurable outcome goals negotiated in collaboration with the client, family, or carer. Measurement instruments can support and monitor the goal-setting process by highlighting individual problems, setting goal priorities, and monitoring and measuring goal achievement (Bovend'Eerdt et al. 2009). Clients' active involvement in goal setting has been shown to increase their motivation, participation, and satisfaction regarding the intervention (Ponte-Allan and Giles 1999). Stevens et al. (2013) identified 11 patient-specific instruments that can support and monitor goal negotiation, goal setting, and evaluation, such as COPM (see Chapter 2) and Goal Attainment Scaling *(GAS)*.

GAS is a method of scoring the extent to which patient's individual goals are achieved in the course of intervention (Kiresuk et al. 2014). Each goal is rated on a 5-point scale, with the degree of attainment captured for each goal area: If the patient achieves the expected level, this is scored at 0. If they achieve more than the expected outcome, this is scored at +1 (somewhat more) or +2 (much more). If they achieve less than the expected outcome, this is scored at: −1 (somewhat less) or −2 (much less; Turner-Stokes 2009).

6. **Action Planning:**
   Sniehotta et al. (2005) described action planning as 'the process of linking *goal*-directed behaviours to certain environmental cues by specifying when, where, and how to act. People who form action plans are more likely to act in the intended way, and they initiate the goal behaviour faster than those who do not form action plans' (p. 567). Figure 3.1 shows the link between goal setting and action planning (Scobbie et al. 2011, p. 577), and has been suggested as a framework to support rehabilitation.

7. **Action or Implementation of Intervention:**
   Once goals and collaborative patient-centred action plans are developed, an AHP needs to implement the chosen intervention. Prior et al. (2008) suggested that didactic education and passive dissemination strategies are ineffective, and that effective implementation of clinical guidelines can support improvement in healthcare outcomes.

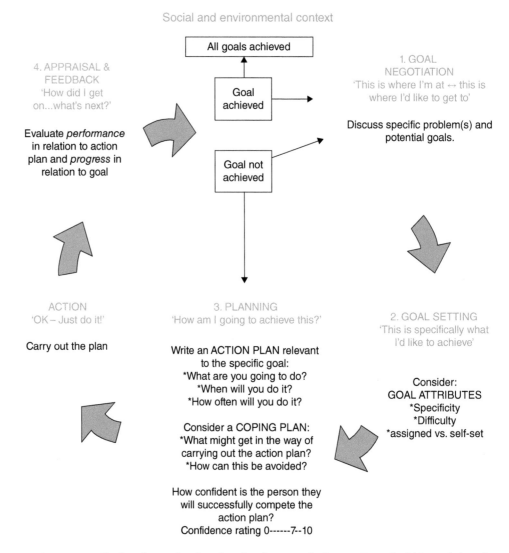

Social and environmental context

All goals achieved

4. APPRAISAL & FEEDBACK
'How did I get on...what's next?'

Evaluate *performance* in relation to action plan and *progress* in relation to goal

Goal achieved

Goal not achieved

1. GOAL NEGOTIATION
'This is where I'm at ↔ this is where I'd like to get to'

Discuss specific problem(s) and potential goals.

ACTION
'OK – Just do it!'

Carry out the plan

3. PLANNING
'How am I going to achieve this?'

Write an ACTION PLAN relevant to the specific goal:
*What are you going to do?
*When will you do it?
*How often will you do it?

Consider a COPING PLAN:
*What might get in the way of carrying out the action plan?
*How can this be avoided?

How confident is the person they will successfully compete the action plan?
Confidence rating 0------7--10

2. GOAL SETTING
'This is specifically what I'd like to achieve'

Consider:
GOAL ATTRIBUTES
*Specificity
*Difficulty
*assigned vs. self-set

FIGURE 3.1   Goal setting and action planning framework. Source: From Scobbie et al. (2011). © 2010, SAGE Publications.

8. **Ongoing Assessment and Revision of Action:**
   Assessment should not stop with the initial assessment but be an integral part of the treatment and assist the AHP's clinical reasoning process as she considers the way in which the person is responding to the treatment plan. Ongoing assessment helps with examining progress and monitoring the effects of the intervention. Government policy now articulates the need for continuing assessment in a number of clinical areas (NHS 2019*)*. Ongoing assessment has been defined as:

Definition of Ongoing Assessment

An integral part of the process of intervention in which information is collected and used to examine the client's progress or lack of progress, to monitor the effects of intervention and to assist the AHP's clinical reasoning process. (Creek 2003, p. 56)

The frequency of evaluative assessment to monitor progress will be related to the anticipated length of contact and the predicted rate of progress (see Figure 3.1). The person's contact with AHP services might last as little as a couple of days, for example, during a short hospital admission for a planned operation, or might last years, for example, with a child who is born with cerebral palsy. Where the AHP is involved over several years and where progress is expected to be gradual, then a monitoring assessment may be carried out at monthly or even six-monthly intervals. Where contact is brief, such as when a client is referred to a Crisis Intervention or Rapid Response Service, or frequent changes are anticipated, then regular evaluation, for example, every couple of days or weekly may be required (Butler et al. 2012; Dibben et al. 2008). When an assessment is re-administered, following a short time period, it is essential that any learning effect related to assessment items is accounted for when interpreting these results. AHPs should examine the test–retest reliability data for the measure; they will find that some assessments, which are influenced by a learning effect, will have parallel forms of the test for evaluation (see the section on parallel form/equivalent form reliability in Chapter 9).

A reduction in lengths of stay in hospital, especially in acute care, is usual (NHS 2019), and AHPs play an important role in *pre-discharge assessment*. A pre-discharge assessment provides information about the person's readiness for discharge (including safety and risk factors), the needed and available physical and social supports, and any requirements for follow-up interventions (Wong et al. 2011).

9. **Outcome and Outcome Measurement:**

The AHP also should conduct an *outcome* assessment when the person is discharged from the service. The final assessment serves to provide an evaluation of the effectiveness of intervention to date and may provide new baseline data to be passed on to other colleagues if the person is being referred to another service provider (see Chapter 10 for further details).

10. **End of Intervention or Discharge**

Preparing *for* discharge or ending an intervention is an important part of any patient contact or episode of care. An AHP needs to consider the requirement for discharge and the timing from the point of initial contact, and throughout an intervention. Discharge planning needs to be individual to each client or patient either leaving hospital or concluding the community or outpatient intervention (Gonçalves-Bradley et al. 2016). Discharge preparation will usually involve the multi-professional team. However, AHPs may have differing perspectives. Tensions between professionals can impede efficient joint working. AHPs need to ensure they have an understanding of the differing roles and expertise each team member can offer (Connolly et al. 2010), to support the best outcome for the patient.

11. **Review:**

Some AHPs offer a review post discharge from a service, face to face in person, by telephone, or through online telecare (such as Skype). This is particularly helpful for clients with a long-term condition. AHPs may decide to book a review where continued **improvement**, or maintenance of improvement, is anticipated following a period of rehabilitation. Some clients experience deterioration in functioning once the support of the AHP is removed, so an AHP may want to check that the client's function has not reached a plateau or declined post discharge, for example because the client has not continued with an exercise programme or is not using equipment and adaptations effectively. A good example is with a service for older people with a history of falls. The client attends a time-limited rehabilitation programme for falls. On discharge from the programme, a number of home modifications are recommended to reduce hazards, and an exercise programme is taught to improve strength, range of movement (*ROM*), and balance. In this case, the AHP reviews the client at home one, three, and six months post discharge from the Falls programme to:

- check the modifications have be made and that no additional hazards are present;
- to observe the exercise routine and ensure that the client continues to do exercises correctly and regularly, and to assess whether the exercises can be upgraded if function has continued to improve or modified if the client finds them too challenging or tiring; and
- in addition, to monitor the outcome in terms of taking a history of any falls that have occurred since discharge or the last review.

Review is also helpful when the person has a condition where a decline in functioning is anticipated over time, such as with dementia or Parkinson's disease, and where the AHP wants to monitor the rate of decline in order to change the medication and/or care package accordingly. The timing of any reviews will vary depending on the nature of the person's condition and the purpose of the service.

DESCRIPTIVE ASSESSMENTS

Most AHP assessments provide some sort of descriptive data. Descriptive assessments are the most frequent type of assessments used by AHPs in day-to-day clinical practice.

Definition of a Descriptive Assessment

A descriptive assessment is an assessment that provides information that describes the person's current functional status, problems, needs, and/or circumstances.

AHP descriptive assessments mostly provide information that describes the person's current functional status, such as the ability to perform activities of daily living (*ADL*), the ROM of a particular joint, or their mobility and transferring. Descriptive assessments often focus on identifying strengths and limitations. They provide a snapshot for the person's function/circumstances/needs at one point in time only and are often used to provide baseline (see definition below) data for treatment planning and clinical decision making. Descriptive assessments may also be used to identify symptoms and problems to help aid diagnosis. In terms of underlying psychometrics, standardised descriptive assessments should have established, adequate content and construct validity (see Chapter 8).

An issue to consider when selecting a *descriptive assessment* is the level of data obtained related to the requirements for accurate treatment planning. For example, ADL assessment might describe the person's ability on a 4-point independence scale; however, a score of 'unable to perform' or 'dependent' does not provide data on the limiting factors in the person's performance within an activity, nor the reason for any observed deficits. The treatment plan will need to be different for a person dependent in dressing because of a motor deficit, from a person who is dependent because of apraxia, or has visual field deficit, or the person has problems with initiation of a task. Most AHPs require more information than a simple description of what the person can and cannot do – they need data that helps them to problem-solve and hypothesise about the reasons behind observed dysfunction. Therefore, when selecting a descriptive assessment, the AHPs needs to think about what behaviours/circumstances she needs to describe, and she may need to use more than one descriptive assessment to answer all the questions that need answers to form an accurate baseline for treatment planning. For example, she may need a description of the person's home environment and social supports at a societal limitation level, as well as a description of the person's ability to mobilise, transfer, and perform ADL at a disability level and also a description of the person's motor and sensory functioning at an impairment level (see Chapter 11).

Many assessments focus on the person's ability to carry out a test item or his degree of independence, but there are other more qualitative aspects of performance that AHPs may want to describe as the basis for treatment planning, which include:

- the physical effort that the client exerts to perform the assessment, which indicates the magnitude of physical difficulty or fatigue;
- the efficiency with which the client carries out the assessment, which indicates the extent of any unnecessary use of time, space, or objects or evidence of disorganisation; and
- safety issues, as AHPs often need to consider the risk of personal injury or environmental damage (Heyman et al. 2010).

An example of an assessment that provides descriptive data at different levels of function is the Structured Observational Test of Function (*SOTOF*; Laver-Fawcett and Powell 1995). The SOTOF is a standardised, valid, and reliable measure with established clinical utility and face validity (Laver-Fawcett 1994) that enables the AHP to describe the person's ability to perform four basic self-care tasks (washing, dressing, eating, pouring a drink, and drinking). Each ADL scale is broken down into small subcomponents, and so the AHP also obtains detailed descriptive data about the aspects of the task the person finds difficult. For example, the SOTOF enables the AHP to answer questions about how the different components of the task are undertaken:

- Can he recognise the objects required for the task?
- Does the client reach accurately for the item of clothing?
- Can he organise the garment to put on?
- Does he sequence the task correctly?
- Has he the fine motor skills to do up the buttons?

From data collected about how the person attempted each task, the AHP is then guided through a diagnostic reasoning process to hypothesise about the underlying impairment level deficits (see Chapter 6). Some test items are also included to directly assess impairment level functioning, such as:

- sensory functioning (e.g. tactile, taste, and temperature discrimination),
- perceptual functioning (e.g. colour recognition, right/left discrimination, figure ground discrimination, depth, and distance perception), and

- visual functioning (visual acuity, field loss, neglect, and scanning) and motor functioning (muscle tone, dexterity, bilateral integration, and ideo-motor apraxia).

(See International Classification of Functioning (*ICF*) – https://www.who.int/classifications/icf/en.)

DISCRIMINATIVE ASSESSMENTS

AHPs use discriminative assessments to distinguish between individuals or groups. For this purpose, comparisons are usually made against a normative group or another diagnostic group. Comparisons may be made for reasons such as making a diagnosis, matching a client against referral criteria or for prioritising referrals, deciding on appropriate placement, or evaluating a person's level of dysfunction in relation to expectations of performance of other healthy people of that age, for example, to see if a child is developing skills at the expected stage versus has a developmental delay.

Definition of a Discriminative Test

A discriminative test is a measure developed to distinguish between individuals or groups on an underlying dimension when no external criterion or gold standard is available for validating these measures (Kirshner and Guyatt 1985).

Depending on their precise purposes, both descriptive and discriminative tests can be labelled as 'diagnostic indices' which are used to assist clinical diagnosis and to detect impairment and/or disability in a diagnostic group. AHPs, often working in a multidisciplinary team setting, use discriminative assessments to help with accurate diagnosis. For example, to assess whether a person has dementia versus depression, or dementia versus cognitive decline associated with the normal ageing process, or to diagnose a specific type of dementia, such as Lewy Body dementia (Saxton et al. 1993). In an ageing population, changes occur because of normal ageing, for example, in the cognitive-perceptual system. Therefore, comprehensive normative data for older populations is required so that AHPs can evaluate test results in the context of normal ageing processes to discriminate pathology from expected change.

When selecting standardised tests for discriminative assessment, the value of the test is dependent on the adequacy of, and the ability to generalise from, the normative sample or client population used to obtain reference data. The lack of normative or comparative test standardisation with a population similar to the specific client restricts the AHP's ability to make accurate and valid comparisons. An example of this is assessments initially developed and standardised for child populations used with adult populations or where tests developed in another country for a different cultural group are used without considering potential differences. In addition, test developers should undertake validity studies to explore the value of test items for discriminating between groups of interest. Discriminative validity relates to whether a test provides a valid measure to distinguish between individuals or groups (see Chapter 8).

An example of a test that has a discriminative purpose is the Infant and Toddler Symptom Checklist (DeGangi et al. 1995). This is a proxy measure developed for use with parents of 7-to-30-month-old infants and toddlers. The Symptom checklist can be used to discriminate between infants and toddlers who are developing normally and those who have sensory-integrative disorders, attentional deficits, and emotional and behavioural problems. The checklists are provided in five age bands (7–9, 10–12, 13–18, 19–24, and 25–30 months), and normative data giving expected score ranges and a cut-off to discriminate an expected from a deficit score is provided for each age band.

Many AHP services are struggling to deal with waiting lists and have more demand for their service than capacity to deliver a service promptly to all referrals (Seabrook et al. 2019). AHPs should consider the use of discriminative assessments as screening tools to help identify the appropriateness of referrals and prioritise them in order to prioritise their referrals and offer a prompt service to those children in greatest need. Green et al. (2005) carried out a study to explore whether screening tools could differentiate between children with a developmental coordination disorder (*DCD*) who needed a full assessment and children with only a low risk of DCD. They compared the results of a parent-completed assessment, The Development Coordination Disorder Questionnaire (DCDQ; Wilson et al. 2000), and a teacher-completed Checklist for the Movement Assessment Battery for Children (*C-ABC*; Henderson and Sugden 1992) with the results of AHPs' observational assessment. The AHP assessment comprised standardised tools including the Assessment of Motor Process Skills (AMPS; Fisher 2003) and the C-ABC (Henderson and Sugden 1992). The researchers found that there was a strong relationship between the parent report using the DCDQ and the AHPs' classification of a child as having, or being at risk of, DCD following observation assessment. They concluded that 'the sensitivity of the DCDQ in this instance suggests that it performs well in screening those children most likely to have coordination difficulties' (p. 7). However, the Checklist version of the C-ABC used with teachers was found to have 'poor discriminative ability … as a screening measure for a clinically referred population' (p. 8).

PREDICTIVE ASSESSMENTS

Predictive tests can also be labelled as *prognostic* measures. AHPs use predictive assessments to classify persons into predefined categories of interest in an attempt to predict an event or functional status in another situation based on the person's performance on the assessment. For example, a kitchen assessment in an occupational therapy department might be used to predict whether the person should be independent and safe in meal preparation once discharged home, or a work assessment may be used to predict current and future employment potential. A predictive test is a measure designed to classify individuals into a set of predefined measurement categories either concurrently or prospectively: to determine whether individuals have been classified correctly (Kirshner and Guyatt 1985).

Definition of a Predictive Assessment

Predictive assessment is undertaken by AHPs to predict the future ability or state of a client or to predict a specific outcome in future (Adams 2002).

It is critical that a test used for predictive purposes has established predictive validity (see Chapter 8). Predictive validity has been defined as 'the accuracy with which a measurement predicts some future event' (McDowell 2006, p. 714). Predictive assessments can be used to identify patients at risk for a particular factor such as suicide, abuse, or falling. In premature or young infants, a predictive assessment may be used to identify those children at risk of developing a problem such as a developmental delay or emotional and behavioural problems; this can enable AHPs to target limited resources for those children most at risk and most likely to benefit from an early intervention. For example, in addition to meeting a discriminative purpose, the *Infant and Toddler Symptom Checklist* (DeGangi et al. 1995) also aims to predict infants and toddlers 'who are at risk for sensory-integrative disorders, attentional deficits, and emotional and behavioural problems' (p. 1).

Bouwstra et al. (2019) have shown how the **Barthel Index** as an observer-based instrument is sufficient for measuring and interpreting changes in physical function of older people. De Wit et al. (2014) suggested that a predictive tool, the Barthel Index, can be used for targeting inpatient stroke rehabilitation and early identification of those who need intensive follow-up.

EVALUATIVE ASSESSMENT

Definition of Evaluative Assessment

Evaluative assessment is used to detect change in functioning over time and is undertaken to monitor a client's progress during rehabilitation and to determine the effectiveness of the intervention.

Evaluative tests are commonly known as **outcome measures**. When measuring outcomes, an AHP explores whether any change in the client has occurred because of a specific intervention. An evaluative test is a measure that can detect and measure the amount of change of the desired outcome overtime (Adams 2002). Evaluative tests are used to measure the magnitude of longitudinal change in an individual or group on the dimension of interest (Kirshner and Guyatt 1985). Evaluative tests should have established test–retest and inter-rater reliability (see Chapter 9).

Responsiveness to change refers to the measure of efficiency with which a test detects clinical change (Wright et al. 1998). When selecting an evaluative measure, AHPs should consider how responsive the test is to detecting the type of clinical change you wish to measure. AHPs should look for reference to psychometric studies that demonstrate responsiveness, specificity, and sensitivity as an evaluative measure needs to be a specific and sensitive measure that can pick up the type and degree of change in function that is anticipated (for more information on responsiveness, sensitivity, and specificity, see Chapter 9). Improvements in function may be small and slow, and many assessments lack sensitivity because they do not have sufficient graduations to measure change, or because they do not include test items that are the focus of rehabilitation. There is also a paucity of test–retest reliability (see Chapter 9) data for many current assessments. It is critical to use objective and sensitive measures because 'any subjective estimate, especially if made by the clinician who has invested time, effort and perhaps more in treating the client, is likely to be unreliable' (de Clive-Lowe 1996, p. 359).

Therapy Outcomes Measures (*TOMs*; Enderby et al. 2013) enable AHPs to describe the comparative abilities and difficulties of a client in four categories: (a) impairment, (b) participation, (c) activity, and (d) well-being (see below for more detail on TOMs).

It is critical to identify the aim of your intervention, because if your goal were to improve performance of a daily living activity, measurement of an underlying component would not measure your outcome. You might learn that the person had increased in strength or ROM, but you would not know if these improvements, at an impairment level, had resulted in the change or improvements in function in the person's daily activities (see Chapter 12 for further exploration of levels of function). In the same way, a measure of level of independence in ADL would not enable you to measure the person's level of social inclusion or their experience of emotional distress.

An outcome measure should be used at the start of intervention to provide a baseline, and then re-administered when intervention ceases in order to ascertain the effects of the intervention (AHP Outcome Measures UK Working Group 2019). The process for measuring outcomes includes the following:

- Establish a baseline from which to measure change.
- Agree on realistic, desired outcomes.
- Define those outcomes as observable and measurable items of performance.
- Implement treatment for an agreed period.
- Carry out the same assessment again.
- Review goals and, if appropriate, revise desired outcomes.

A baseline assessment is often the first assessment completed by the AHP, from which changes are then reviewed.

Definition of a Baseline Assessment

A baseline assessment is the initial data gathered at the start of an intervention. Baseline data can be used to guide the nature of the required intervention. A baseline forms the basis for comparison when measuring outcomes to evaluate the effects of the intervention.

An example of an evaluative test is the TOM (Enderby et al. 2013). This measure was developed in the United Kingdom, initially as a measure of speech therapy outcomes. It was adapted for use by AHPs and rehabilitation nurses. A TOM provides a global measure of health outcomes and can be used with clients of different ages and with a wide variety of diagnoses. The conceptual foundation of the TOM was based on the World Health Organisation (WHO 1980) 'International Classification of Impairments, Disabilities and Handicaps' (ICIDH-1). (See Chapter 11 for a description of the updated ICF model.)

The AHP records baseline and post-test scores for four test domains: impairment, disability, handicap, and distress/well-being. Scoring is undertaken using an 11-point ordinal scale (see Chapter 4 for a definition of an ordinal scale). Research has been conducted in Australia to develop outcome measures based on the revised WHO ICF model (2002), which provides a greater focus on health rather than on disease. Commonwealth Government funding has enabled researchers to adapt the TOM to be compatible with the ICF and to produce separate scales for occupational therapy, physiotherapy, and speech pathology (Perry et al. 2004).

The occupational therapy version, Australian Therapy Outcome Measures for Occupational Therapy (*AusTOMs-OT*; Unsworth and Duncombe 2004, Unsworth et al. 2018), comprises four domains, with the first three drawn from the ICF model: impairment, activity limitation, participation restriction, and distress/well-being. It is made up of 12 scales (for a list of these scale items, see Chapter 9) of which the AHP selects only those that relate to agreed outcomes; in practice, between 1 and 5 outcome scales tend to be used per client (Unsworth 2005).

The updated reliability studies for the AusTOMs-OT look favourable, with moderate to very high reliability across the 12 scales (Unsworth et al. 2018). Previously, 33 of the 48 test items (12 scales by four domains in the total test) were found to have test–retest reliability levels of at least 70% agreement, with the lowest level for the remaining items being 50%. A further reliability study that just focused on the self-care scale (found to be the most frequently applied scale) showed better levels of reliability (Wiseman 2004 cited by Unsworth 2005), with 'inter-rater interclass correlation coefficients (*ICCs*) over 0.79 for the three domains of activity limitation, participation restriction and distress/wellbeing, and over 0.70 for impairment. Test-retest reliability was also reported to be quite high, with ICCs of 0.88 for activity limitation, 0.81 for participation restriction, 0.94 for distress/wellbeing and 0.74 for impairment' (p. 356). Figure 3.2 shows an example of scoring the AusTOM-OT.

Unsworth (2005) also reports on a study to examine the sensitivity of the AusTOM-OT to detect change in client status over time. A large sample of 466 clients was assessed across 12 health facilities, and the results indicated 'that all scales were successful in demonstrating statistically significant client change over time' (p. 354).

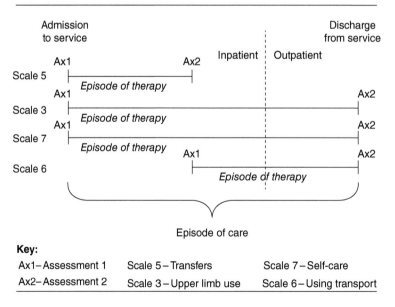

FIGURE 3.2   Scoring AusTOM-OT scales with Josef. Source: From Unsworth and Duncombe (2004). © 2004, La Trobe University.

Table 3.1 provides a summary of the four types of assessment for clinical purposes.

TABLE 3.1   Summary of four clinical purposes of assessment.

Purposes of assessment	Description
Descriptive Assessment	• Undertaken to provide a description of the person's current circumstances, past history, roles, habits, interests, level of occupational engagement, performance component skills, and deficits and desired outcomes. May be used to identify symptoms and problems to help aid diagnosis. • A descriptive assessment may be undertaken to gain information about environmental (physical, social, cultural- institutional) barriers and facilitators, which need to be optimised or overcome to ensure a successful intervention. • The assessment may be undertaken on one occasion or over a period of time until sufficient information has been obtained to inform clinical decision making. • Data is used to inform the development of aims and goals, negotiate outcomes, and formulate intervention planning. • Standardised descriptive tests should have adequate content, construct, and face validity. • If they are to be administered by more than one AHP, a high level of inter-rater reliability is also important.
Discriminative Assessment	• Used to distinguish between individuals or groups. • Comparisons are usually made against a normative group or another diagnostic group. • Discriminative assessment can be useful to refine a differential diagnosis, assess a client against referral criteria, prioritise referrals, assess the person against criteria related to service provision or placement options, or evaluate a person's level of dysfunction in relation to expectations of performance of other healthy people of that age. • Standardised discriminative tests should have established discriminative validity; this may include data on concurrent validity.
Predictive Assessment	• Undertaken when AHPs need to make predictions about a person's future function or behaviour. • The AHP may use the results of an assessment undertaken in one environment to predict likely function in another environment. • In psychosocial practice areas, AHPs may undertake predictive assessment for a number of reasons, including prediction of: likely function when discharged home as part of a pre-discharge assessment (e.g. level of independence, ability to safely use appliances); and risk assessment (e.g. of harm to self or others, abuse, wandering, falls). • Standardised predictive tests should have established predictive validity.
Evaluative Assessment	• Undertaken to evaluate changes in symptoms over time and/or the effectiveness of the intervention or management plan. • Needed to establish whether the level and nature of expected changes (outcomes) have been achieved. • Requires at least two assessments undertaken at different times. The baseline assessment data is used for comparison at the review, discharge, or when a perceived significant change needs to be explored further. • Qualitative and/or quantitative data may be used to inform evaluative decisions. • Standardised evaluative tests are also known as outcome measures. • Standardised evaluative tests should have high levels of test–retest reliability and established responsiveness to change.

Source: From Laver-Fawcett (2012). © 2012, Cengage Learning.

ASSESSMENT FOR PARTICULAR PURPOSES

Care pathways in the UK have particular assessment processes and tools associated with them (De Luc 2001), and have been described as complex interventions (Seys et al. 2019). Assessment for particular purposes may include a formal contract assessment, an overview assessment, a specialist assessment, a comprehensive assessment, and or a capacity assessment. In addition, risk assessments will be undertaken in many services, and sometimes assessments for tribunals.

A **contact assessment** does not have to be undertaken for every contact. In some cases, an AHP could be the first point of contact and will need to judge how a 'contact' assessment is recorded. Where the presenting needs or requests are straightforward and people have indicated there are no other needs or issues, it would usually be inappropriate for professionals to prolong the assessment. Some people may request only pieces of assistive equipment such as grab rails or bath equipment. These requests are often quick, provided there are no other needs, the equipment is appropriate to the assessed or eligible need, and its safe use is explained. As part of this type of assessment, these seven key issues help identify needs:

1. the nature of the presenting need
2. the significance of the need for the older person
3. the length of time the need has been experienced
4. potential solutions identified by the older person
5. other needs experienced by the older person
6. recent life events or changes relevant to the problem(s)
7. the perceptions of family members and carers.

The second type of assessment is an **overview assessment**. The purpose of an overview assessment is to provide a broad, contextual assessment of the person's situation and problems. Professionals carry out an overview assessment if, in their judgement, the individual's needs are such that a more rounded assessment should be undertaken (Curtin et al. 2009).

Definition of an Overview Assessment

An overview assessment is required if the presenting problem is not clear-cut or if there is evidence of potential wider health and/or social care needs.

The third type of assessment is labelled **specialist assessment.** A specialist assessment is undertaken when a domain needs to be explored in detail. From the specialist assessment, professionals should be able to confirm the presence, extent, cause, and likely development of a health condition or problem or social care need, and establish links to other conditions, problems, and needs (Goodwin et al. 2010). AHPs can offer a specialist contribution to the assessment of mobility, transfers, eating, drinking, and functional capacity, and the impact of the home and wider environment on assessed needs. In particular, AHPs are skilled in the assessment of potential for rehabilitation and quality of independence.

A specialist assessment as an assessment undertaken by a clinician or other professional who specialises in a branch of medicine or care, e.g. stroke, cardiac care, or bereavement counselling.

The use of standardised assessments is of particular importance for both specialist and comprehensive assessments. AHPs should ensure that assessment scales to identify physical and personal care problems have a prominent role in assessment procedures, not losing sight of the value of professional judgement (Goodwin et al. 2010).

The fourth and last type of assessment is labelled a **Comprehensive Assessment.** A comprehensive assessment may be required for several reasons.

A comprehensive assessment provides an assessment that is both broad and deep. A comprehensive assessment should be completed for people where the level of support and treatment likely to be offered is intensive or prolonged, including permanent admission to a care home, intermediate care services, or substantial packages of care at home.

As stated earlier, AHPs have a key role to play in providing comprehensive assessment; this will often be as part of a specialist or multidisciplinary team. A coordinated multidisciplinary approach is seen to be crucial for accurate and timely diagnoses of treatable and other health conditions, without which wider assessment and subsequent care planning are likely to be flawed. For a comprehensive assessment, it is also critical that any specialist assessments, particularly if a number of different professionals have conducted these, are coordinated, compared, and interpreted.

These four types of assessment should not be considered as sequential. The four types are distinguished by the breadth and depth of information collected. AHPs have to use their judgement as to how broad (number of domains covered) and how specific (the depth to which a particular domain is assessed) the assessment should be for each client.

For older people and those with long-term conditions, comprehensive assessment reviews should:

- establish how far the support and treatment have achieved the outcomes set out in the care plan;
- re-assess the needs and issues of individual service users;
- help determine users' continued eligibility for support and treatment;
- confirm or amend the current care plan, or lead to closure; and
- where appropriate, comment on how individuals are managing direct payments, personalised care, and personal health budgets (Anderson et al. 2020).

CAPACITY ASSESSMENT

AHPs may need to consider capacity issues. First, does the client have the capacity to consent to the proposed intervention? Second, an AHP might be asked to contribute to an assessment of the person's capacity in a particular situation, for example, to assess whether someone remains competent to drive following a stroke or the onset of dementia.

AHPs may be asked to make an informed judgement about a person's capacity or lack of capacity (Mental Capacity Act 2005). Lack of capacity is defined as follows: 'For a person to lack capacity, he or she must have an impairment of or disturbance in the functioning of the brain or mind, and this defect must result in the inability to understand, retain, use, or weigh information relevant to a decision or to communicate a choice' (Nicholson et al. 2008, p. 324). The Mental Capacity Act (2005, 2019) provides a detailed consideration of capacity issues. AHPs should be aware of its implications.

The Mental Capacity Act states factors that decision makers must explore when deciding what is in a person's best interests. AHPs will need to explore whether the person has made an 'Advanced wishes' statement and must consider any written statement in which the person has articulated his wishes and feelings when making a determination about the person's best interests. Carers and family members also have a right to be consulted.

The Act is underpinned by a set of five key principles (https://www.nhs.uk/conditions/social-care-and-support-guide/making-decisions-for-someone-else/mental-capacity-act accessed 17.02.20).

The Mental Health Act Five Key Principles

1. Assume a person has the capacity to make a decision themselves, unless it is proved otherwise.
2. Wherever possible, help people to make their own decisions.
3. Do not treat a person as lacking the capacity to make a decision just because they make an unwise decision.
4. If you make a decision for someone who does not have capacity, it must be in their best interests.
5. Treatment and care provided to someone who lacks capacity should be the least restrictive of their basic rights and freedoms.

Source: NHS, Mental Capacity Act.

The Mental Capacity Act (2005) clarifies that where a person is providing care or treatment for someone who lacks capacity, then the person can provide the care without incurring legal liability. The key will be proper assessment of capacity and best interests, so AHPs must ensure that a thorough assessment of capacity has been undertaken and that the process and decision made from this assessment are clearly and thoroughly documented. This assessment and documentation serves to cover any actions that would otherwise result in a civil wrong or crime if someone has interfered with the person's body or property in the ordinary course of caring. Jayes et al. (2019) have recently identified that mental capacity assessment practice varies across England and Wales and that the training and practical resources to support professionals in decision making should be used in improve consistency.

ASSESSMENT FOR TRIBUNALS

AHPs (for example, as members of the care team) may be required to provide information for tribunals that includes baseline assessment data, treatment plans, evaluation of the effectiveness of the treatment, and plans for continuing care/review post discharge. AHPs may be involved in providing information that enables a tribunal to judge whether the criteria for compulsory powers are met; the proposed care plan is consistent with the principles set out in the law; and the interventions are appropriate to the treatment of the person's disorder or diagnosis.

RISK ASSESSMENT

Assessment of risk is a big part of AHPs' clinical work. It can range from a small and straightforward risk decision, for example:

- *What is the risk that this elderly person will trip on their loose mat and should I advise that it is taken up before their discharge home?*

To decisions that relate to potentially life-threatening events, such as:

- *What is the risk that this person will become violent and hurt another person?*
- *What is the risk that this child is being physically abused by his parent?*
- *What is the risk that this person will forget to turn the gas cooker off?*

Systematic risk assessment is an approach to identifying and assessing risks using explicit risk management techniques. More tools are now available to assess aspects of risk. The following factors are particular areas to be considered as part of a risk assessment:

- Autonomy and freedom to make choices
- Health and safety including freedom from harm, abuse, and neglect, and taking wider issues of housing circumstances and community safety into account
- The ability to manage personal and other daily routines
- Involvement in family and wider community life, including leisure, hobbies, unpaid and paid work, learning, and volunteering.

AHPs also consider risks faced by people close to their clients, such as carers. AHPs need to identify which risks cause serious concern, and which risks may be acceptable or viewed as a natural and healthy part of daily living and discuss these with clients and carers so that informed choices can be made.

In response to care pathways and assessment guidance, a number of tools have been developed, such as evidence summaries from various professional associations, and government departments (see National Institute for Health and Care Excellence [*NICE*] Evidence search https://www.evidence.nhs.uk).

Two of the most important areas of risk that an AHP might need to assess are risk of harm to self and risk of harm to others. Blank (2001) undertook a systematic review of 10 studies related to the assessment of risk of violence in a community mental health setting. She focused on both clinical and contextual factors in the prediction of violence risk. This is an area where the predictive validity (see Chapter 8)

of any measure of risk is very important. Blank explored two main approaches to the assessment of risk of violence. The first approach involves clinical judgement and the AHP's assessment of the person's predisposition to violence based on available data about the person and his background, diagnosis, history, and social situation. The second approach is called 'actuarial prediction of violence' and 'involves the assigning of a numerical value to factors known to contribute to being violent. For example, being male, falling within a certain age group or having a coexisting diagnosis of substance misuse would all attract certain scores. Risk is then calculated by the overall score' (p. 585).

One measure used for the assessment of suicidal ideation is the Beck Scale for Suicide Ideation (BBS; Beck and Steer 1991). This is a 21-item self-report assessment that is used with adolescents and adults 'to detect and measure the severity of suicidal ideation'. AHPs might presume that such a test would provide a predictive assessment of suicide, but should look carefully at any predictive validity data to justify this presumption. In the BSS manual, the authors refer to a predictive validity study of the Scale for Suicide Ideation (SSI) and Beck Hopelessness Scale (*BHS*) that was a longitudinal study with 207 people. They 'found that the SSI did not predict eventual suicide' but that another measure in their study – the BHS – did (Beck and Steer 1991, p. 21). In a further study, they found that the predictive validity for the SSI improved if people were asked to rate the items in terms of 'their feelings at the worst period in their psychiatric illness' (p. 21). In this study of 72 outpatients, the eight people who went on to commit suicide had a mean SSI score of 21.75 (standard deviation = 10.43) compared to the remaining 64 patients, who had a SSI mean score of only 9.7 (s.d. = 9.98); this was found to be a significant difference (p < 0.01). The BSS was built upon earlier studies and is a self-report version of the SSI that has been developed to be used either alone or with the clinical (interview/observational) rating version. At the beginning of the BSS, the authors note a number of cautions and limitations of the measure, including the following:

1. 'The BSS scores are best regarded as indicators of suicide risk rather than as predictors of eventual suicide in a given case' (p. 1)

   Therefore, AHPs need to be aware that the BSS does not actually predict who will go onto to commit suicide, but it may help them identify people at risk of committing suicide.

2. 'The BSS systematically covers a broad spectrum of attitudes and behaviours that clinicians routinely consider in judging suicidal intention. The BSS measures suicide ideation: as such, it should not be used as a sole source of information in the assessment of suicide risk. Any endorsement of any BSS item may reflect the presence of suicide intention and should be investigated by the clinician'.

   AHPs should use the test as a starting point and should undertake more detailed assessment of those areas of suicidal ideation that are shown up on the BSS. The 21 BSS items comprise 19 items that measure facets of suicide and 2 items that relate to the number of previous suicide attempts and the seriousness of the person's intention to die when the last suicide attempt was made.

3. The BSS is a self-report instrument and contains no mechanism to detect dissimulation or confusion. Suicidal patient may deliberately conceal their intentions from others and may distort their BSS responses'.

A person who is very serious in his intention to commit suicide may not want help and may deliberately under-rate himself on the self-report scale. In the previous chapter (Chapter 2) on sources of data and methods of assessment, we considered the value of obtaining assessment data from three different sources (self-report, proxy report, and AHP observation) and then triangulating data to explore consistencies and inconsistencies in the results obtained from each source. For the assessment of risk of suicide, such an approach is very valuable, and a measure such as the BSS would form just one part of your total assessment.

Another more common area of risk assessment involves the assessment of the person's home environment, such as at a pre-discharge home visit (Lockwood et al. 2019). The purpose of a pre-discharge home visit, made for example, by an occupational therapist is to ensure that an individual is safe and can manage in their own home (Lannin et al. 2007). Standardised assessments that can make such an assessment more rigorous, for example the Safety Assessment of Function and the Environment for Rehabilitation (*SAFER* Tool, Letts et al. 1998).

NEEDS ASSESSMENT – CONSIDERING WIDER POPULATIONS

AHPs have an important role to play as advocates and lobbyists for people with disabilities. For example, AHPs may be asked to undertake an assessment to evaluate the accessibility of their local community. Even if we are not asked, as professionals embracing the health promotion and inclusion agendas, we should put ourselves forward with this assessment purpose. Many communities still pose severe challenges for people with disabilities, and even the simplest of needs, such as an accessible toilet, is sadly lacking in many environments.

SHARING YOUR PURPOSE

It is critical that you not only clarify the purpose(s) of your assessment for yourself but that you also share the purpose with the client and where appropriate their family/carer and the multidisciplinary team. In sharing your assessment purposes with the client, it is also essential that you ask what he wants to gain in general and what he would like to learn from any assessment. An excerpt from Bonnie Sherr Klein's book *Slow Dance*, in which she describes her experience of having a stroke, helps to illustrate the pitfalls of not sharing our purpose or seeking that of our client:

> *The [AHP] spent weeks 'assessing' me: measuring every minute angle of movement; testing and timing my reactions to hot and cold, sharp and dull. The testing seemed irritatingly pointless to me, but it was also tiring, and I needed many rest stops when I would just lie still on the mattress, which seemed irritatingly pointless to the [AHP]. At the very end of our time, she would stretch my arms and legs, and do some passive range-of-motion exercises. After a few weeks of this and a few awkward weekends in bed at home, I asked her if she could stretch my groin so it would be possible to have intercourse. She pretended not to hear me. No one ever talked to me about sex: no physio, no doctor, no OT, no psychologist. Michael [her husband] and I figured it out ourselves, not without pain.*
>
> (Sherr Klein 1997, p. 220)

Case Study

Mr Smith by Alison Laver-Fawcett

This case study is based on my experience of working for a couple of years as an AHP in a geriatric day hospital setting and on my research experience with people with stroke. It is not based on one particular case, but is rather an imaginary case developed to illustrate the application of explicit thinking about purposes of assessment to a clinical setting.

Mr Smith is a 66-year-old man who has been discharged home from a Stroke Rehabilitation Unit (*SRU*) at his local the District Hospital. He was admitted to the SRU five weeks previously with a right parietal infarct. The AHP in this scenario is a senior occupational AHP working as a member of a community-based intermediate care team. Mr Smith has been referred for continuing occupational therapy and physiotherapy for up to six weeks to help him adjust to community living post stroke. The referral information states that Mr Smith has a mild hemiplegia of his left upper and lower limbs and can transfer and mobilise with the assistance of one person. He also has some unilateral neglect. The AHP plans her assessment process by reflecting on the following questions:

Why Am I Doing This Assessment?

I need to understand the impact of the diagnosis (stroke) and impairment (left-sided hemiplegia and unilateral neglect) on Mr Smith's functioning in everyday tasks in his home environment so I can develop a client-centred treatment plan and to provide baseline information so I can monitor the effects of my intervention. I also want to assess the couple's affect and coping skills, as clients often fully realise the impact of the stroke when they return home and try to function outside an inpatient environment, and they can become depressed at this stage. For family members, also, the full impact of their loved one's stroke is realised on discharge home and the change of role to a carer becomes apparent, so I need to consider carer burden.

What Information Do I Need to Collect?

I will need information about Mr Smith's lifestyle prior to his stroke: I want to know what were his roles and interests, and what kind of lifestyle does he want to create post stroke? I need to know his pre-stroke and current level of independence in personal and domestic ADL, leisure, and productive activities. I need his viewpoint on which activities are most important to him to achieve independently and what his priorities are for improving his function. I require information about his mood. I should seek information about how his wife is coping in her new role as a carer and about her priorities.

What Decisions Will I Need to Make from This Information?

I will use the information to identify problem areas relevant to occupational therapy intervention and then to negotiate treatment goals with the client in order to prioritise areas for intervention and develop a treatment plan.

What Will Be the Benefit to the Client (and Where Relevant the Carer) from Undertaking This Assessment?

Accurate assessment will enable a realistic and effective intervention to be implemented. As self-report and proxy data collection methods will be implemented, the couple will become active partners in the therapeutic process as their views and priorities will be taken into account when identifying problems, setting outcome goals, and prioritising the treatment plan. By undertaking a re-assessment, I will be able to demonstrate any changes in function following my intervention – this helps the client and family to see improvements and should help boost morale and confidence. If I identify carer burden, I will signpost Mrs Smith to supporting agencies, such as the Carers' Resource.

Articulating the answers to these questions enables me to focus my assessment and to select an effective and efficient assessment approach. In summary:

- To collect the information needed, I will have to use several data collection methods, including the informal and standardised use of client self-report, carer proxy report, and observation, and I plan to triangulate assessment data to get a comprehensive picture.
- I require a descriptive assessment of functioning in everyday tasks, but I also need this to be an outcome measure as I want to be able to evaluate outcomes to monitor the effects of my intervention.
- I also need to understand what problems are most significant for the client and his carer, so that we can select relevant mutually agreed outcome goals for intervention.
- I want to assess his mood in order to identify any depression; this will need to be an evaluative test so I can monitor any depression over time.
- I want to assess whether Mrs Smith is experiencing any carer burden and monitor the degree of burden over time.

There are quite a few standardised tests which I could use but I do not want to waste too much intervention time as my intermediate care service is only for six weeks and I do not want to over-assess the client, which might lead to fatigue or him disengaging from the therapeutic process. Therefore, I need to select assessments that will meet more than one purpose wherever possible.

I will start the assessment with an **informal interview.** I find this helps to build rapport and establish a therapeutic relationship. I will explain my role and the purpose of this first assessment home visit; for example, I might say:

I want to get to know about your previous lifestyle so I can help you work towards regaining as much of that lifestyle as possible and I need to understand any problems you are experiencing now you are back home so that we can develop strategies to try to overcome these problems.

During the informal interview, I would ask how the couple have been managing since discharge, and about their lifestyle prior to his stroke, what are his roles and interests, and, what kind of lifestyle do they want to lead in future.

On the first visit, I plan to use the COPM (Law et al. 1994), which is a self-report assessment that provides an individualised measure of a client's self-perception in occupational performance and covers the constructs of self-care, productivity, and leisure. The area of self-care includes personal care, functional mobility, and community management. The area of productivity includes paid or unpaid work, household management, and school or play. Leisure includes quiet recreation, active recreation, and socialisation. Function is rated in terms of importance, performance, and satisfaction on three 10-point scales. I selected this as my first standardised assessment for the following reasons:

- The COPM identifies information about the activities from across a person's lifestyle (personal ADL, domestic ADL, transportation, shopping, and leisure) and it incorporates the roles and role expectations of the client.
- It is a person centred tool that considers the importance of activities to the person and his level of satisfaction with current ability, as well as how well he can do each of the activities discussed, this will help me to prioritise client-centred areas for treatment.
- The COPM focuses on the client's own environment, thereby ensuring the relevance of the problems to the client. This is relevant because Mr Smith has now been discharged home, and previous assessments were undertaken in an inpatient setting.
- It is a well-researched measure with published psychometric properties.
- It is good for evaluating clinical change and has acceptable levels of test–retest reliability so that I will be able to re-assess using the COPM and measure the effectiveness of my intervention.
- Moreover, it can be used as a self-report or proxy-report measure. This allows for input from members of the client's social environment if the client is unable to answer on his or her own behalf. This will be useful if Mr Smith is unable to comprehend the assessment. I could use the tool with both Mr and Mrs Smith, as his wife may have different perspectives about his level of performance and about the importance Mr and Mrs Smith place on them.

On the home visit, I explain the purpose of COPM to the couple and describe how we will do the assessment. I clarify that I need their independent viewpoints initially, and that then we will discuss the results together. I then administer the COPM to Mr Smith in the living room as an interview, as I anticipate that he will need extra explanation and prompting to complete the test. At the same time, Mrs Smith completes the COPM individually in the kitchen (I tell her to pop back to me in the living room if anything is unclear or she has any questions). I then review the two sets of data while Mrs Smith makes us all a cup of tea, and the three of us sit down to discuss the results and identify similarities and differences in their scores to negotiate the mutually agreed priority areas for treatment.

In order to examine carer burden, I decide to use a self-report measure, the **Zarit Burden Interview** (Zarit et al. 1980). The Zarit Burden Interview was developed to report the burden experienced by the carer in managing the person with cognitive impairment. Factor analysis revealed two important variables: (a) emotion-focused stress; and (b) demand stress. The assessment can be completed in an interview or a survey format by the carer. The test is scored on a 5-point scale according to how the carer feels about the item presented. The score 0 indicates no feeling; 1, they feel a little; 2, they feel moderately; 3, feel quite a bit; and 4, feel extremely. I selected this tool because:

- it was developed to report the burden experienced by the carer, and it considers both emotion-focused stress and demands placed by the physical tasks associated with caregiving;
- it can be administered either as an interview or as a survey;
- it is quick to complete; and
- it is easy to score.

I decide to use the survey version and leave it with Mrs Smith at the end of the first home visit for her to complete in her own time and return to me when I visit two days later.

From the COPM, Mr and Mrs Smith both identify that feeding, washing, and dressing are areas where he cannot manage without her help. Mr Smith feels very strongly that he does not want to be dependent on his wife for these self-care tasks. When I question the couple further about what help he needs, it sounds like the unilateral neglect might be more problematic than the hemiplegia. I feel I need to observe Mr Smith doing these tasks to identify the main problems, assess the level of physical help and cueing he requires, and select appropriate treatment strategies. I, therefore, decide that I will administer a standardised observational test, the **SOTOF** (Laver-Fawcett and Powell 1995), on my next home visit. SOTOF gives data about the level of independence, the behavioural skill components of the tasks, and the underlying motor, sensory, cognitive, and perceptual functioning. This is a standardised assessment that can be used as for both my descriptive and evaluative purposes. I selected this measure for the following reasons:

- It provides a structured diagnostic reasoning tool that involves the observation of feeding, pouring, and drinking, handwashing, and dressing tasks, the kind of personal ADL tasks identified as problematic and important by Mr Smith and his wife.
- The test provides a simultaneous assessment of both self-care function, residual and deficit skills, and abilities within ADL performance (for example, reaching, scanning, grasping, and sequencing) and underlying neurological deficit, thus eliminating the necessity to administer two separate tests and showing the explicit relationship between functional performance dysfunction and underlying neurological deficit.
- SOTOF allows the AHP to prompt the person and observe responses to any prompts.
- The test has good face validity with clients who have a primary diagnosis of stroke.
- The test has been shown to have good clinical utility; it is age-appropriate and is quick and simple to administer.
- SOTOF has acceptable levels of test–retest reliability, so I could use it as an evaluative measure.
- The SOTOF self-care tasks are broken down into discrete skill components, so the test is very sensitive to small changes in function within the task performance. For example, if the subject does not change from dependent to independent feeding but can complete some aspects of the feeding task more easily, this will be shown. This is important because progress following

a stroke can be slow, and when working in an intermediate care setting, my intervention period is short (usually about six weeks).

The SOTOF allows me to address four related assessment questions simultaneously:

- How well does Mr Smith perform basic personal ADL tasks, independently or dependently, and how much help and prompting does he need?
- What skills and abilities does Mr Smith have intact, and what skills and abilities have been affected by the neurological damage caused by his stroke?
- Which of the perceptual, cognitive, motor, and sensory performance components have been affected by the neurological damage (based on referral information, I am anticipating that the motor and perceptual components are impaired)?
- Why is function impaired? (I will be able to identify the cause by naming the specific neurological deficits and underlying pathology; in this case, I am expecting unilateral neglect to be one of these deficits).

The SOTOF was administered on the second home visit, and the results formed the basis of the treatment approach for two agreed intervention goals:

- To get dressed independently, he agreed that to begin with his wife would lay out clothes ready on their bed.
- To eat independently using adapted cutlery and crockery to enable one-handed feeding. Mr Smith conceded his wife would need to cut up some food for him and agreed to work on strategies to overcome his neglect.

At the beginning of the third visit, the results of the Carer burden measure were discussed with Mrs Smith, and she agreed to referral to Carers' Resource for advice on benefits and to attend a carers' support group. At the end of the six-week intervention, Mr Smith was revaluated on the COPM for the agreed dressing and feeding goals, and the two SOTOF scales related to feeding and dressing were re-administered.

Reflecting on Purposes of Assessment in Your Own Practice

At the end of each chapter, you will find templates of worksheets designed to assist you in applying principles of assessment and outcome measurement to your own practice. See **Worksheet 3.1** found on p. 125.

For this reflection, you will need to review the range of un-standardised and standardised data collection methods and outcome measures used within a service or by a multidisciplinary team. If you are a student, reflect on the range of assessments and outcome measures that you have seen used on one of your clinical placements. The worksheet takes you through a series of questions related to each of the four main assessment purposes: descriptive, evaluative, predictive, and discriminative. There is

WORKSHEET 3.1   Reflecting on the Purposes of Assessment.

Purpose of assessment	What data do you currently collect related to each purpose?	What decisions do you need to make from this data?	What assessments (standardised or un-standardised) do you currently use to collect data for this assessment purpose?	Is this assessment method adequate? YES or NO	List potential assessments that you could use to collect data for this assessment purpose
Descriptive Assessment					
Evaluative Assessment (outcome measure)					
Discriminative Assessment					
Predictive Assessment					
Service Evaluation					

also a section related to service evaluation. You will be asked to think about the data currently collected for each purpose and to reflect on how this data is used (for example, to make decisions about the client's problems, symptoms, and need for further intervention). There is then space to list the standardised and un-standardised assessments that currently provide data for this purpose and to reflect upon whether these are adequate. Finally, there is space to list other potential measures that can yield data for a specific purpose.

REVIEW QUESTIONS

3.1   What factors should you consider when selecting a discriminative assessment for your service?

3.2   Define predictive assessment.

3.3   Why do AHPs undertake evaluative assessment and why should they use standardised outcome measures for this purpose?

3.4   Why should AHPs evaluate their service?

You will find brief answers to these questions at the back of this book on p. 445.

REFERENCES

Adams, J. (2002). The purpose of outcome measurement in rheumatology. *British Journal of Occupational Therapy* 65 (4): 172–174. https://doi.org/10.1177/030802260206500404.

Allied Health Professions (AHP) Outcome Measures UK Working Group (2019) Key questions to ask when selecting outcome measures: a checklist for allied health professionals London: Royal College of Speech and Language Therapists. https://www.rcslt.org/-/media/docs/selecting-outcome-measures.pdf?la=en&hash=12ECB2CFDA0B2EFB1979E592A383D24E792AB9DD

Anderson, M., Charlesworth, A., and Mossialos, E. (2020). Understanding personal health budgets. *BMJ* 2020: 368. https://doi.org/10.1136/bmj.m324.

Beck, A.T. and Steer, R.A. (1991). *Manual for the Beck Scale for Suicide Ideation*, 63. San Antonio, TX: Psychological Corporation.

Blank, A. (2001). Patient violence in community mental health: a review of the literature. *British Journal of Occupational Therapy* 64 (12): 584–589. https://doi.org/10.1177/030802260106401202.

Bouwstra, H., Smit, E.B., Wattel, E.M. et al. (2019). Measurement properties of the Barthel Index in geriatric rehabilitation. *Journal of the American Medical Directors Association* 20 (4): 420–425. https://doi.org/10.1016/j.jamda.2018.09.033.

Bovend'Eerdt, T.J., Botell, R.E., and Wade, D.T. (2009). Writing SMART rehabilitation goals and achieving goal attainment scaling: a practical guide. *Clinical Rehabilitation* 23 (4): 352–361. https://doi.org/10.1177/0269215508101741.

Butler, C., Holdsworth, L.M., Coulton, S., and Gage, H. (2012). Evaluation of a hospice rapid response community service: a controlled evaluation. *BMC Palliative Care*, 11 11 (1) https://doi.org/10.1186/1472-684X-11-11.

de Clive-Lowe, S. (1996). Outcome measurement, cost-effectiveness and clinical audit: the importance of standardised assessment to occupational therapists in meeting these new demands. *British Journal of Occupational Therapy* 59 (8): 357–362. https://doi.org/10.1177/030802269605900803.

Colquhoun, H.L., Letts, L.J., Law, M.C. et al. (2012). Administration of the Canadian occupational performance measure: effect on practice. *Canadian Journal of Occupational Therapy* 79: 120–128. https://doi.org/10.2182/cjot.2012.79.2.7.

Connolly, M., Deaton, C., Dodd, M. et al. (2010). Discharge preparation: do healthcare professionals differ in their opinions? *Journal of Interprofessional Care* 24 (6): 633–643. https://doi.org/10.3109/13561820903418614.

Creek, J. (2003). *Occupational Therapy Defined as a Complex Intervention*. London: College of Occupational Therapists (COT).

Curtin, M., Molineux, M., and Webb, J.A. (2009). *Occupational Therapy and Physical Dysfunction E-Book: Enabling Occupation*, 6e. Elsevier Health Sciences.

De Luc, K. (2001, e-book 2018). *Developing Care Pathways: The Handbook*. Routledge https://doi.org/10.4324/9781315379166.

De Wit, L., Putman, K., Devos, H. et al. (2014). Long-term prediction of functional outcome after stroke using single items of the Barthel Index at discharge from rehabilitation centre. *Disability and Rehabilitation* 36 (5): 353–358. https://doi.org/10.3109/09638288.2013.793411.

DeGangi, G.A., Poisson, S., Sickel, R.Z., and Santman, W.A. (1995). *Infant/Toddler Symptom Checklist: A Screening Tool for Parents*. San Antonio (TX): Therapy Skill Builders, Psychological Corporation.

Dibben, C., Saeed, H., Stagias, K. et al. (2008). Crisis resolution and home treatment teams for older people with mental illness. *Psychiatric Bulletin* 32 (7): 268–270. https://doi.org/10.1192/pb.bp.107.018218.

Enderby, P., John, A., and Petheram, B. (2013). *Therapy Outcome Measures for Rehabilitation Professionals: Speech and Language Therapy, Physiotherapy, Occupational Therapy*. Wiley. 13:978-0-470-0262-2.

England, N. H. S (2016). *Commissioning Guidance for Rehabilitation*. London: NHS England https://www.england.nhs.uk/wp-content/uploads/2016/04/rehabilitation-comms-guid-16-17.pdf.

Fisher, A. G. (2003). Assessment of motor and process skills. Administration and Scoring Manual.

Gonçalves-Bradley, D.C., Lannin, N.A., Clemson, L.M. et al. (2016). Discharge planning from hospital. *Cochrane Database of Systematic Reviews* 1 https://www.cochranelibrary.com/cdsr/doi/10.1002/14651858.CD000313.pub5/abstract.

Goodwin, N., Curry, N., Naylor, C., Ross, S., & Duldig, W. (2010). Managing people with long-term conditions. The King's Fund 2010. www.kingsfund.org.uk/sites/default/files/field/field_document/managing-people-long-term-conditions-gp-inquiry--research-paper-mar11.pdf

Green, D., Bishop, T., Wilson, B.N. et al. (2005). Is questionnaire-based screening part of the solution to waiting lists for children with developmental coordination disorder? *British Journal of Occupational Therapy* 68 (1): 2–10. https://doi.org/10.1177/030802260506800102.

Henderson, S. E., & Sugden, D. A. (1992). Movement Assessment Battery for Children. London: The Psychological Corporation. *Movement ABC—Batteria per la Valutazione Motoria del Bambino*, 2000.

Heyman, B., Alaszewski, A., Shaw, M., and Titterton, M. (2010). *Risk, Safety and Clinical Practice: Health Care Through the Lens of Risk*. Oxford University Press.

Holdsworth, L., Webster, V., and Judge, P. (2018). *Patient Self Referral: A Guide for Therapists*. CRC Press.

Jayes, M., Palmer, R., Enderby, P., and Sutton, A. (2019). How do health and social care professionals in England and Wales assess mental capacity? A literature review. *Disability and Rehabilitation* 42: 1–12. https://doi.org/10.1080/09638288.2019.1572793.

Johnstone, L. and Dallos, R. (2013). *Formulation in Psychology and Psychotherapy: Making Sense of people's Problems*. Routledge.

Kiresuk, T.J., Smith, A., and Cardillo, J.E. (2014). *Goal Attainment Scaling: Applications, Theory, and Measurement*. Psychology Press.

Kirshner, B. and Guyatt, G. (1985). A methodological framework for assessing health indices. *Journal of Chronic Diseases* 38 (1): 27–36. https://doi.org/10.1016/0021-9681(85)90005-0.

Lannin, N.A., Clemson, L., McCluskey, A. et al. (2007). Feasibility and results of a randomised pilot-study of pre-discharge occupational therapy home visits. *BMC Health Services Research* 7 (1): 42. https://doi.org/10.1186/1472-6963-7-42.

Laver-Fawcett, A. J. (1994). The development of the Structured Observational Test of Function (SOTOF) (Doctoral dissertation, University of Surrey). https://ethos.bl.uk/OrderDetails.do?uin=uk.bl.ethos.259917

Laver-Fawcett, A.J. and Powell, G.E. (1995). *The Structured Observational Test of Function (SOTOF)*. Windsor: NFER-Nelson.

Laver-Fawcett, A.J. (2012). Chapter 18. Assessment, Evaluation and Outcome Measurement. In: *Psychosocial Occupational Therapy: An Evolving Practice*, 3e (eds. E. Cara and A. MacRae). Hingham Massachusetts: Cengage Learning.

Law, M. (1987). Measurement in occupational therapy: scientific criteria for evaluation. *Canadian Journal of Occupational Therapy* 54 (3): 133–138. https://doi.org/10.1177/000841748705400308.

Law, M., Polatajko, H., Pollock, N. et al. (1994). Pilot testing of the Canadian Occupational Performance Measure: clinical and measurement issues. *Canadian Journal of Occupational Therapy* 61 (4): 191–197.

Letts, L., Scott, S., Burtney, J. et al. (1998). The reliability and validity of the safety assessment of function and the environment for rehabilitation (SAFER tool). *British Journal of Occupational Therapy* 61 (3): 127–132. https://doi.org/10.1177/030802269806100309.

Lockwood, K.J., Harding, K.E., Boyd, J.N., and Taylor, N.F. (2019). Predischarge home visits after hip fracture: a randomized controlled trial. *Clinical Rehabilitation* 33 (4): 681–692. https://doi.org/10.1177/0269215518823256.

McDowell, I. (2006). *Measuring Health: A Guide to Rating Scales and Questionnaires*. USA: Oxford University Press.

Mental Capacity Act. (2005). Mental Capacity Act. London: The Stationery Office. https://www.nhs.uk/conditions/social-care-and-support-guide/making-decisions-for-someone-else/mental-capacity-act

Mental Capacity Act Amendment (2019). https://www.nhs.uk/conditions/social-care-and-support-guide/making-decisions-for-someone-else/mental-capacity-act/

NHS (2019). *The NHS Long Term Plan*. NHS https://www.longtermplan.nhs.uk.

Nicholson, T.R., Cutter, W., and Hotopf, M. (2008). Assessing mental capacity: the mental capacity act. *BMJ* 336 (7639): 322–325. https://doi.org/10.1136/bmj.39457.485347.80.

Perry, A., Morris, M., Unsworth, C. et al. (2004). Therapy outcome measures for allied health practitioners in Australia: the AusTOMs. *International Journal for Quality in Health Care* 16 (4): 285–291. https://doi.org/10.1093/intqhc/mzh059.

Ponte-Allan, M. and Giles, G.M. (1999). Goal setting and functional outcomes in rehabilitation. *American Journal of Occupational Therapy* 53 (6): 646–649. https://doi.org/10.5014/ajot.53.6.646.

Prior, M., Guerin, M., and Grimmer-Somers, K. (2008). The effectiveness of clinical guideline implementation strategies–a synthesis of systematic review findings. *Journal of Evaluation in Clinical Practice* 14 (5): 888–897. https://doi.org/10.1111/j.1365-2753.2008.01014.x.

Saxton, J., McGonigle, K.L., Swihart, A.A., and Boller, F. (1993). *The Severe Impairment Battery Manual.* Pisttsburgh: Thames Valley Test Company.

Scobbie, L., Dixon, D., and Wyke, S. (2011). Goal setting and action planning in the rehabilitation setting: development of a theoretically informed practice framework. *Clinical Rehabilitation* 25 (5): 468–482. https://doi.org/10.1177/0269215510389198.

Seabrook, M., Schwarz, M., Ward, E.C., and Whitfield, B. (2019). Implementation of an extended scope of practice speech-language pathology allied health practitioner service: an evaluation of service impacts and outcomes. *International Journal of Speech-Language Pathology* 21 (1): 65–74. https://doi.org/10.1080/17549507.2017.1380702.

Seys, D., Panella, M., VanZelm, R. et al. (2019). Care pathways are complex interventions in complex systems: New European Pathway Association framework. *International Journal of Care Coordination* 22 (1): 5–9. https://doi.org/10.1177/2053434519839195.

Sherr Klein, B. (1997). *Slow Dance: A Story of Stroke, Love and Disability.* Toronto: Vintage Canada.

Sniehotta, F.F., Schwarzer, R., Scholz, U., and Schüz, B. (2005). Action planning and coping planning for long-term lifestyle change: theory and assessment. *European Journal of Social Psychology* 35 (4): 565–576. https://doi.org/10.1002/ejsp.258.

Stevens, A., Beurskens, A., Köke, A., and van der Weijden, T. (2013). The use of patient-specific measurement instruments in the process of goal-setting: a systematic review of available instruments and their feasibility. *Clinical Rehabilitation* 27 (11): 1005–1019. https://doi.org/10.1177/0269215513490178.

Turner-Stokes, L. (2009). Goal attainment scaling (GAS) in rehabilitation: a practical guide. *Clinical Rehabilitation* 23 (4): 362–370. https://doi.org/10.1177/0269215508101742.

Unsworth, C.A. (2005). Measuring outcomes using the Australian Therapy Outcome Measures for Occupational Therapy (AusTOMs-OT): data description and tool sensitivity. *British Journal of Occupational Therapy* 68 (8): 354–366. https://doi.org/10.1177/030802260506800804.

Unsworth, C.A. and Duncombe, D. (2004). *AusTOMs for Occupational Therapy.* Melbourne, Australia: La Trobe University.

Unsworth, C.A., Timmer, A., and Wales, K. (2018). Reliability of the Australian Therapy Outcome Measures for Occupational Therapy (AusTOMs-OT). *Australian Occupational Therapy Journal* 65 (5): 376–386. https://doi.org/10.1111/1440-1630.12476.

Volkmer, A., Spector, A., Warren, J.D., and Beeke, S. (2018). Speech and language therapy for primary progressive aphasia: referral patterns and barriers to service provision across the UK. *Dementia* 19 (5): 1349–1363. https://doi.org/10.1177/1471301218797240.

Wilson, B.N., Kaplan, B.J., Crawford, S.G. et al. (2000). Reliability and validity of a parent questionnaire on childhood motor skills. *American Journal of Occupational Therapy* 54 (5): 484–493. https://doi.org/10.5014/ajot.54.5.484.

Wiseman, F. (2004). Reliability of the Occupational Therapy Australian Therapy Outcome Measure (OT- AusTOM) Self Care Scale. (Honours thesis.) Melbourne, VIC: La Trobe University.

Wong, E.L., Yam, C.H., Cheung, A.W. et al. (2011). Barriers to effective discharge planning: a qualitative study investigating the perspectives of frontline health-care professionals. *BMC Health Services Research* 11 (1): 242. https://doi.org/10.1186/1472-6963-11-242.

World Health Organization. (1980). International classification of impairments, disabilities, and handicaps: a manual of classification relating to the consequences of disease, published in accordance with resolution WHA29. 35 of the Twenty-ninth World Health Assembly, May 1976. https://apps.who.int/iris/handle/10665/41003

Wright, J., Cross, J., and Lamb, S. (1998). Physiotherapy outcome measures for rehabilitation of elderly people: responsiveness to change of the Rivermead Mobility Index and Barthel Index. *Physiotherapy* 84 (5): 216–221. https://doi.org/10.1016/S0031-9406(05)65552-6.

Zarit, S.H., Reever, K.E., and Bach-Peterson, J. (1980). Relatives of the impaired elderly: correlates of feelings of burden. *The Gerontologist* 20 (6): 649–655.

RESOURCES

Allied Health Professions (AHP) Outcome Measures UK Working Group (2019) Key questions to ask when selecting outcome measures: a checklist for allied health professionals London: Royal College of Speech and Language Therapists, 2 White Hart Yard, London SE1 1NX https://www.rcslt.org/-/media/docs/selecting-outcome--measures.pdf?la=en&hash=12ECB2CFDA0B2EFB1979E592A383D24E792AB9DD

GAS now available as a mobile app – GOALed

International Classification of Function (ICF) - https://www.who.int/classifications/icf/en

Mental Capacity Act, 2005 and Amendment 2019 - https://www.nhs.uk/conditions/social-care-and-support-guide/making-decisions-for-someone-else/mental-capacity-act

National Institute for Health and Care Excellence (NICE) Evidence search https://www.evidence.nhs.uk

Practical Guide of GAS from Kings College London by Professor L Turner-Stokes www.kcl.ac.uk/cicelysaunders/attachments/tools-gas-practical-guide.pdf

CHAPTER 4

What Is Measurement?

In this chapter, we consider what measurement is. In the Introduction, we defined measurement as follows: 'A measurement is the data obtained by measuring'. Measuring is undertaken by allied health professionals (AHPs) to ascertain the dimensions (size), quantity (amount), or capacity of a trait, attribute, or characteristic of a person that is required by the AHP to develop an accurate picture of the person's needs and problems to form a baseline for therapeutic intervention and/or to provide a measure of outcome. A measurement is obtained by applying a standard scale to variables, thus translating direct observations or patient/proxy reports to a numerical scoring system.

QUESTIONS TO CONSIDER

1. What is measurement?
2. What are levels of measurement?
3. What are patient-related outcome measures?
4. How do I select measures for my practice?

WHAT IS MEASUREMENT?

Sarle (1997) provides a simple example to explain the concept of measurement:

Suppose we have a collection of straight sticks of various sizes and we assign a number to each stick by measuring its length using a ruler. If the

Principles of Assessment and Outcome Measurement for Allied Health Professionals:
Practice, Research and Development, Second Edition. Alison J. Laver-Fawcett and Diane L. Cox.
© 2021 John Wiley & Sons Ltd. Published 2021 by John Wiley & Sons Ltd.

number assigned to one stick is greater than the number assigned to another stick, we can conclude that the first stick is longer than the second. Thus a relationship among the numbers (greater than) corresponds to a relationship among the sticks (longer than).

Sarle (1997) goes on to use the same example of measuring sticks to show how more complex measurements can be made:

> If we lay two sticks end-to-end in a straight line and measure their combined length, then the number we assign to the concatenated sticks will equal the sum of the numbers assigned to the individual sticks (within measurement error). Thus, another relationship among the numbers (addition) corresponds to a relationship among the sticks (concatenation). These relationships among the sticks must be empirically verified for the measurements to be valid.

WHAT IS MEASUREMENT THEORY?

A basic understanding of measurement theory (sometimes referred to as test theory) is important for all AHPs. AHPs have to consider a number of issues when measuring human behaviour, in particular, when they are attempting to measure psychological attributes (referred to as constructs) that cannot be directly observed (Crocker and Algina 1986):

- Measurements obtained are always subject to some degree of error (p. 6). This error may occur for a wide variety of reasons; for example, errors may occur because the person is more fatigued than usual, or he is feeling anxious about being tested, or is having to perform in a strange environment instead of his own home. A big problem for AHPs is how to establish the amount of error that is present in the person's test results.
- Measurements are usually based on limited samples of behaviour (p. 6). AHPs often have a limited amount of time in which to undertake assessment. Therefore, a measurement may only be taken at one point in time, or functional ability may have to be judged on a limited observation of performance.
- No single approach to the measurement of any construct is universally accepted (p. 6). AHPs are faced by a wide range of published tests all purporting to measure the same thing, such as depression or pain or independence in activities of daily living (ADL).
- Units on a measurement scale may not be well defined (p. 6). Many therapy scales use labels like 'independent', 'severe', or 'frequently', but what do these labels mean and do they mean the same thing to each person rating the test?
- When measuring a psychological construct, such as memory, 'the construct cannot be defined only in terms of operational definitions but must also have demonstrated relationships to other constructs or observations' (p. 7). To

understand processes that we cannot directly observe, we turn to theoretical explanations. Such theories will postulate relationships between different observed behaviours and the construct of interest (such as attention) and between different constructs (such as attention and short-term memory).

Measurement theory can help AHPs to understand and reduce the impact of such problems. It encourages AHPs to reflect on the meaning of the data they obtain through testing, and it supports a critical examination of the assumptions behind the analysis of test data. Sarle (1997) provides the following definition of measurement theory:

> Measurement theory is a branch of applied mathematics that is useful in measurement and data analysis. The fundamental idea of measurement theory is that measurements are not the same as the attribute being measured. Hence, if you want to draw conclusions about the attribute, you must take into account the nature of the correspondence between the attribute and the measurements ... Mathematical statistics is concerned with the connection between inference and data. Measurement theory is concerned with the connection between data and reality. Both statistical theory and measurement theory are necessary to make inferences about reality.

There are three types of measurement theories discussed in the literature; these are generally referred to as:

- representational measurement theory
- operational measurement theory
- classical measurement theory, also sometimes known as traditional measurement theory (see Crocker and Algina 1986).

Sarle (1997) distinguishes these three approaches to measurement in the following way:

1. **The representational theory** assumes that a 'reality' being measured exists, and that scientific theories are about this reality.
2. **The operational theory** requires only that measurement should consist of precisely specified operations; scientific theories concern only relationships among measurements.
3. **The classical theory** holds that only quantitative attributes are measurable, and measurement involves the discovery of the magnitudes of these attributes. Meaningfulness comes from empirical support for scientific theories describing the interrelationships of various measurements.

THE ASSIGNMENT OF NUMBERS FOR THE PURPOSES OF ASSESSMENT

In Chapter 2, we saw that there are many different methods, both qualitative and quantitative, that can be used to collect and record assessment data. Using numbers adds to the range of evidence at an AHP's disposal (Eva and Paley 2004). Numbers are a tool AHPs can use to aid their understanding and documentation of their client's problems, functioning, and situation. Lord Kelvin (1824–1907) talked about the benefit of using numbers to define a construct: 'When you can measure what you are speaking about, and express it in numbers, then you know something about it, and when you cannot express it in numbers, then your knowledge is of a meagre and unsatisfactory kind' (Ratcliffe 2016 https://www.oxfordreference.com/view/10.1093/acref/9780191826719.001.0001/q-oro-ed4-00006236).

However, in some healthcare disciplines, there is considerable distrust of quantification. Many AHPs are wary of using numbers to quantify aspects of human function because they believe that there is something limiting about numbers and that numbers cannot adequately describe the psychological, social, and spiritual dimensions of human life (Eva and Paley 2004). The AHP must 'select the most relevant permutation of facts and figures in any given situation, where relevance is determined by the specific purpose that we have or the specific question that we are trying to answer' (p. 48). Although it is true that assigning numbers will not offer a complete description of function, and cannot illustrate every aspect of a client of interest, numerical scoring systems offer a useful permutation in assessment, particularly in the measurement of outcome in order to evaluate whether an intervention has achieved the desired results. Numbers are used in very different and not always appropriate ways in therapy assessments. In order to be able to interpret and handle appropriately any numerical scores, it is critical that you are able to determine and understand the type of numerical scale and level of measurement being used.

Many standardised and non-standardised assessments score the person's performance on some sort of scale. Scaling methods vary in complexity, and the AHP needs to judge whether the scaling method used provides at least an adequate measurement system and at best the ideal level of measurement for the construct or behaviour being measured.

WHAT ARE LEVELS OF MEASUREMENT?

The level of measurement of a variable in mathematics and statistics describes how much information the numbers associated with the variable contain (Gershkoff 2011). In statistics, the kinds of descriptive statistics and significance tests that are appropriate depend on the level of measurement of the variables concerned (Bowling and Ebrahim 2005; Norman 2010).

Fundamental to all scaling methods is a distinction between four ways of applying numbers in measurement. These four applications of numbers to scales 'lie in a hierarchy of mathematical adequacy' (McDowell 2006, p. 18). Stanley Smith Stevens (1946) described this model of four levels of measurement scales back in the 1940s, and his model is still widely used today in order classify scoring systems. Stevens' system identified scales that differ in the extent to which their scale values retain the properties of the real number line. The four levels of measurement data are called *Nominal*, *Ordinal*, *Interval*, and *Ratio*. Some authors refer to the mnemonic NOIR to help remember the names and order of the levels of measurement.

The type of scoring that an assessment tool, measurement instrument, or outcome measure is based on must be taken into account depending on whether it yields:

- **Nominal data**: Numbers are used simply for classification (e.g. 'died', 'survived').
- **Ordinal scale data**: Scale items stand in some kind of relation to each other (e.g. 'very difficult' through to 'not very difficult').

- **Interval scale data**: The characteristics are those of an ordinal scale, but the distances between any two numbers on the scale are of a known size (e.g. temperature).
- **Ratio scale data**: The characteristics are those of an interval scale with the addition of a true – not arbitrary – zero point (e.g. weight) (Bowling and Ebrahim 2005, p. 22).

NOMINAL SCALES

Nominal scales are the lowest level of measurement (see Figure 4.1, Carman 2012). In fact, the nominal level does not provide a system of measurement at all, but rather a system of classification. A nominal scale simply uses numbers to classify a characteristic and is used to identify differences without quantifying or ordering those differences. This means that no inferences can be drawn from the numbers used; whether one category is allocated a higher or lower number than another is arbitrary. These scales are sometimes referred to as **categorical scales** because numbers are used simply as labels for categories (McDowell 2006). Nominal scales can be used for any information that contains mutually exclusive categories. Numbers are assigned to nominal scales to either aid data entry, for example, when medical and therapy records are entered onto a computer database, or to aid analysis for research. In the research literature, you may see the terms *categorical data* or *nominal data* used. Stevens (1946, cited in Crocker and Algina 1986) described a nominal scale as a scale in which:

- numbers are used purely as labels for the elements in the data system;
- numbers assigned to a nominal scale do *not* have meaningful mathematical qualities; this means numerical scores do not have the properties of meaningful order within the scale, items within the scale do not have equal distances between them, and there is no fixed origin or zero point;
- any set of numbers may be used;

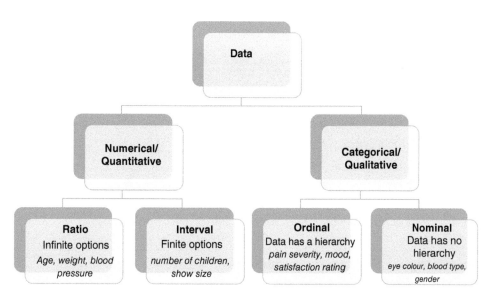

FIGURE 4.1   Levels of measurement data.

- each unique object or response in the data system must be assigned a different number; and
- any other set of numbers could be substituted as long as one-to-one correspondence between members of the sets is maintained; this is called isomorphic transformation.

Nominal level information provides us with some descriptive information, but has no hierarchical value (Lewis and Bottomley 1994). In a nominal scale, numbers are assigned to mutually exclusive categories (Fisher and Marshall 2009). Numbers used in a nominal scale are not meaningful in a quantitative sense and do not have any meaning except in the context in which they are being used (Kielhofner and Coster 2006). There are no 'less than' or 'greater than' relations among nominal scores, and operations such as addition or subtraction are not possible. Nominal scales are useful if the frequencies or proportions of a particular characteristic within a sample need to be recorded. The scores indicate that qualitative differences between categories exist, and the scores serve as shorthand labels. This can be useful when entering information into a database. When data is collected using a nominal scale, non-parametric statistical techniques (e.g. chi square) are used if statistical analysis is needed (Scott and Mazhindu 2014).

Healthcare Example of a Nominal Scale

The International Classifications of Disease (ICD) produced by the World Health Organization (WHO) uses numbers as a code for classification of health disorders and to aid reliability of diagnosis. The ICD system of nominal labels uses a numeric or alphanumeric code that represents a clinical description and diagnostic guideline for a wide range of disorders for clinical, educational, research, or service use worldwide. For example, the ICD-10 Classification of Mental and Behavioural Disorders (WHO 1993) uses an alphanumeric code involving a single letter followed by two numbers at the three-character level; for example, F00 is used to label Dementia, F00.0 = Dementia in Alzheimer's Disease with early onset, F00.1 = Dementia in Alzheimer's Disease with late onset, and F06.0 = organic hallucinations. ICD-9 uses numeric codes ranging only from 000 to 999.

Examples of Nominal Scales Used by AHPs

Some scales used in AHP assessments are nominal scales. Nominal scores can be applied to categories such as diagnosis, type of living accommodation, equipment provided, and discharge destination. For example, discharge destination of service users might be recorded as follows:

1 = discharged to own home

2 = discharged to a relative/friend's home

3 = discharged to an intermediate care setting for further rehabilitation

4 = discharged to long-term residential care

5 = discharged to long-term nursing home care

6 = transferred to another unit/ward

7 = died while undergoing treatment/during admission

ORDINAL SCALES

An ordinal scale can be applied when data contains information that has relative magnitude or a rank order (first, second, third, etc.). Numbers are allocated depending on the ordering of the property assessed, from *more to less* or *first to last,* and so they have real meaning beyond being used simply as labels. This means that the numbers allocated reflect the ascending order of the characteristic being measured (McDowell 2006). Numbers indicating position in a series or order are called ordinals. The ordinal numbers are first (1st), second (2nd), third (3rd), and so on. Variables measured using an ordinal scale are called ordinal variables or rank variables. Stevens (1946, cited in Crocker and Algina 1986) described an ordinal scale as a scale in which:

- the elements in the scale can be ordered on the amount of the property being measured;
- the scaling rule requires that values from the real number system must be assigned in the same order; and
- scores may be converted to other values, as long as the original information about the rank order is preserved; this is called monotonic transformation.

So, like a nominal scale, an ordinal scale does *not* have the properties of equal distance between units nor a fixed origin.

An ordinal scale is used to rank the order of the scores assigned to the characteristics being measured. The numbers represent values relative to each other (Lewis and Bottomley 1994). The order of scores indicates that the parameter being measured is either greater (better) or less (worse) than the other scores, but the AHP cannot make inferences about the magnitude of the difference between scores (McDowell 2006; Scott and Mazhindu 2014). Non-parametric techniques are used if statistical analysis of ordinal level data is needed. The Wilcoxon or Mann–Whitney U test is used if groups are being compared. To examine hypotheses, correlation coefficients (such as Spearman or Kendall rank correlations) are used.

Examples of Ordinal Scales Used by AHPs

Many assessments used by AHPs are based on ordinal scales. Fisher (1993) states that 'virtually all functional assessments, even timed tests, yield ordinal raw scores' (p. 322). Lewis and Bottomley (1994) explain that ordinal level information is provided by scales indicating a continuum, such as stronger to weaker or faster to slower. A frequently used example of an ordinal scale is where scores are assigned to describe levels of independence or amount of assistance required to complete an activity:

1 = independent
2 = needs verbal prompting
3 = needs physical assistance
4 = dependent and unable to perform activity.

Another example is the assessment of severity of a symptom (Hunter 1997), for example:

1 = none
2 = mild

3 = moderate

4 = marked

5 = severe.

Ordinal scales are also used for the measurement of pain and pain relief (Turk and Melzack 2011), for example:

4 = complete relief

3 = good relief

2 = moderate relief

1 = slight relief

0 = no relief.

Likert scales (numerical rating scales) are also used frequently for the measurement of pain. These are often given as a 100 mm line and give 7 or 11 points along the line to choose on a continuum which is defined at the two ends, for example, between least possible pain to worst possible pain or no relief of pain to complete relief of pain (Turk and Melzack 2011).

AHPs should be aware that some ordinal rating scales are open to a considerable degree of subjectivity. People use the same adjectives, such as 'frequently', in different ways. This means that AHPs should not assume that what frequently means to one client or carer or colleague is the same for all the people who may be using that assessment. This means that the term *frequently* cannot indicate the same frequency for the occurrence of a symptom or behaviour of interest to the AHP (McDowell 2006). Fisher (2003) warns that:

> *There is a general misconception that scales which describe a client's ADL task performance in terms of level of independence are objective ... in actual practice, any rating scale that relies on professional judgement of a client's ADL performance is subjective. While the use of scales that reflect a client's level of independence is common and widely accepted as 'objective', it is likely that we have confused familiarity and common usage with objectivity.*
>
> (p. 136)

The issue of subjectivity is illustrated by the common assessment of the level of assistance required for ADL. For example, when assessing the level of independence a person demonstrates for transfers and mobility, the level of assistance might be rated in terms of the type of assistance required, such as

1. a 3-point scale: standby, verbal prompts, physical assistance),
2. the level of assistance needed (e.g. 3-point scale: minimal, moderate, maximum), or
3. the amount of assistance (e.g. given as a percentage: 10% of the time, 25% of the time, 50% of the time).

Subjectivity can impact the assessment as different AHPs may have varying judgements as to what behaviour represents each definition of assistance, for example, rating minimum versus moderate assistance. Evidence of strong inter-rater reliability is, therefore, particularly important when using assessments with these types of scales.

INTERVAL SCALES

An interval scale is the level where the scale is truly quantitative (as opposed to numbers being used as codes to categorise qualitative data). From a purist point of view, this is the level of data at which measurements can be taken. Wright and Linacre (1989), for example, argue that measurements must be taken at least at an interval level, whereas observational assessments produce ordinal level data. The interval level of measurement goes beyond either nominal or ordinal scaling as interval scores are classified by both order and by a known and equal interval between points (McDowell 2006). Stevens (1946, cited in Crocker and Algina 1986) described an interval scale as follows:

- An interval scale has rank order, and the distances between the numbers have meaning with respect to the property being measured.
- If two scores at the low end of an interval scale are one unit apart, then two scores at the high end are also one unit apart, and the difference between these two high scores and two low scores represents the same amount of the property.
- Transformation of values in an interval scale is restricted and must contain the information in the values of the original scale.

An interval scale describes, provides a hierarchy, and ascribes a numerical difference (Lewis and Bottomley 1994). Interval scales have a constant, common unit of measurement, and the gap, or 'interval', between each position on the scale is kept the same. However, the units of measurement and the zero point on an interval scale are arbitrary (Scott and Mazhindu 2014). Statistical analysis of data collected using interval scales can be undertaken with parametric statistics, including mean, standard deviation, and Pearson correlation coefficients. Statistical tests of significance, such as the t-test, can be used if the data are normally distributed (Scott and Mazhindu 2014).

In rehabilitation, some AHPs have tried to convert ordinal scales to interval scales by weighting the value attached to particular scores. McDowell (2006) describes the 'equal-appearing interval' scaling method, which is used by some test developers:

... a sample of people is asked to judge the relative severity of each response category ... Items such as 'Pain prevents me from sleeping', 'I have aches and pains that bother me', and 'I require prescription medicines to control my pain' are sorted by each judge into rank-ordered categories of severity ... This scaling approach has been used in instruments such as the Sickness Impact Profile.

(p. 20)

The Sickness Impact Profile (SIP; Bergner et al. 1981) was developed to assess perceived health status to provide a descriptive measure of changes in a person's behaviour that have resulted owing to sickness. The test developers wanted to provide a measure that could be used with a broad population of people experiencing a wide range of illnesses of varying degrees of severity. The SIP has a number of purposes including evaluating a patient's progress and measuring outcomes of healthcare to inform service planning and policy development (for a critique of SIP, see McDowell 2006).

RATIO SCALES

A **ratio scale** is also a truly quantitative scale; it has a constant unit of measurement, a uniform interval between points on the scale, and a true zero at its origin (Scott and Mazhindu 2014). Stevens (1946, cited in Crocker and Algina 1986) described a ratio scale as follows:

- A ratio scale has the properties of order, equal distance between units, and a fixed origin or absolute zero point.
- Once the location of the absolute zero is known, non-zero measurements can be expressed as ratios of one another.
- Transformation of values is very restricted.
- Parametric statistics can be used to analyse ratio scales.

Examples of Ratio Scales Used by AHPs

When evaluating a therapy service, many measures used in health economics, such as cost per case, are ratio scales. Lewis and Bottomley (1994) also give the examples of timed scores and goniometric measurements. In physiotherapy, speed (measured as distance over time) is a useful ratio scale. An example of a ratio scale used by AHPs is joint range of movement assessment using a goniometer. A goniometer has a scale from 0° to 180° with zero indicating a total absence of movement around the joint. As a ratio scale can be used to provide a quantitative measure of change, meaningful comparisons can be made between people, and between individual measurements taken over time, using measurement tools like a goniometer. For example, if a person improves from 40° to 80° of shoulder movement, he can be said to have twice as much movement at the shoulder joint than before. Recently, this approach has developed with smartphone digital technology and electronic applications (Mitchell et al. 2014). Grip strength can also be measured using a ratio scale.

McDowell (2006) describe a method called **magnitude estimation**, which is used by some test developers to produce a ratio scale estimate: 'a more sophisticated approach to scaling statements about health ... has people judge the relative severity implied by each statement on scales with no limits placed on the values' (p. 19). With the equal-appearing interval scaling method (described earlier in the section on interval scales), the raters sort verbal descriptions of the construct or behaviour being measured into a defined number of categories. There have been objections to category scaling, derived from this application of a fixed number of categories, because it is thought that people are able to make more refined and accurate judgements of relative magnitude than the fixed categories method permits. An example of a test that has been developed following magnitude estimation procedures is the Pain Perception Profile (Tursky et al. 1982). For a description and critique of the Pain Perception Profile, see McDowell (2006).

APPLICATION OF DIFFERENT LEVELS OF MEASUREMENT – ISSUES TO CONSIDER

The four levels of measurement are in a hierarchy of sophistication (see Figure 4.1), with nominal scales being the least sophisticated and ratio scales being the most sophisticated level of measurement. In this order, the scale above contains the properties of the scale below; i.e. values meeting the requirements of a ratio scale may be regarded as meeting the requirements for an interval scale, and data collected on an interval scale may be regarded as providing ordinal level information. To summarise, nominal measurement shows difference in type, ordinal in rank, and interval or ratio in amount.

The first three levels of measurement are used to measure abilities, attitudes, or intelligence (Salkind 2017). Most variables can only be measured at one of the four levels of measurement. However, some common types of scales, such as Likert scales, can be found in the literature as examples of both ordinal and interval scales (Norman 2010). In our opinion, in the majority of cases the construct measured by AHPs using Likert scales do not have equal intervals between properties and should be treated as ordinal scales. This is particularly important when conducting clinical research, as different statistical analyses can be applied to interval scales which are not appropriate for ordinal scales (Norman 2010). When you are in doubt about the level of measurement being used, it is wise to assume the lower level of measurement until you have sought clarification.

Another debate with Likert-type scales centres around how many points the scale should have to achieve the best levels of sensitivity and reliability. There is no one best solution, and factors such as the age of the client group need to be taken into consideration. For example, Sturgess et al. (2002) found that three categories/scale points were most frequently used on self-report scales designed for young children. They acknowledge that statistical analysis of 3-point scales cannot produce the same power as 5-, 7-, or 10-point scales and that 3-point scales are less likely to be sensitive to small clinical changes. However, test developers for paediatric populations have found that young children can only discriminate between a few responses, making 3-point scales more reliable in children whose cognitive functioning is predominately at the level of dichotomous thought; therefore, if you are seeking a measure for a children's service, you may decide to compromise statistical power and responsiveness for reliability.

It is very important that AHPs should not handle scores in a manner that is inconsistent with the level of measurement used. This is a particular problem with ordinal scales. The values of numbers used in an ordinal scale and the numerical distance between each point in an ordinal scale have no intrinsic meaning. Therefore, a change between scale points at one level in the scale (such as from 1 to 2) is not necessarily equivalent to a change between other neighbouring scale points (such as from 5 to 6, or from 8 to 9) elsewhere in the scale. McDowell (2006) makes it clear that mathematical calculations using such scores cannot be meaningfully undertaken and should be used with caution. Fisher (1993) agrees that summing of ordinal scores to provide a total score 'does not result in a number that is a valid means of making quantitative comparisons of performances, whether it be between two different persons or the same person on different occasions' (p. 319). So, summed ordinal scores just result in numerical values that are 'assigned to qualitative differences in ability' (p. 319). Despite these limitations, a significant number of AHP assessments are based on ordinal level data and sum item or sub-scale scores to provide an overall score. The Barthel Index (BI; Mahoney and Barthel 1965) is a well-known measure that has an ordinal level scale and that requires the addition of scores to provide a total score from the test items. Summing scores is possible with interval level scales where the unit of measurement between each scale items in known and equal. However, summing scores is dubious because independence in one activity, such as in making a cup of tea, does not imply the same level of function as independence in another activity, such as cooking a meal. McAvoy (1991) states that one reason why AHPs may not use existing standardised assessments is that AHPs find 'a global score is difficult to interpret. For example, a patient may achieve a "totally independent" score, that is, 100 with the BI, but still be unable to live independently at home because, for example, he/she is unable to cook for himself or is unsafe or unsteady, or independence may not be the ideal aim where energy conservation or safety are important' (p. 385). Several other authors (for example, Hogan and Orme 2000) have argued against the use of the BI because the total score has no real meaning and the same total score does not carry the same meaning for all people with that particular score. In addition, two people might show equal increases in their total scores when re-tested following treatment, but their specific gains in functional status might be very different. Bouwstra et al. (2019) have shown that the structural validity, reliability, and interpretability of the BI are considered sufficient for measuring and interpreting changes.

Another practice to avoid when implementing an ordinal level scale is presuming that an increase in function indicated by moving from needing verbal prompting (score 2) to being independent (score 1) equals the same amount of change as moving from dependence (score 4) to physical assistance (score 3). The presumption of equal change occurring between two scores can be made only when using interval or ratio level scales.

Addition and subtraction is permissible at the top two levels of measurement (interval and ratio scales) because the unit of change between each item in the scale remains constant across the whole scale. With this level of measurement, it is possible to calculate differences in scores and to calculate averages. Because a ratio scale has a zero point, it is only at this highest level of measurement that you can calculate how many times greater one score is compared to another score (McDowell 2006).

AHPs need to identify the level of measurement used when critiquing a potential measure for use in their service or when reading journal articles describing research to explore the psychometric properties of potential therapy assessments. For example, in a study examining the responsiveness to change of the Rivermead Mobility Index (RMI) and the BI the authors (Wright et al. 1998) explore the pros and cons of different statistical procedures for calculating responsiveness to change related to the level of measurement used in the two tests:

> *Disadvantages of using effect sizes to estimate the responsiveness of ordinal scales like the RMI and BI are that they assume that each successive point on the score represents an equal amount of change (which is not strictly the case for the BI and RMI) and that the data are normally distributed (referred to as parametric assumptions) ... to overcome these difficulties both parametric and non-parametric methods of calculations were used.*
>
> (p. 217)

AHPs need to be discerning readers when critiquing a research article and deciding whether the results reported should lead to changes in clinical practice.

When an AHP undertakes assessments, they do not want to bore clients by presenting them with lots of very easy items nor discourage them by forcing them to attempt test items that are too demanding. (Note: The influence of the demands of the assessment task has already been discussed in Chapter 1.) Some assessments do provide scales where the level of difficulty of a task is taken into account and provide a hierarchy that represents level of difficulty/demand, for example, the Assessment of Motor Process Skills (AMPS; Fisher 2003). Two methods have been applied to therapy and health measures to provide these types of scales. The first method is Guttman scaling and the second is Rasch analysis. For further information, please see Chapter 14.

Reflecting on Levels of Measurement.

Level of measurement	What level of measurement is provided by each of the assessments (standardised and un-standardised) that you are using in your clinical practice? List the tests/assessment methods for each level:	Are you using data in an appropriate way for the level of measurement? Identify any issues or limitations in current assessment practice:	List potential assessments that you could use to collect data at this level of measurement. This is particularly important if the majority of your assessment data is collected at the lower nominal and ordinal levels:
Nominal			
Ordinal			
Interval			
Ratio			

APPLYING CONCEPTS OF LEVELS OF MEASUREMENT TO YOUR OWN PRACTICE

At the end of this and other chapters, you will find templates for a series of worksheets designed to assist you in applying the principles of assessment and outcome measurement to your own practice.

Please now turn to **Worksheet 4.1: Reflecting on Levels of Measurement** found on p. 143. The first column of this worksheet lists the four levels of measurement (nominal, ordinal, interval, and ratio). In the second column, you are asked to consider the level of measurement that is provided by each of the assessments (standardised and un-standardised) that you are using in your practice or which you have observed being used by AHPs while on placement. List the tests/ assessment methods you identify in the row for that level of measurement. The third column is used to reflect on whether you are using data in an appropriate way for the level of measurement. Look at the way scores are used, and identify any issues or limitations in current assessment practice. In the last column, you are encouraged to list potential assessments that you could use to collect data at the different levels of measurement. This is particularly important if the majority of your assessment data is collected at the lower nominal and ordinal levels.

REVIEW QUESTIONS

4.1   Describe the similarities and differences between nominal and ordinal scales.

4.2   What property does a ratio scale have that is not present in the other three types of scale?

4.3   Define an interval scale.

You will find brief answers to these questions at the back of this book on p. 445.

REFERENCES

Bergner, M., Bobbitt, R.A., Carter, W.B., and Gilson, B.S. (1981). The sickness impact profile: development and final revision of a health status measure. *Medical Care*: 787–805. http://www.jstor.org/stable/3764241.

Bouwstra, H., Smit, E.B., Wattel, E.M. et al. (2019). Measurement properties of the Barthel Index in geriatric rehabilitation. *Journal of the American Medical Directors Association* 20 (4): 420–425. https://doi.org/10.1016/j.jamda.2018.09.033.

Bowling, A. and Ebrahim, S. (2005). *Handbook of Health Research Methods: Investigation, Measurement and Analysis*. McGraw-Hill Education (UK) https://pdfs.semanticscholar.org/783f/b94571f0529c6c2a17b25e75270ca722a6a0.pdf.

Carman, C.A. (2012). Levels of measurement. In: *Encyclopedia of Research Design* (eds. J. Neil and N.J. Salkind), 709–712. Thousand Oaks: SAGE Publications, Inc. https://doi.org/10.4135/9781412961288.

Crocker, L. and Algina, J. (1986). *Introduction to Classical and Modern Test Theory*. Orlando, FL: Holt, Rinehart and Winston.

Eva, G. and Paley, J. (2004). Numbers in evidence. *British Journal of Occupational Therapy* 67 (1): 47–49. https://doi.org/10.1177/030802260406700107.

Fisher, A.G. (1993). The assessment of IADL motor skills: an application of many-faceted Rasch analysis. *American Journal of Occupational Therapy* 47 (4): 319–329. https://doi.org/10.5014/ajot.47.4.319.

Fisher, A. (2003). *AMPS Assessment of Motor and Process Skills*. Colorado: Fort Collins.

Fisher, M.J. and Marshall, A.P. (2009). Understanding descriptive statistics. *Australian Critical Care* 22 (2): 93–97. https://doi.org/10.1016/j.aucc.2008.11.003.

Gershkoff, A.R. (2011). Level of measurement. In: *Encyclopedia of Survey Research Methods* (ed. P.J. Lavrakas), 422–423. Thousand Oaks: Sage Publications, Inc. Print ISBN: 9781412918084 Online ISBN: 9781412963947. doi:https://doi.org/10.4135/9781412963947.

Hogan, K. and Orme, S. (2000). Measuring disability: a critical analysis of the Barthel Index. *British Journal of Therapy and Rehabilitation* 7 (4) https://doi.org/10.12968/bjtr.2000.7.4.13885.

Hunter, J. (1997). Outcome, indices and measurements. In: *Rehabilitation of the Physically Disabled Adult* (eds. C.J. Goodwill, J. Goodwill, M.A. Chamberlain and C. Evans). Nelson Thornes.

Kielhofner, G. and Coster, W.J. (2006). *Developing and Evaluating Quantitative Data Collection Instruments*. Philadelphia: FA Davis.

Lewis, C.B. and Bottomley, J.M. (1994). *Geriatric Physical Therapy: A Clinical Approach*. Prentice Hall.

Mahoney, F.I. and Barthel, D.W. (1965). Functional evaluation: the Barthel Index: a simple index of independence useful in scoring improvement in the rehabilitation of the chronically ill. *Maryland State Medical Journal* 14: 61–65. https://psycnet.apa.org/record/2012-30334-001.

McAvoy, E. (1991). The use of ADL indices by occupational therapists. *British Journal of Occupational Therapy* 54 (10): 383–385. https://doi.org/10.1177/030802269105401009.

McDowell, I. (2006). *Measuring Health: A Guide to Rating Scales and Questionnaires*. USA: Oxford University Press.

Mitchell, K., Gutierrez, S.B., Sutton, S. et al. (2014). Reliability and validity of goniometric iPhone applications for the assessment of active shoulder external rotation. *Physiotherapy Theory and Practice* 30 (7): 521–525. https://doi.org/10.3109/09593985.2014.900593.

Norman, G. (2010). Likert scales, levels of measurement and the "laws" of statistics. *Advances in Health Sciences Education* 15 (5): 625–632. https://link.springer.com/article/10.1007/s10459-010-9222-y.

Ratcliffe, S. (ed.) (2016). *Oxford Essential Quotations*. Oxford: Oxford University Press.

Salkind, N.J. (2017). *Tests & Measurement for People Who (Think they) Hate Tests & Measurement*. Sage Publications.

Sarle, W.S. (1997). Measurement theory: Frequently asked questions. *Disseminations of the International Statistical Applications Institute* 1 (4): 61–66. http://www.medicine.mcgill.ca/epidemiology/courses/EPIB654/Summer2010/EF/measurement%20scales.pdf accessed 31.10.19.

Stevens, S.S. (1946). On the theory of scales of measurement. *Science*, New Series 103 (2684): 677–680.

Sturgess, J., Rodger, S., and Ozanne, A. (2002). A review of the use of self-report assessment with young children. *British Journal of Occupational Therapy* 65 (3): 108–116. https://doi.org/10.1177/030802260206500302.

Turk, D.C. and Melzack, R. (eds.) (2011). *Handbook of Pain Assessment*. Guilford Press.

Tursky, B., Jamner, L.D., and Friedman, R. (1982). The pain perception profile: a psychophysical approach to the assessment of pain report. *Behavior Therapy* 13 (4): 376–394. https://doi.org/10.1016/S0005-7894(82)80002-6.

World Health Organization (1993). *The ICD-10 Classification of Mental and Behavioural Disorders: Diagnostic Criteria for Research*, vol. 2. World Health Organization.

Wright, B.D. and Linacre, J.M. (1989). Observations are always ordinal; measurements, however, must be interval. *Archives of Physical Medicine and Rehabilitation* 70 (12): 857–860. https://europepmc.org/article/med/2818162.

Wright, J., Cross, J., and Lamb, S. (1998). Physiotherapy outcome measures for rehabilitation of elderly people: responsiveness to change of the Rivermead Mobility Index and Barthel Index. *Physiotherapy* 84 (5): 216–221. https://doi.org/10.1016/S0031-9406(05)65552-6.

CHAPTER 5

Test Administration, Reporting, and Recording

OVERVIEW

This chapter will consider factors to ensure the most efficient and effective assessment process, such as:

- building rapport,
- constructing your test environment, and
- communicating the results of the assessment.

We will discuss the importance of obtaining informed consent from clients prior to undertaking an assessment. The importance of following standardised procedures and of recording and reporting test results is explored. Suggested content for a report format for standardised test administration is described. The chapter concludes with an example report for a standardised test administration. There are eight steps in a rigorous test administration process; we provide information on some of these steps and direct you to other chapters in this book pertinent to the process. The chapter ends with a case study example.

QUESTIONS TO CONSIDER

1. How do I prepare for an efficient and effective test administration?
2. How do I build rapport with my client?
3. How do I ensure that my test administration remains standardised?
4. How do I communicate the results of my assessment?

TEST ADMINISTRATION

The eight steps in a rigorous test administration process are shown in Figure 5.1.

Principles of Assessment and Outcome Measurement for Allied Health Professionals:
Practice, Research and Development, Second Edition. Alison J. Laver-Fawcett and Diane L. Cox.
© 2021 John Wiley & Sons Ltd. Published 2021 by John Wiley & Sons Ltd.

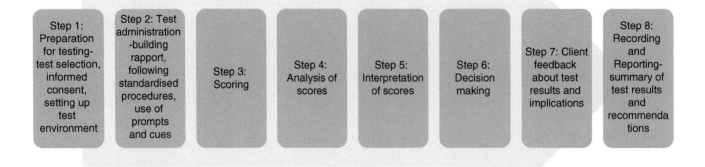

FIGURE 5.1   Steps in the test administration process.

Step 1: Preparation for Testing

Informed Consent

Allied health professional (AHP) interventions are rarely as invasive or risky as many other medical procedures, such as general anaesthesia or drug treatments, but they can still be intrusive, stressful, and tiring. Before undertaking an assessment or treatment intervention, AHPs have to obtain consent and need to ensure that this consent is valid. Just because the person has signed a consent form does not guarantee that the consent is valid. To be valid, consent must be given voluntarily and in full understanding and agreement of the proposed assessment or intervention. Clients must be given sufficient information to enable them to make an informed decision. The person must be able to understand and weigh up the information provided. The person must be given the space to act under his own free will (Data Protection Act 2018). The AHP needs to be aware if consent is being given reluctantly, especially if this is under the strong influence of another person, whether that other person is a professional or a relative. Consent can be given either verbally, non-verbally, or in writing. Consent forms are used by some services (although generally written consent forms are used for more invasive procedures, such as general anaesthesia). AHPs should be aware that the person can withdraw consent at any time, even after signing a consent form. Before embarking on an assessment process and/or a specific test administration, you should take time to give the person details of the proposed assessment/measurement and to answer any questions the client may have. To gain informed consent this discussion should cover:

- The purpose of the proposed assessment/standardised test/measurement.
- A description of how the assessment results will be used; especially talk about how any decisions or treatment plans will be guided by the results. Some assessments lead to decisions that have a very profound effect on the person's future life; for example, results may to lead to a decision that the person requires long-term care or a decision that the person is no longer competent to drive.

- Details as to who will be given access to the results of the assessment/test/ measurement and what form the results will take. For example:
  - 'a copy of the test form will be placed in your medical notes and will be seen by the doctors, nurses, and AHPs involved in your care' or
  - 'a letter summarising the results will be sent to your GP'.
- A description of what will be involved, for example, an interview, observations, and tasks to undertake. Especially mention if the person will be required to remove clothing. If the person will be required to undress, a chaperone should be offered.
- Explain who will be involved in the assessment: the AHP and client, or whether the AHP planning to interview/survey the person's spouse, children, other healthcare professionals or social care providers, or a child's teacher.
- Tell the client where the assessment/test/measure will be undertaken. For example:
  - 'we will need to go down to the AHP department' or
  - 'I will come to assess you at home' or 'we will observe your son at school in his classroom'.
- Estimate how long the assessment/test/measure should take. For example:
  - 'it usually takes about 30 minutes to complete the tasks involved'.
- If it is going to be a lengthy assessment, let the person know that he can ask for a break if he starts to feel fatigued.
- Sometimes, photographs and videos are taken as part of the assessment; this can be useful to monitor change over time and to demonstrate progress to the client. If photographs or video is to be taken, then make sure to explain the purpose and proposed use of these to the person and gain consent to use this media as part of the assessment.

Your clients should be given the opportunity to ask more questions about any proposed assessment and also be given more time to make the decision if they appear uncertain. The client may choose to agree to part but not all of the proposed assessment. For example: he may agree to be interviewed but not want to undertake standardised tests; he may be happy to be assessed on the ward or in the AHP department but not want a home assessment; or he may not want you to interview a particular family member. Under these circumstances, you undertake the best assessment you can within the parameters agreed to by the client. If you use an assessment pathway in your service, you should document that the pathway was not followed completely in respect of the client's wishes and detail the parts of the pathway for which consent was not granted.

You may decide to develop a consent form for your AHP service. This may seek to gain consent to administer a specific outcome measure, or could seek consent to undertake a more generic assessment process. For example, a consent form for a joint AHP service for children with physical disability might state the following:

AHP assessments provide information used to assist in the determination of the need for services and in the planning of intervention and the monitoring of progress. The assessment of your child may include any or all of the following elements:

- use of standardised assessment tools (these are published and validated tests);
- a structured physical examination including measurements of joint range of movement, balance, gait, and mobility and

- other manual activities requiring that the AHP touch the child and in some cases requiring the child to remove some items of clothing;

- observation of the child doing everyday activities at home or at school (such as getting dressed, playing, preparing a snack, eating lunch, doing school work); interviews with the child, parents, family members, and/or school staff;

- examination of the child's equipment or equipment needs (special items such as wheelchairs, walkers, adapted desks, etc.);

- photographs and videotape may be taken as part of the assessment (for example, to set a baseline and then monitor improvements in gait and mobility, or to monitor a contracture during a course of splinting)

Results of the assessments will be recorded in the child's AHP notes, and a summary report will be sent to the referring doctor.

Once consent has been given, you should document this. If written consent has been obtained, include a copy of the consent form in the person's notes. If verbal or non-verbal consent is granted, then document that you have explained the reason for the assessment and described the procedure to be followed and that you have obtained consent. Also, note that the person was given the opportunity to ask questions about the proposed assessment. Remember to sign and date your entry.

There are a few situations when informed consent cannot be sought or is not sought from the person. The AHP might be part of a multidisciplinary team assessment of an inpatient detained under the Mental Health Act (1983, 2007), or the person may not possess the cognitive capacity to understand what is proposed and make an informed decision as to whether or not to agree to the assessment. See the section on capacity assessment in Chapter 3.

The AHP will need to judge whether the client has the capacity to consent to the proposed AHP assessment and intervention. The Mental Capacity Act (Act 2005) is designed to protect and empower people aged 16 and over who may lack the mental capacity to make their own decisions about their care and treatment. Adults are assumed to be competent unless demonstrated otherwise. For example, cognitive capacity might be reduced following a stroke, head injury, or with the onset of dementia. If you have doubts about a person's competence to give consent, then ask yourself *'can this person understand and weigh up all the information required to make this decision?'*

If cognitive capacity might be an issue, the AHP should consult with medical colleagues, and a formal evaluation of capacity may need to be made before the proposed assessment can proceed. Cognitive capacity is not a clear-cut issue; a person may be competent to make some decisions, such as whether to talk to a AHP or allow the AHP to observe him prepare a meal, but not others, such as whether to have an internal investigation involving general anaesthesia and potential risk for a negative outcome. The more complex the decision and the greater potential for negative outcomes, the greater the degree of cognitive competency required for informed decision making. Where a person no longer has the cognitive capacity to provide informed consent, the AHP should check whether the person has made a statement of Advanced Wishes, or a Living Will, or an advanced refusal for a particular intervention (Tamayo-Velazquez et al. 2010). Where this is available, it should be used to judge whether the person would have wanted the proposed assessment or intervention. No one can give consent on behalf of an individual who has been assessed as incompetent to consent, but family members may have useful information about the person's advanced wishes that can assist in making a decision in the person's best interest. Best interests refer to the person's wishes and beliefs when he was still cognitively competent related to his well-being, his medical state, and his spiritual and religious beliefs.

If a person feels unable to make a decision about consent, or feels unhappy about an assessment being undertaken without him fully understanding what was involved, then the Patient Advocacy and Liaison Service (*PALS*) may be of support. The person might also be put in touch with an advocate; for example, some voluntary agencies provide advocacy for people with specific conditions, and some areas have local advocacy services. The Department of Health and Social Care (2009) has produced guidelines on consent, which is available on the UK government website at https://www.gov.uk/government/publications/reference-guide-to-consent-for-examination-or-treatment-second-edition.

It is very important to remember that obtaining consent is rarely a one-off process, particularly if you will be working with the client over a period of time. Each time you undertake a new assessment or intervention you should fully explain what you propose to do and gain consent for that specific assessment/intervention. It is good practice when undertaking a re-assessment to remind the person of the rationale for the original and follow-up assessment, and to check that the person still consents to this assessment.

Test Selection

Advice on how to select the best test(s) for your client and service is provided in Chapter 12.

Organising the Environment

The environment and conditions required for an optimum assessment will depend on the purpose of the assessment, the person, and the nature of any presenting problems. In Chapter 1, in the section titled 'The Influence of Environment upon Performance', we discussed how familiarity with an environment might influence assessment results. People will usually behave differently in a familiar environment, such as their home, workplace, or school, than in an unfamiliar AHP department, ward, or day hospital setting. However, assessment in a familiar environment is not always possible or necessary.

Wherever the assessment is to be undertaken, the AHP should ensure the basics are addressed:

- The room is accessible to the client and any carer who may also be attending the assessment, e.g. lift if not on the ground floor, doorways wide enough for wheelchair or walking aids, clearly sign-posted (especially if it is in a large district hospital).
- The room is free from hazards, such as a slippery floor, loose mats, toxic substances, or potentially dangerous equipment.
- There is sufficient room for the person to move around to the degree required for the assessment.
- Any furniture or large equipment to be used is appropriate (e.g. the correct height or adjustable height chair, table, bed, commode, frame).

- There is good lighting; this is particularly important if the person has any visual impairment and/or the task has a visual component such as reading, writing, drawing, or construction.
- The room is a comfortable temperature for the nature of the assessment; it will need to be warmer if the person has to undress for a physical assessment.
- You have taken steps to limit interruptions; for example, you put an *'Assessment in progress – please do not interrupt', 'Quiet please testing in progress'* type notice on the door, have turned your mobile phone off or to silent or turned the phone to answer-phone and the ringer volume down.
- You have ensured the required level of privacy, for example, curtains pulled round a cubicle or bed provide visual privacy, but the person can still be heard by others outside the curtain.
- If a parent or carer is to be present, ensure there is sufficient space and a suitable chair for them to sit on.

If the person has any hearing loss or the assessment requires a significant degree of concentration, then background noise levels should be considered and limited. Remember to check whether the person usually wears a hearing aid, and if so ensure that it is with them and in good working order and switched on. If the person has any visual impairment, the AHP will need to check whether visual aids (contact lenses, glasses, magnifying glass) are used, and ensure that these are clean and being worn. The assessment setting should have good lighting, and the AHP should check there is no glare. For example, a shiny, white table top might reflect a long strip light, and the glare could impede the person's ability to read instructions, fill out a survey, or see test materials. Also, be aware of the impact of colour uniformity versus colour contrast; for example, a white paper on a white table top may be difficult for the person to see. In a home setting, check what lighting the person would normally have on during the task to be observed and assess first with this level of lighting; and then if necessary increase the lighting and see if this has an impact on function.

Preparing Tools, Materials, and Equipment

It is important to be well organised ahead of any assessment. Allow time for setting up, not just for organising the environment but for ensuring you have the required tools, materials, and/or equipment for the assessment. This means you will be organised and professional, and it will save unnecessary time wasting during the assessment:

- Do you need a checklist, test form, blank/lined paper?
- If it is a standardised test, do you have the instructions and/or questions?
- Do you have pens/pencils, etc. for you and if relevant for the client – are these working/sharp?
- Do you need a stopwatch or calculator; if so, is the battery working?
- If you are administering a battery of tests, are all the component parts present and in their correct bags/places?
- Do you need ingredients for a cooking assessment?
- If you are assessing the suitability of an aid, do you have the right one or a range of models to try out?

Timing Your Assessment

Think about the optimum time for conducting your assessment, and try to schedule the assessment accordingly. The optimum time will mostly be when the person is able to perform at his best. However, sometimes you may need to evaluate what the person can manage when their performance is at its most compromised, for example, when they are fatigued at the end of the day or when the effects of medication are wearing off just before the next dose is taken. You may need this information to judge the level of risk or the maximum level of care the person will need. If you are not able to conduct the assessment at the optimum time for the purpose of the assessment, be aware of how a different timing could impact the results, and remember to take this into account and document any impacts. When thinking about optimum timing, consider the following factors:

- Does the person's function fluctuate because of medication?
- Is the person more agitated at a particular time of day?
- Does the person fatigue easily, and if so, what will he be doing before the planned assessment?
- When is the environment you plan to use for the assessment available?
- When is it most free from interruptions and background noise?
- If a carer, parent, teacher, or other care provider is required for the assessment, when are they available?

Undertaking an assessment immediately following a large meal is not recommended due to changes in blood flow to the brain after a large meal (Liu et al. 2000), which is a particular issue for older patients.

Clarifying Expectations

It is important to be aware of your own expectations. To ensure the client's expectations are of the assessment are realistic, you must be very clear about the purpose, nature, and format of any planned assessment with the client, and if appropriate, the carer. If you have ensured that the person has sufficient information to provide informed consent for the proposed assessment or measurement, then you are likely to have ensured that the person's expectations about the purpose and nature of the assessment are realistic. Your expectations as to how long you will be able to conduct the assessment and what you will be able to undertake also need to be realistic, and these will depend on the person (age, diagnosis, anticipated impairments, and stamina) and the environment.

If you are changing work from one client group to another or from one service to another, your expectations about the timing, nature, or pacing of assessment will almost certainly need to adjust accordingly. This can take time and lead to some initial frustrations. When you are a visitor in a person's home, or at a child's school or client's workplace, you need to allow time for some informal conversation and be cognisant of the fact that you are the visitor. The person may want to give you a guided tour, and it may be their culture to serve you a drink or food before you can proceed with a more formal interview or assessment. You may arrive at the environment to discover that you do not have the furniture, equipment, or space to conduct the assessment as planned. AHPs have to be flexible and ingenious!

Step 2: Test Administration

Developing Rapport

Rapport is a critical ingredient to ensuring that your assessment process or test administration is effective and efficient. However, what exactly do we mean by rapport? Online dictionaries give several useful definitions. Rapport has been defined as:

- 'a good understanding of someone and an ability to communicate well with them' (https://dictionary.cambridge.org/dictionary/english/rapport)
- 'a relationship characterized by agreement, mutual understanding, or empathy that makes communication possible or easy' (https://www.merriam-webster.com/dictionary/rapport)
- 'a good sense of understanding and trust' (https://www.vocabulary.com/dictionary/rapport).

Rapport is very important to ensure a successful assessment. If the person is going to be required to share personal informal and feelings, then they are going to need to trust and respect the AHP. Test anxiety can have a big impact on test results and can be alleviated by a positive therapeutic relationship (Taylor et al. 2009). Therefore, it is important to think about the need for developing rapport and to plan strategies for how you will build rapport with the person, and if relevant the carer, both before and during an assessment.

Mosey (1981) identified the *conscious use of self as a key therapeutic tool:* 'conscious use of self involves a planned interaction with another person in order to alleviate fear or anxiety; provide reassurance; obtain necessary information; give advice; and assist the other individual to gain more appreciation, expression, and functional use of his or her latent inner resources' (p. 95). Developing a therapeutic relationship involves the conscious use of self to build and maintain rapport with the client.

An AHP can apply a number of techniques to facilitate building rapport; these include leading attention by matching, mirroring, or verbal and non-verbal behaviours. Many of these techniques are described in the literature on neuro-linguistic programming (*NLP*). For example, see Clabby and O'Connor's (2004) article on teaching medical students to use physical and verbal mirroring techniques from NLP for building rapport with patients:

- *Physical mirroring*: Physical mirroring requires the conscious and subtle use of body language to put a client at ease. It is important to differentiate between imitating and mirroring. Overt imitation might make a person feel mocked and can decrease rapport. Mirroring is much more subtle. It might involve using the same gesture or tilting your head in the same way as the client. If you are sitting opposite the client, you should echo the person's movements so that your position will look similar to the person's if he were looking in a mirror. For example, if the client crosses his right leg over his left, the AHP sitting opposite would cross their left leg over their right. The AHP should leave a little time (seconds to minutes) before mirroring the client's movements and should try to make her position and movements seem as natural as possible (Clabby and O'Connor 2004).
- *Eye contact:* The use of eye contact is very important to building rapport. The amount of eye contact the AHP should use will vary depending on what is culturally acceptable for the client. In general, maintaining eye contact is helpful for conveying that the AHP is actively listening to the client.

- *Verbal mirroring*: Verbal mirroring requires the conscious use of word selection, pace of communication, and tone of voice. With verbal mirroring, the AHP tries to echo the person's tone of voice and exactly repeats the person's last phrase or word. It can also be helpful to repeat the phase or word with a questioning inflexion (Clabby and O'Connor 2004), thus inviting the person to clarify that was what he meant or to elaborate on what was said. For example, an interview between a AHP and client might go:
  - **AHP**: *'Do you have any problems with getting dressed?'*
  - **Client**: *'No! I can get dressed just fine on my own!'*
  - **AHP**: *'Okay, you can get dressed fine on your own, can you bathe or shower on your own too?'*
  - **Client**: *'I can manage, but I'm a bit scared'*
  - **AHP**: *'You can manage, but you're a bit scared?'*
  - **Client**: *'Yes, I'm scared I'm going to slip and fall again'*
  - **AHP**: *'You're scared you are going to slip and fall again, what happened when you slipped and fell?'*
- *Matching Client's Pace of Speech*: In addition to mirroring the client's choice of words, mirroring the pace of a client's speech can also aid communication. If the client is speaking fast, with energy and animation, then the AHP should mirror this communication pace and style with quick, animated responses. However, if a client speaks slowly and quietly and leaves gaps between sentences, then the AHP should likewise speak slowly and softly and allow gaps between questions, phrases, or sentences.
- *Use of metaphors in building rapport*: People often speak in metaphors to describe their feelings and experiences. AHPs are becoming more aware of how the conscious exploration of metaphors can help build rapport and can facilitate an understanding of the person's perspective on his condition or problem (Landau et al. 2018; Lawley and Tompkins 2000). A metaphor is a direct comparison between two or more seemingly unrelated subjects. The metaphor is used because the person associates implicit and/or explicit attributes from the concept with the subject they are discussing.

Examples of Metaphors Include

'The pain is like someone is stabbing me repeatedly with a sharp knife'.

'I've got butterflies in my stomach'.

'There's a black cloud hanging over me'.

Clients especially use metaphors to explain feelings (such as pain, anxiety, depression, and grief) and experiences (such as discrimination, dependence, and loss). AHPs need to be attuned to the use of metaphors because they are not 'throw-away' comments. People often use leading phrases, such as 'You know it's like …'? The AHP should pay particular attention to the description the person puts in the '…', because this is the metaphor, and the choice of metaphor will have significant meaning for the client.

AHPs learn to *converse within the frame of the metaphor* (Lawley and Tompkins 2000). One technique used by AHPs to un-package metaphors are **Clean Language questions** (Rees and Ioan Manea 2016). Clean Language questions are simple questions that follow a particular syntax and delivery. The questions are used to prompt and encourage clients to use and explore metaphor to describe their symptoms and problems. James Lawley and Penny Tompkins, who developed the Metaphor Model in 1997 and related Clean Language questions after studying the work of David Grove, an AHP from New Zealand, have described Clean Language. Clean Language is applied to both validate the client's experience and facilitate the description and exploration of the person's symbolic ideas, which are normally outside the person's explicit everyday awareness. The aim of using Clean Language early in a therapeutic relationship is to allow an understanding of the client's problems and symptoms to emerge into the client's awareness by exploring *his* coding of *his* metaphor.

Tompkins and Lawley (1997) describe nine basic Clean Language questions, each of which has a specific purpose for helping the client to un-package and understand his use of metaphor further:

Two questions are used to request information about the metaphoric symbol's attributes:

1. And is there anything else about ...? e.g. 'Is there anything else about that sharp knife?'
2. *And what kind of ... is that ...?* e.g. 'And what kind of black cloud is that black cloud?', from which the AHP may obtain more information about how big, or dark, or constant that 'black cloud' feels to the client.

Two questions are used to ask for locational information:

3. *And where is ...?* e.g. 'And where is that black cloud hanging above you', which could help the client identify whether this 'black cloud' feels very oppressively just above his head or much further away up in the sky.
4. *And whereabouts?* e.g. 'And whereabouts are the butterflies in your stomach?', which may help the AHP to understand whether the person feels this 'butterflies' sensation in a very specific spot or more generalised over the centre of his body.

Two questions which reference the future (from the client's perceptual present):

5. *And what happens next?* e.g. 'And what happens next when you feel butterflies in your stomach?' might prompt the person to describe his feelings of mounting anxiety further: 'and then I start to feel the butterflies are fluttering up my throat and I think I'm going to be sick'.
6. *And then what happens?* e.g. 'And then what happens after the sharp knife repeatedly stabs you?' can help the AHP to understand whether the pain sensation continues, or how the person feels when it stops: 'It feels like I'm stabbed again and again for an eternity and I wait in agony for it to stop'

Two questions which reference the past:

7. *And what happens just before ...?* e.g. 'And what happens just before you get butterflies in your stomach?' can help the AHP understand what triggers the sensation.
8. *And where does/could ... come from?* e.g. 'And where does that black cloud come from?' could prompt a wide variety of responses: 'It comes down from the sky', 'It comes out of my head', 'It just appears out of nowhere'.

The last question offers the client the opportunity to make a lateral, and therefore metaphorical, shift in perception:

9. *And that's ... like what?* e.g. 'And that butterflies in the stomach is like what?' could lead to further descriptions of sensations ('it's like a gentle fluttering feeling', 'it's like lots of wings beating fast to get out') to the use of an alternative metaphor 'it's like lots of worms wriggling inside me'.

Note: The article *'Less is More ... The Art of Clean Language'* by Tompkins and Lawley (1997) article can be found at www.cleanlanguage.co.uk/articles/articles/109/1/Less-Is-More-The-Art-of-Clean-Language/Page1.html.

Source: Based on Tompkins and Lawley (1997).

Some of the techniques described above take considerable practice in order for them to become a refined and habitual part of the AHP's 'conscious use of self'. However, some very simple actions can also help to build rapport. For example, it can be useful to make a phone call to book an assessment yourself, as opposed to delegating this to a team secretary. Ten minutes spent popping up to see a person on the ward the day before you bring him down to the AHP department for an hour's worth of standardised testing can also be 10 minutes well spent. You can use this time to explain the proposed purpose, nature, and format of the assessment and obtain informed consent, and this more informal time can help to build rapport and trust between AHP and client. It can also be helpful to collect a person yourself, for example, from the ward or waiting area and use the time walking down the corridor or waiting for a lift to chat informally and put the person at ease.

Using Standardised Tests

Prior to using any new standardised test, AHPs should take enough time to 'be fully conversant with the test content, use, reliability, and validity before administering the test in order that this is done correctly and that any interpretation of test findings be accurate' (Jones 1991, p. 179). In addition to reading the test manual and examining the test materials and forms, it can be very helpful to role-play test administration with a colleague to familiarise oneself with the test materials and instructions before undertaking the test with a client.

Following Standardised Procedures

See Chapters 7 and 15 for more details and definitions on what is meant by a standardised test and the advantages of using standardised tools.

The use of standardised tests can facilitate objectivity, and this is very important because it is virtually impossible to obtain complete accuracy and objectivity when assessing human functioning. Any standardised assessment should have detailed instructions detailing how and when it should be administered and scored, and how to interpret scores. You should not consider modifying a test in any way unless you are prepared to go through validation and reliability studies again. This is very time consuming and should not be undertaken lightly (Pynsent 2004). Following standardised procedures means that you should:

- follow instructions exactly;
- repeat instructions to be given to the client word for word;

- use the standardised materials and forms provided; and
- follow precisely the instructions for the test environment, conditions, and equipment that should be used.

Use of Prompting and Cues

The majority of standardised tests have verbal and/or visual instructions. Some standardised tests permit the repetition of instructions, and allow the use of prompts and/or cues, but many do not. Most test protocols define and, therefore, impose limitations on the phrasing and repetition of instructions. Sometimes a person may not understand your standardised instruction. You need to have established in advance whether the repetition of instructions or the use of prompts and cues is permissible with that particular test.

Often, standardised instruction formats do not account for people with multisensory deficits. If instructions are not heard or seen correctly, then the purpose of the task can be misunderstood; the patient could fail the test item because of limited comprehension. In such cases, the individual could be considered to have a deficit in the area evaluated by the test item, and this could lead to unreliable test results. For example, the Rivermead Perceptual Assessment Battery (*RPAB*; Whiting et al. 1985) involves the timing of the written and drawn sub-tests. Many patients with stroke (who are a primary population for this test) experience hemiparesis to an upper limb; in some cases, this affects a previously dominant hand. In these circumstances, the patient has to perform the sub-tests using a non-dominant hand to hold the pen. As assessment usually occurs as soon as possible after diagnosis, and precedes intervention, the patient rarely has had an opportunity to practice writing with the non-dominant hand prior to testing. Therefore, many patients were found to fail these tests as a consequence of the length of time taken rather than due to lack of actual ability (Cramond et al. 1989).

Further limitations to the RPAB include the difficulty of administering the test to clients with severe cognitive impairment (short-term memory, attention, and concentration are required) or aphasia. The formality of the test administration procedures increases test anxiety and can have detrimental effects on performance. Many older clients have visual and auditory acuity loss because of ageing. The RPAB protocol does not permit the repetition of instructions or the use of additional verbal and visual cues; some clients fail sub-tests as they do not comprehend the instructions. Furthermore, the colour-matching task has been criticised (Laver 1990). There is poor differentiation between the colours of some items on the tasks. Colour vision alters with ageing owing to yellowing of the lens; this affects the perception of the blue-green end of the spectrum. RPAB involves the differentiation of several pieces in blue and green shades. Many older clients failed this sub-test but could name and point to colours on command. The task requires more complex functioning than the simple identification of colour.

The use of prompts and non-verbal cues is particularly important for some client groups, for example, people with communication difficulties associated with problems with visual and auditory acuity, learning disability, or cognitive impairment. The use of prompts, cues, and repeated instructions may even be part of what is scored on the test, especially in tests of comprehension and cognitive functioning; for example, see the Severe Impairment Battery (*SIB*; Saxton et al. 1993). AHPs working with people with dementia often need to identify which type(s) of prompts and cues are most successful in supporting the person to achieve maximum functioning.

Culler (1993, 2003) provided an overview of the types of prompts and cues that might be provided. These include:

- printed materials (such as prompt cards, written instructions, diagrams, and photographs);
- tactile cueing by touching the person to modify or guide their performance; e.g. the AHP could touch the client's lower back to encourage a more upright posture or touch the client's arm to remind him to use a hemiplegic limb following a stroke;
- verbal prompts to repeat the original instruction or guide the person further in the performance of the test item or task; and
- visual prompts, such as pointing.

Culler (1993, 2003) also broke verbal cues into two categories: direct cues and indirect cues. She provided an example of the observation of a shopping assessment: 'a direct cue provides the patient with a specific instruction, such as "the spaghetti is here" [whilst] an indirect cue provides assistance to the patient in a less directive manner, such as "can you find the foods listed on your [shopping] list"' (Culler 1993, p. 218).

In any assessment, whether it is standardised or informal, AHPs should record the number and nature of any repeated instructions or supervision, prompts, or cues provided. Some tests allow for physical assistance and include a score to represent that physical assistance was provided. The nature and amount of physical assistance should be described in sufficient detail so that another AHP repeating the assessment could ascertain whether more or less physical assistance was given during re-testing. AHPs should also record any equipment or environmental modifications made to the prescribed testing method that may impact the test results.

Step 3: Scoring

When a scoring system has been specified, then an AHP must use it. Pynsent (2004) notes that 'inventing a new system will make the results incomparable, and also greatly detract from the value and efforts made to collect the data' (p. 6). AHPs should also ensure that the instructions for dealing with and recording missing data are followed (Pynsent 2004). Examples of different types of scoring systems are provided for each of the four levels of measurement (nominal, ordinal, interval, and ratio) in Chapter 4.

Step 4: Analysis of Scores

Where the AHP needs to convert a raw score, for example, by referring to normative data, then the AHP needs to be careful to select the correct table for reference. Where individual test item scores need to be totalled to provide a summary score, the AHP needs to ensure that their calculation is accurate. Some standardised tests provide recommendations based on test results, and the scoring method may involve cross-checking the score with a cut-off point that indicates the requirement for further testing or referral to another service.

Step 5: Interpreting Test Scores

Test scores are rarely sufficient on their own and must be interpreted within the wider context of the specific testing situation and influences of the test environment and the client's current situation and personal idiosyncrasies (de Clive-Lowe 1996).

AHPs should not just report results; rather, to add value, an AHP should offer an interpretation of what these results mean in context. The AHP needs to pose a series of questions when examining test scores, such as:

- *Do I think these scores are a true reflection of the person's function?*
- *If not, did test anxiety, fatigue, lack of motivation, distractions, etc. influence the test results?*
- *How do these scores compare with other data I have collected about this person (e.g. through interview, proxy report, non-standardised observations)?*
- *Is there consistency in the data or discrepancies in the picture I am building about this person's ability and needs?*

Step 6: Decision Making in Light of the Interpretation of Test Scores

Information on decision making and reasoning is provided in Chapter 6.

Step 7: Client Feedback About the Test Results and Implications

It is very important that you share the results and your interpretations of assessment data with the client, and where appropriate with the carer/significant other(s). This should be done in a way that the client and carer can easily comprehend. AHPs must be aware of the need to avoid professional jargon and explain any abbreviations or technical or theoretical terms. This feedback enables the client and carer to understand the relevance of the assessment process, the nature of the problems that have been identified, and to make informed choices and become actively involved in decision making about any further assessment, intervention, or care package.

Step 8: Recording and Reporting Results

It should be remembered that a good test administration is just a beginning, and it is critical to document and interpret the results and to share the conclusions drawn from the assessment with the client and other relevant people. When reporting on standardised test results, the AHP should state the rationale for administering this particular standardised test. In the report, the AHP should also include a description of the person's responses to and behaviour during testing (for example, whether the person was anxious, if they complied with requests, or were restricted by pain or fatigue). These additional qualitative observations will provide a context for the AHP's hypotheses about the meaning of the test scores (de Clive-Lowe 1996). Suggested headings for reporting on a standardised test administration and an example test report are provided below.

Suggested Headings for Writing a Report on a Standardised Test Administration

Personal details: Client's name, date of birth, age, diagnoses, address

Date(s) of assessment: It is important to give the date of an initial assessment and any re-assessment. If appropriate, also state the time of day. For example, if one test was given first thing in the morning and the re-assessment was conducted in the afternoon, fluctuating levels of fatigue or stiffness might influence the test results.

Referral information: The name of the person who made the referral.

The reason for referral: This should influence the selection of assessment focus and methods and have implications for how the test results are interpreted. For example, the referral might be a request to assess the person's safety to be discharged home.

Relevant background information: This includes brief information relevant to the selection and interpretation of the assessment, for example, the person's occupational history, hobbies and interests, medication (especially if this leads to varying function), and how the person came to be in the present situation. In the example of a home safety assessment, details such as whether the person lives alone would be useful to include here.

Previous assessment results (if any): Previous assessment might influence the choice of current assessment and will also be useful for comparison to interpret whether the person's function has improved or deteriorated. If no previous assessment data is available, state 'none known'

Reason for this assessment: State your rationale for assessing this client with this test at this time. How does this assessment fit into the overall AHP process or service pathway? Do you need descriptive, discriminative, predictive, and/or evaluative assessment data?

Test(s) administered: State the title of the test(s) given and provide a brief description of the test and its purpose. This is particularly important if the person reading the report is not familiar with the test(s) used.

Behaviour during testing: Describe any behaviour that might have influenced the test results. This information is needed so that anyone reading the report can decide whether the results represent a reliable estimate of the person's ability. Keep descriptions as concise and objective as possible. Include information about apparent fatigue, anxiety, level of cooperation with testing, ability to follow instructions, any distractions or interruptions to the test, etc.

Results: Give a concise summary of the results. If appropriate, attach a copy of the assessment form and/or summary table or graph to the report. If any parts of the test were not assessed, make a note of this and state the reasons for the omission. If using percentile or standard scores, state which norms have been used so that anyone re-assessing the person can use the same norms for future comparison (e.g. give the date of the test manual and the page reference for the table). This is very important where there are several editions of an assessment with updated normative data.

Discussion: Consider what the results of the assessment mean, whether the results represent a reliable picture of the person's function, and hypothesise about what might account for the results. Relate the discussion back to the reason for referral. Give brief examples of observable behaviour and/or specific test results to justify your reasoning. Also refer back to the 'Behaviour during testing section' if this has a bearing on how the results should be interpreted.

Recommendations: These should derive directly from the assessment results and should relate back to the reason for the referral and the person's current situation. This may include the need for further assessment to confirm provisional hypotheses. If you recommend further intervention, give timelines and state an appropriate time for re-assessment in order to monitor progress. This may also involve referral to other professionals or services for further assessment, intervention, or care packages. Consider whether this same test could be used as an outcome measure to monitor the effectiveness of the proposed intervention. If not, then note that another assessment will be required for monitoring progress during intervention and for measuring final outcomes, and recommend an appropriate measure (if possible).

Group Analyses

It can be useful to aggregate data for groups of clients who have been tested on a particular measure. This can be of particular value when reviewing the appropriateness of referrals or examining outcomes from a specific intervention (see the section titled 'What Is Evaluation?' in Chapter 13). Pynsent (2004) noted that feedback and sharing of group results can encourage staff compliance with the administration of a measure, as they can see the benefit to the client group as a whole and to the service.

Step 8: Recording and Reporting Results – Record Keeping

AHPs are required to maintain detailed and accurate records of any assessment, plan, intervention, care package, and of the person's condition over time.

Accurate records are an essential part of the provision of evidence-based AHP, and they support effective clinical decision making, improve client care through a clear communication of the intervention rationale and progress, and facilitate a consistent approach to team working and continuity of care (RCOT 2018). Records are also required to meet legal requirements. In the United Kingdom, all health professionals registered with the Health and Care Professions Council (*HCPC*) must keep accurate records as parts of the standards of care (https://www.hcpc-uk.org/registration/meeting-our-standards/information-on-record-keeping) including requests from clients to access their own records and in cases of complaint or litigation. When AHPs are working under heavy demands, such as high caseloads and waiting list pressures, record keeping can be delayed or compromised. The Chartered Society of Physiotherapy (*CSP*) notes that a record is only useful if it is correctly recorded in the first place, regularly updated, and easily accessible when it is needed (www.csp.org.uk/publications/record-keeping-guidance#overview).

AHPs should remember that record keeping is a useful and critical part of an assessment process and not just a requirement. Sitting down to write a report or note in the person's records provides time to reflect upon and summarise the assessment or standardised test process and results. Accurate records serve a number of important functions (RCOT 2018). They:

- provide an objective basis to determine the appropriateness of, need for, and effectiveness of intervention;
- demonstrate the AHP's professional reasoning and the rationale behind any care provided (see Chapter 6 for more information on clinical reasoning);
- highlight problems and changes in the client's condition at an early stage;
- facilitate better communication and dissemination of information between members of health and social care teams; and
- protect the welfare of clients by promoting high standards of care.

Some services require AHPs to follow a set format for record keeping. One example is SOAP notes. SOAP stands for:

- S = subjective
- O = objective
- A = assessment (the analysis of data to formulate an understanding of the client's problems)
- P = plan (for intervention/management/treatment).

Pynsent (2004) defined subjective as 'pertaining to a perceived condition within the patient's own consciousness' (p. 3) and objective as 'a condition of the mind or body as perceived by another' (p. 3). Standardised test scores would be reported as an 'objective' entry. Comments that the client has made about the standardised testing experience, for example, 'I'm feeling very tired today', would be recorded as a 'subjective' entry, whereas the AHP's interpretation of the test scores within the wider context of their knowledge of the client, the testing environment, and circumstances would be recorded as an 'assessment' entry. SOAP notes were described in Chapter 2.

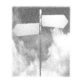

Electronic Care Records

Many health and social care services are moving to integrated records on an electronic care record systems (Garner and Rugg 2005), rather than on paper. However, the nationwide spread across the United Kingdom of integrated health and care records has been a complex process (Robertson et al. 2010). Halford and colleagues (2010) noted the multiple and complex relations between record keeping, healthcare work, and healthcare professionals.

Data Protection and Confidentiality

The **Data Protection** Act 2018 is an Act of Parliament which updates data protection laws in the United Kingdom. It is a national law, which complements the European Union's General Data Protection Regulation (*GDPR*) and updates the Data Protection Act 1998 (https://ico.org.uk/for-organisations/guide-to-data-protection). Data protection is the fair and proper use of information about people, and their fundamental right to privacy. As AHPs, we need to ensure that the information (data) we are collecting is required, and necessary for our assessment, any intervention, and recording and reporting.

The HCPC provide guidance on confidentiality as a key aspect of health and care (https://www.hcpc-uk.org/registration/meeting-our-standards/guidance-on-confidentiality). AHPs have a professional and legal responsibility to respect and protect the confidentiality of service users at all times. You need to ensure that you have taken reasonable steps to keep identifiable information related to the person's care or treatment safe. This may include personal details such as name and address, photographs, videos, and information a family member provides you. You should seek the person's permission and consent before sharing any information.

Case Study

Case Study Example: James' Assessment of Motor and Process Skills (AMPS) Report
by **Rachel Hargreaves**

About the AHP: The AHP completing the assessment and report has worked as an occupational therapist for eight years, practising in a variety of clinical settings including Neurology and Mental Health Services for Working Age Adults and Older Adults. She became an Assessment of Motor and Process Skills (*AMPS*) calibrated AHP 18 months ago. AMPS is an assessment which is used in the Multi-Disciplinary Specialist Memory Clinic service and also in the Community Mental Health Team for Older Adults in which she is based.

Test Report

Assessment of Motor and Process Skills (AMPS)

NAME:	James
AGE:	**
DIAGNOSES:	Parkinson Disease, Bowel Cancer, treated surgically three years ago. Under investigation for cognitive impairment
REFERRED BY:	Memory Clinic Consultant Psychiatrist
ASSESSED BY:	Memory Clinic Occupational AHP
DATE OF ASSESSMENT:	** ** **

Reason for Referral

Assessment of quality in activities of daily living (*ADL*).

- Identification of areas of ability and deficit in ADL.
- Recognition of areas that would benefit from restorative interventions using occupation and adaptation.

Referral Information

James has an 11-year history of Parkinson's disease, with a 1-year history of visual hallucinations and gradually deteriorating memory. All physical causes for memory problems have been ruled out by GP prior to the referral to the memory clinic. Referred for Multi Disciplinary Team assessment as per Memory Clinic protocol, with a view to introduction of cholinesterase inhibitors in line with National Institute for Health and Care Excellence (NICE) guidance. The Occupational AHP assessment is identified as being required owing to James's physical health difficulties, along with problems with his memory, which are increasing his dependency on his carer. The referral requests that other appropriate interventions to assist James and his wife with community living are explored.

Relevant Background Information

James has lived with his supportive wife in their isolated owner-occupied, three-bedroom, detached property for the last four years. After their retirement, both James and his wife were active members in the local community, being volunteers for several community services. They have found it difficult adjusting to being 'on the other side', and they have resisted asking for help themselves until this time. Up until the memory clinic appointment, the only service they had accessed was a respite stay for James in a local Residential Home. James's wife is considering a similar arrangement to allow her to take a holiday with friends later this year, owing to increasing levels of carer stress. James spends the majority of his time in his bedroom, sitting on the bed watching television. His room is ensuite, with a raised toilet seat/freestanding toilet frame in situ. He prefers to use the shower in the house bathroom.

Previous Assessment Results

Mini Mental State Examination (*MMSE*) score 24/30. No previous Multi Disciplinary Team assessments completed, no specific Occupational AHP assessments, including AMPS administered.

Reasons for Use of AMPS

The AMPS (5th Edition; Fisher 2003) was selected by the specialist Occupational AHP Team within the Memory Clinic as the best-researched and most robust available tool to measure ADL qualities/deficits in older people reporting cognitive impairment. The occupational AHP that picked up James' referral identified that AMPS would provide data regarding James's possible process deficits owing to his memory problems and would also illustrate the impact of his Parkinson's disease on his motor skills.

Test Administered

AMPS (Fisher 2003) is an observational assessment enabling simultaneous evaluation of motor and process skill areas. Motor skills are those observable actions enabling a person to move himself/herself or task objects. Process skills are the observable actions that are used to logically organise and adapt behaviour in order to complete a task. The person chooses two or three daily living tasks to perform, is observed carrying them out, and then rated by the occupational AHP. The results are computer-analysed to provide profiles of performance and measures for motor and process skill ability. The cut-off points on the AMPS motor skill scale (2.00 logits $\pm$ 0.3 logits) and AMPS process skill scale (1.0 logits $\pm$ 0.3 logits) are the levels at which the skill deficit begin to impact the performance of daily living tasks. The majority of people at this level begin to experience difficulties with independent community living.

The tasks negotiated with James for completion within the AMPS contract were:

1. P-4: Putting on socks and shoes
2. P-2: Brushing teeth.

Both the tasks chosen for the AMPS test administration were within the very easy/much easier than average categories. They were selected as the tasks which were performed regularly. Owing to his Parkinsonian symptoms, James had identified that he limited his performance of ADLs.

Behaviour During Testing

Throughout the assessment, there was no evidence of psychotic symptoms. James cooperated with the occupational AHP throughout the assessment, including negotiating the tasks and then the completion of both tasks. He reflected on feelings of self-worth and purposefulness in being encouraged to undertake tasks to his own standards, as opposed to relying on others, which caused subsequent feelings of powerlessness.

Results

James scored −1.16 logits on the AMPS motor skills scale, which demonstrates a severe level of impairment, with the cut-off being 2.00 logits. He scored 0.07 logits on the process skills scale, which is well below the cut-off point of 1.0 logits. In motor skills areas, a moderate level of disruption was noted throughout all skills, except the items of *flows* and *calibrates*, where there was a marked disruption. In process skill areas, James demonstrated no deficit in chooses, heeds, inquires, continues, sequences, searches, gathers, and restores. In the remaining 12 areas, there was evidence of moderate disruption, specifically *energy* and *adaptation* (the ability to appropriately respond to and modify actions in an environment, to overcome problems and/or prevent them occurring).

Discussion

The results show that James has trouble with both motor and process skills, which impact his ability to sustain independent community living. The motor skills score indicate that James needs physical support when completing ADLs. James's wife is currently providing this physical assistance, but is finding this increasingly difficult. The process skills score means that James needs less support in this area, but that when confronted with a problem, he finds it difficult to overcome. Support is, therefore, required to assist James with problem solving; again, his wife is providing this.

James's wife states she was considering the option of respite/day care, during which time her husband would require the support of carers for both his motor and process skills deficits. James highlighted that mealtimes were 'particularly trying', due to dribbling, dropping food, and difficulty applying sufficient pressure to facilitate food onto a fork (when brushing teeth, James also experienced difficulty applying the correct pressure effectively). James's wife explained that she was reviewing the option of employing a private cleaner and gardener, as she completes all domestic tasks.

James identified that he perceived himself as a failure in domestic ADL, following a number of incidents and accidents (e.g. dropping crockery), stating he is 'banned' from the kitchen. This has compounded to reduce his confidence in himself and his abilities. During the latter part of the assessment, James became tearful when acknowledging all the things he had lost (i.e. hobbies/interests/roles). He also reported several falls over the last four weeks. The AMPS showed impairment with mobility owing to a marked short shuffling gait, with difficulty initiating forward movement. At times during the visit, James had problems transferring in and out of the chair, having a poorly controlled descent into the chair.

James became easily frustrated when he initiated a task but was unable to complete it, as he forgot the sequence. He recalled statements made by the occupational AHP during the assessment, including equipment recommendations.

Recommendations

Motor Skills

Poor Grip (manipulates, calibrates, grips, flows, and lifts skill areas):

- Adaptive cutlery assessed for and provided.
- Advice given regarding alternative methods for brushing teeth, other equipment highlighted to assist, e.g. electric toothbrush.

Poor mobility (stabilises, aligns, positions, and walks skill areas):

- Referral made for assessment.
- Referral sent for the fitting of a second banister rail.

General Motor Deficits (reaches, bends, calibrates, and lifts skill areas):

- Respite services to be informed of difficulties, ensuring provision of appropriate equipment.
- Previously provided equipment to be checked.

Process Skills

Problem Solving (uses, initiates, organises, and adaptation skill areas):

- Education for James's wife regarding management skills/techniques.
- Identification of the areas that produce the greatest difficulties; also, grading of activities, to be pursued during further occupational AHP visits.

Support/Other

Carer Stress: Referrals to Crossroads, Carers Resource, and Social Services

- James's negative outlook: Identification and participation in meaningful tasks with appropriate support as required
- Medication: Liaison with Consultant Psychiatrist to feedback findings, for consideration in prescribing cholinesterase inhibiters

Worksheet

At the end of this chapter (p. 168), you will find a worksheet (Worksheet 5.1) designed to assist you in *preparing for an assessment*. The worksheet takes you through a 'To do list' and can be used by students on placement or AHPs to ensure that they have prepared thoroughly for an assessment or test administration (see p. 168).

REVIEW QUESTIONS

5.1 What factors should you discuss with the client prior to assessment to ensure you have gained informed consent?

5.2 What factors should you consider to ensure you achieve an effective and efficient assessment?

5.3 What techniques could you apply to help build rapport with your client?

You will find brief answers to these questions at the back of this book on p. 445.

WORKSHEET 5.1   Checklist for Preparing for an Assessment.

To do list	Tick when completed or mark as not applicable (N/A)	Notes
• Discussed purpose of assessment/measurement with client		
• Discussed purpose of assessment/measurement with carer		
• Obtained informed consent		
• Identified optimum timing for the assessment		
• Contacted and liaised with other people who need to be involved (colleagues for joint assessments, carer, parent, teacher, etc.)		
• Organised time, date, and venue and informed client and any others involved		
• Checked the environment (hazards, lighting, temperature, furniture), and set the environment up ready for the assessment		
• Got the test instructions and test materials		
• Got pens/pencils for recording and if needed for assessment		
• Got a stopwatch and checked that it is working		
• Got a calculator and checked that it is working		
• Battery of tests: checked all the component parts are present and in their correct bags/places		
• Got any consumables required (paper, food, drink, ingredients for a cooking assessment, etc.)		
• Have the right aids/equipment needed for assessment		
• Checked if the person uses a hearing aid and checked that it is on and working		
• Checked if the person uses visual aids and checked that these are being used		
• (left blank for any other things you need to add)		

REFERENCES

Act, D. P. (2018). Data Protection Act. HM Government. https://www.legislation.gov.uk/ukpga/2018/12/contents/enacted

Act, M.C. (2005). *Mental Capacity Act.* London: *The Stationery Office* https://www.legislation.gov.uk/ukpga/2005.

Act, M.H. (1983) Mental Health Act 1983, Chapter 20: An Act to consolidate the law relating to mentally disordered persons. [9th May 1983]. https://www.legislation.gov.uk/ukpga/1983/20/contents

Act, M.H. (2007) Mental Health Act. HM Government. https://www.legislation.gov.uk/ukpga/2007/12/contents

Clabby, J. and O'Connor, R. (2004). Teaching learners to use mirroring: rapport lessons from neurolinguistic programming. *Family Medicine* 36 (8): 541–543. https://pdfs.semanticscholar.org/64ed/7000ffe02ba311bac945514690e3d830e7d1.pdf.

de Clive-Lowe, S. (1996). Outcome measurement, cost-effectiveness and clinical audit: the importance of standardised assessment to occupational therapists in meeting these new demands. *British Journal of Occupational Therapy* 59 (8): 357–362. https://doi.org/10.1177/030802269605900803.

Cramond, H.J., Clark, M.S., and Smith, D.S. (1989). The effect of using the dominant or non-dominant hand on performance of the Rivermead Perceptual Assessment Battery. *Clinical Rehabilitation* 3 (3): 215–221. https://doi.org/10.1177/026921558900300306.

Culler, K.H. (1993). Occupational therapy performance areas: home and family management. In: *Willard and Spackman's Occupational Therapy*, 8e (eds. H.L. Hopkins and H.D. Smith), 207–269. Philadelphia: *Lippincott Williams & Wilkins.*

Culler, K.H. (2003). Home management. In: *Willard and Spackman's Occupational Therapy* (eds. E.B. Crepeau, E.S. Cohn and B.A.B. Schell), 534–541. Philadelphia: Lippincott Williams & Wilkins.

Fisher, A.G. (2003). Assessment of motor and process skills. In: *Administration and Scoring Manual, Vol. 2: User Manual.* Three Star Press. *ISBN:* 0964512785.

Garner, R. and Rugg, S. (2005). Electronic care records: an update on the Garner Project. *British Journal of Occupational Therapy* 68 (3): 131–134. https://doi.org/10.1177/030802260506800306.

Halford, S., Obstfelder, A., and Lotherington, A.T. (2010). Changing the record: the inter-professional, subjective and embodied effects of electronic patient records. *New Technology, Work and Employment* 25 (3): 210–222. https://doi.org/10.1111/j.1468-005X.2010.00249.x.

Jones, L. (1991). The standardized test. *Clinical Rehabilitation* 5 (3): 177–180. https://doi.org/10.1177/026921559100500301.

Landau, M.J., Arndt, J., and Cameron, L.D. (2018). Do metaphors in health messages work? Exploring emotional and cognitive factors. *Journal of Experimental Social Psychology* 74: 135–149. https://doi.org/10.1016/j.jesp.2017.09.006.

Laver, A. J. (1990). Test review: the Rivermead Perceptual Assessment Battery. Assessment of the Elderly. Windsor, NFER-Nelson.

Lawley, J., & Tompkins, P. (2000). Metaphors in mind. Transformation through Symbolic Modelling.

Liu, Y., Gao, J.H., Liu, H.L., and Fox, P.T. (2000). The temporal response of the brain after eating revealed by functional MRI. *Nature* 405 (6790): 1058–1062. https://doi.org/10.1038/35016590.

Mosey, A.C. (1981). *Occupational Therapy: Configuration of a Profession*, vol. 63, 67–69. New York: Raven Press.

Pynsent, P. (2004). Choosing an outcome measure. In: *Outcome Measures in Orthopaedics and Orthopaedic Trauma* (eds. P. Pynsent, J. Fairbank and A. Carr). CRC Press.

Rees, J. and Ioan Manea, A. (2016). The use of clean language and metaphor in helping clients overcoming procrastination. *Journal of Experiential Psychotherapy* 19 (3): 30–36.

Robertson, A., Cresswell, K., Takian, A. et al. (2010). Implementation and adoption of nationwide electronic health records in secondary care in England: qualitative analysis of interim results from a prospective national evaluation. *British Medical Journal* 341: c4564. https://doi.org/10.1136/bmj.c4564.

Royal College of Occupational Therapists (2018). *Keeping Records: Guidance for Occupational Therapists*, 4e. London: Royal College of Occupational Therapists.

Saxton, J., McGonigle, K.L., Swihart, A.A., and Boller, F. (1993). *The Severe Impairment Battery Manual*. Bury St. Edmunds: Thames Valley Test Company.

Tamayo-Velazquez, M.I., Simon-Lorda, P., Villegas-Portero, R. et al. (2010). Interventions to promote the use of advance directives: an overview of systematic reviews. *Patient Education and Counseling* 80 (1): 10–20. https://doi.org/10.1016/j.pec.2009.09.027.

Taylor, R.R., Lee, S.W., Kielhofner, G., and Ketkar, M. (2009). Therapeutic use of self: a nationwide survey of practitioners' attitudes and experiences. *The American Journal of Occupational Therapy* 63 (2): 198. https://doi.org/10.5014/ajot.63.2.198.

Tompkins, P. and Lawley, J. (1997). Less is More: The Art of Clean Language. *Rapport Magazine* 35.

Whiting, S., Lincoln, N.B., Bhavnani, G., and Cockburn, J.E. (1985). *Rivermead Perceptual Assessment Battery*. Windsor: NFER-NELSON.

RESOURCES

The Department of Health and Social Care (2009) Guidelines on consent, https://www.gov.uk/government/publications/reference-guide-to-consent-for-examination-or-treatment-second-edition (accessed 09.11.2019).

CHAPTER 6

The Importance of Clinical Reasoning and Reflective Practice in Effective Assessment

OVERVIEW

The aim of this chapter is to highlight to you as an allied health professional (AHP) the importance of reflecting upon how you and others think about and make clinical decisions related to assessment and measurement. This chapter will:

- define clinical reasoning, show how it is an essential component of assessment and is required for interpreting measurement data;
- define and describe different types of reasoning, for example, diagnostic reasoning, procedural reasoning, interactive reasoning, conditional reasoning, ethical reasoning, and narrative reasoning;
- discuss the importance of reflective practice; and
- provide a case study example as an illustration of how an AHP thinks in practice when assessing a client.

Johns (2017) has suggested that to be an effective professional practitioner, we require a strong sense of vision to guide us. We need expert clinical judgement. We then need to evaluate and reflect in order to learn from the situation and apply such learning and new experiences within a reflexive spiral of being and becoming. Within that spiral, we draw on relevant theory to inform us, theory that we then assimilate into our personal knowing. So how do AHPs develop expert clinical judgement?

Principles of Assessment and Outcome Measurement for Allied Health Professionals: Practice, Research and Development, Second Edition. Alison J. Laver-Fawcett and Diane L. Cox.
© 2021 John Wiley & Sons Ltd. Published 2021 by John Wiley & Sons Ltd.

QUESTIONS TO CONSIDER

1. How do I combine the best available evidence, with my clinical experience and my knowledge of my client's preferences?
2. How do we learn to reflect upon and improve our clinical practice?
3. How do we form this 'strong sense of vision' to guide our practice wisely?

The following text provides some basic answers to these questions, but as professional judgement, clinical reasoning, and reflective practice are complex areas of study, this chapter can only serve as a basic introduction.

CLINICAL REASONING AS AN ESSENTIAL COMPONENT OF PRACTICE

Problem solving in therapy can be directed, as in medicine, to problem identification and diagnosis, but it also often refers to 'the invention of the unique solutions for the complex problems and issues the client faces' (Unsworth 1999, p. 53). Therefore, problem solving by AHPs involves reasoning directed towards solving a goal, the goal usually being to understand the nature of the problem *and* to organise a response that will be therapeutic (Rogers 1983). The problems identified by AHPs during assessment are usually framed as problems of understanding, for example, identifying the cause of the observed behaviour. Information from several assessment sources is gathered to research the presenting problem(s). It is then integrated into a single clinical image through clinical reasoning processes. Fleming (1994) identified and described a variety of reasoning strategies used by AHPs to determine clients' problems and select appropriate treatments. Both the explicit and tacit reasoning that guides therapy problem-solving processes has been called 'clinical reasoning' (Mattingly 1991). Other synonymous phrases seen in therapy, healthcare, and social care literature include clinical expertise, clinical judgement, clinical decision making, and reflective thinking.

Donaghy and Morss (2000) recommend that physiotherapists should focus their attention on problem solving and clinical reasoning and engage in systematic critical enquiry. They stress the importance of linking reflection to higher-order cognitive processes, such as memory schema, illness scripts, and clinical knowledge. Although Jones et al. (2008) suggest that clinical decision making is linked inextricably to the therapist and patient interaction and to the reflective and analytic phase of clinical reasoning which takes place during and after contact.

In Chapter 1, we examined the demand for AHPs to deliver an evidenced-based practice. Clinical reasoning plays a critical role in enabling an AHP to connect practice based on best evidence with practice that is client centred and centred upon a person's unique presentation of problems and needs. Sackett et al. (1996) emphasised that practitioners undertaking evidence-based practice cannot take a 'cookbook' approach. Evidence-based practice requires an 'approach that integrates the best external evidence with individual clinical expertise and patients' choice, it cannot result in slavish, cookbook approaches to individual patient care' (p. 71).

External clinical evidence is used to inform clinical decisions, but should not replace individual clinical expertise. Clinical reasoning is the process through which clinical expertise is applied to individual client problems; the AHP engages in clinical reasoning to decide whether available external evidence applies to the individual client's presentation. When the clinician decides that external evidence does apply, clinical reasoning is required to establish how this evidence should be applied in this particular case and underlies clinical decision making around how the evidence should be integrated into this client's assessment, management, and/ or intervention.

The underlying knowledge base and experience that an AHP brings to an assessment is critical, but it is not sufficient to address the complexity of assessment. Kielhofner (2009) suggested that the use of theory is not a simple mapping of theory onto reality; it is a much more complex process. Each assessment requires the AHP to engage in original thinking:

> *[AHPs] must recognize the unique conditions presented by each patient and make careful observations and interpretations to find the best strategies for resolving each patient's particular set of problems. Clinical reasoning takes place as [AHPs] attempt to understand the nature of patients' problems and develop individualized therapy directed towards the future life for each patient*

> (Cohn and Czycholl 1991, p. 161)

Clinical judgement should be informed by the use of objective, preferably standardised, assessment processes. The AHP needs to address a number of assessment questions. These will vary depending upon the nature of the referral, service, and diagnosis but may include the following:

- What are the person's strengths or abilities?
- What are the person's deficits or needs?
- What is the person's occupational profile?
- What degree of independence does the person have?
- Why is performance affected?
- How does the person perform the task?
- When is the person functioning at his best?

The specific questions to be addressed will vary from person to person and depend upon the diagnosis, presenting problems, and the profession to which the AHP belongs. It is important to recognise the unique conditions presented by each person, and the assessment should involve careful observations and interpretations in order to identify the optimum strategies for resolving each person's particular problems.

CLINICAL JUDGEMENT AND CLINICAL REASONING

Clinical judgement has been defined as 'the ability of professionals to make decisions within their own field of expertise using the working knowledge that they have acquired over time. It is based on both clinical experience and the theoretical principles embedded in their professional knowledge base but it may remain highly subjective' (Stewart 1999, p. 417). Clinical judgement is exercised through both theoretical and clinical reasoning. The differences between theoretical and clinical reasoning are as follows:

- **Theoretical reasoning** is learned from sources such as textbooks and lectures and relates to generalities, to what the AHP can predict (Unsworth 1999).
- **Clinical reasoning** occurs as the AHP works to understand the nature of the person's problems and to construct individualised client-centred interventions (Cohn and Czycholl 1991).

Clinical reasoning has been described as 'the thinking or cognitive processes and decision making that [AHPs] use to guide their work'; it is 'a practical know-how that puts theoretical knowledge into practice' and is concerned 'with deliberating over appropriate action and then putting this in place' (Unsworth 1999, pp. 45–46). Simply put, clinical reasoning is 'the process used by practitioners to plan, direct, perform and reflect on client care' (Schell and Schell 2008, p. 5). So when an AHP is involved in planning, doing, or thinking about therapy, they are engaged in clinical reasoning.

SCIENTIFIC REASONING

The basic process of reasoning is considered to be universal; 'all human beings reason' (Roberts 1996, p. 233). Problem solving is a fundamental process that is undertaken by people who face some sort of problem. However, the precise nature of the problem-solving process can vary depending on the nature of the problem, the context in which problem solving is undertaken, and the expertise of the problem solver. The two most commonly discussed forms of reasoning in scientific literature are deductive and inductive reasoning. Both types of reasoning are used by therapy clinicians and researchers.

DEDUCTIVE REASONING

Discussion about deductive reasoning dates back to Aristotle. Deductive reasoning involves reasoning from the general to the particular (or from cause to effect). The deductive reasoning process begins with statements that are accepted as true and then applies these held 'truths' to a new situation to reach a conclusion. Deduction, therefore, is seen as reasoning based on facts. Deductive reasoning is the process of reaching a conclusion that is guaranteed to follow, if the evidence provided is true and the reasoning used to reach the conclusion is correct. The conclusion must be based only on the evidence previously provided; it cannot contain new information about the subject matter. Deductive reasoning is seen as a top-down approach to reasoning (see Figure 6.1).

AHPs use deductive reasoning in assessment. For example, a clinician may start from theories of perception and the knowledge that perception can be affected by a stroke. One type of perceptual deficit they has seen in previous clients with stroke is figure-ground discrimination deficit. The AHP forms the hypothesis that the client has figure-ground discrimination perceptual deficit. They forms a further more specific hypothesis that states that this figure-ground discrimination deficit will negatively impact the person's ability to retrieve the previously recognised object of a spoon from a drawer full of cutlery. The AHP then sets about to test their hypothesis by presenting the client with a drawer of knives, forks, and spoons and asks him to take out a spoon. The client fumbles about in the drawer, complains that it is such a muddle and finally takes out a fork. He recognises it is a fork once it is the only object of his attention and puts it back. He looks at the drawer again, but struggles to see each individual item of cutlery from the other pieces of cutlery and the background of the base of the drawer. The AHP concludes from these observations that her hypothesis is confirmed and makes a diagnosis of figure-ground discrimination deficit.

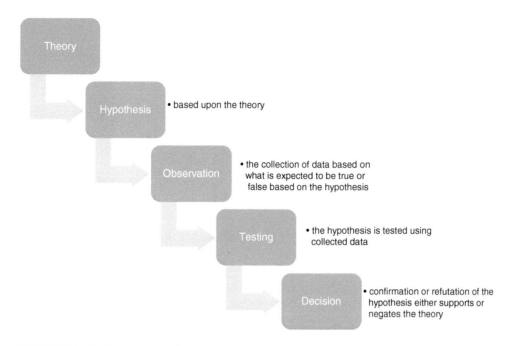

FIGURE 6.1   Deductive reasoning process.

With deductive reasoning, we can make deductive conclusions based on known facts, i.e. that if x is present and x and y are known to occur together, then if x is present then y will also be present. For example, it is known that if it rains then the ground below becomes wet, so if we observe from a window that it is raining we can reliably deduce that the ground below will be wet. However, we cannot necessarily deduce the opposite – i.e. that if the ground is wet it must be raining – because there are a number of other causes of wet ground. If we begin with the observation that the ground is wet, then we would need to use an inductive reasoning process to problem-solve the cause.

INDUCTIVE REASONING

Inductive reasoning is a system of reasoning based on observation and measurement. Inductive reasoning works in the opposite way to deductive reasoning; the reasoning process works from specific observations to broader generalisations and theories. Inductive reasoning involves observing patterns and using those observations to make generalisations. AHPs use inductive reasoning to draw a general conclusion based on a limited set of observations. In inductive reasoning, AHPs begin with specific observations and measurements; from these they detect patterns and regularities, and they then formulate some tentative hypotheses that can be explored and tested; and finally they produce some general conclusions or theories. Inductive reasoning is seen as a bottom-up approach to reasoning (see Figure 6.2).

For example, the person may start with the observation that the ground is wet. There may be several causes for this: a sprinkler may have been on; a river may have flooded; a drain may have overflowed; a container of liquid may have spilt; or it may have been raining. A measurement of how much ground has become wet and observation of the nature of the dampness (e.g. whether it is clear or muddy or smelly) will aid the narrowing of these possible hypotheses. The person may observe over time that whenever it rains the ground is wet; this becomes a pattern. Rain may also be noted as the most frequent reason the ground becomes wet. Other observations may

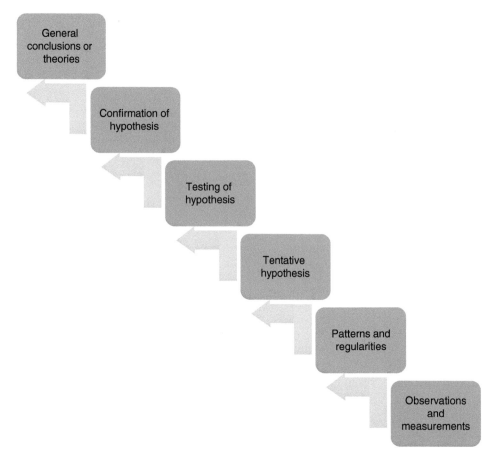

FIGURE 6.2   Inductive reasoning process.

also be associated with this pattern, for example, that other objects higher up, such as trees and buildings, also become wet. This additional information can be used as an observation to be made when narrowing and testing out hypotheses for the causes of wet ground in future. So the inductive process would go as follows: observation that the ground is wet; hypothesis that it has been raining; hypothesis tested by further observation that the ground is wet as far as the eye can see and that the trees and plants are also wet with a clear, clean liquid; general conclusion made that it has been raining.

GENERALISATION

Generalisation is a type of inductive reasoning of relevance to AHPs. It is known as inductive generalisation. This type of reasoning proceeds from a premise about a sample of people to a conclusion about the whole population. Therefore, if a proportion of the sample has a particular attribute, then we generalise that the same proportion of the total population has that same attribute. How accurate these generalisations are depends on two main factors: first, the number of people in the sample group compared to the number in the population; and second, the randomness of the sample. This is of relevance when using normative data obtained from a sample of the population for comparison of a client's score on a normative test (for more information on normative tests, see the section titled 'Normative Data' in Chapter 7). It is also relevant when applying prevalence data for a diagnosis or a problem, drawn from research on a sample, to a wider population; for example, in order to estimate the level of demand on a therapy service.

If an AHP is starting from the position of individual client-based observations, then you start with an inductive reasoning process, but if you receive a referral and read the name of a diagnosis or problem that leads your thinking straight to a theory or frame of reference, then you start your assessment process with deductive reasoning. Both forms of reasoning are useful in clinical practice. How these types of reasoning have been implemented and adapted by AHPs has become the focus of some studies on AHP's clinical reasoning.

In therapy, scientific reasoning is undertaken by clinicians to understand the client's presenting condition and to decide which interventions would produce the best desired effect for removing or reducing the impact of the presenting condition for the client. Scientific reasoning in therapy is a process which parallels scientific inquiry (Tomlin 2008). Two types of scientific reasoning are discussed in the therapy literature: diagnostic reasoning (Rogers and Holm 1991; Rogers 2004) and procedural reasoning (Fleming 1994).

PROCEDURAL REASONING

Procedural reasoning is an 'umbrella term that describes an AHP's thinking when working out what a client's problems are and what procedures may be used to reduce the effect of those problems' (Unsworth 1999, p. 54). AHPs use procedural reasoning to understand the person's problems and to consider ways to alleviate, or reduce the impact of, these problems. Fleming (1994), in her research into procedural reasoning, found the following:

> *In situations where problem identification and treatment selection were seen as the central task, the AHPs' thinking strategies demonstrated many parallels to the patterns identified by other researchers interested in problem solving in general, and clinical problem solving in particular. The typical medical problem-solving sequence – diagnosis, prognosis, prescription – was commonly used. However, the words the AHPs used to describe this sequence were problem identification, goal setting and treatment planning. (p. 121)*

Fleming also found that the AHPs she studied utilised the three problem-solving methods that had been previously described by Newel and Simon (1972, as cited by Fleming 1994): the methods of recognition, generate and test, and heuristic search.

Diagnostic Reasoning and the Therapy Diagnosis

Many professions use the process of diagnosis (Schon 1983) and apply the scientific model, which involves hypothetical reasoning (Fleming 1991). For example, Benner (1984) has described the diagnostic reasoning and treatment decision-making processes in nursing. Diagnostic reasoning becomes a unique occupational therapy process or physiotherapy process when it is applied to profession-specific concepts. For example, in occupational therapy, diagnostic reasoning is applied to profession-specific concepts such as occupational performance, and as diagnosticians, we seek to learn about a patient's functional performance and to describe it so that intervention can be initiated (Rogers and Holm 1991). In a problem-solving process, the problem is some sort of malfunction that you are trying to track down. In therapy, the client comes to you with suboptimal functioning in some area of his life. So, for AHPs, diagnostic reasoning is concerned with clinical problem sensing and problem definition (Schell 2013). It is similar to, although not the same as, medical problem solving (Mattingly and Fleming 1994).The product of an initial therapy assessment is the formulation of a problem statement. AHPs use various clinical reasoning processes to develop problem statements. The case method, for example, is a problem-solving process that fosters the application of knowledge for defining and resolving problems. Data are collected, classified, analysed, and interpreted in accordance with a clinical frame of reference, and transformed into a definition of the problem and subsequently an action plan (Line 1969).

In occupational therapy literature, the problem statement has been called the 'occupational therapy diagnosis' (Rogers and Holm 1991). This is defined as a 'concise summary of a client's disruptions in occupational role that are amenable to occupational therapy' (Rogers 2004, p. 18).

The thinking that leads to a therapy diagnosis is referred to as *diagnostic reasoning*. Diagnostic reasoning involves creating a clinical image of the person through cue acquisition, hypothesis generation, cue interpretation, and hypothesis evaluation (Rogers and Holm 1991). It has developed from scientific reasoning, following the process of hypothesis generation and testing (Unsworth 1999). The diagnostic reasoning process can be explained in two ways, in terms of the steps taken and in terms of strategies used (Rogers and Holm 1991). The *steps* involved in functional assessment are, for example, data collection and the analysis and synthesis of that data, such as the steps in a problem-orientated reasoning process (see the description later on in this chapter). The *principles* and *strategies* that AHPs use to collect, analyse, and synthesise data include the use of hypothesis generation, testing and validation, and the application of heuristics (the use of hypotheses and heuristics will be explored below).

If a patient is unable to perform activities independently, the AHP will note not only a lack of mastery or independence, but will also need to explore the underlying causes for the dysfunctional interaction. Therefore, the function of performance components will need to be evaluated. In order to do this, the AHP has to understand what the requirements of the interaction were. When an AHP analyses an activity, both the individual and non-human components of the activity are unpackaged.

Many AHPs draw upon models that are founded upon general systems theory and view the person as an open system. *Open systems theory* is an interdisciplinary approach used by AHPs. In Alison's doctoral work (Laver 1994) on assessment and diagnostic reasoning, she drew upon early work on systems theory from von Bertalanffy (1951), Allport (1968), and Mackay (1969) to form an understanding of open systems theory and explored the later work of Kielhofner (e.g. 1978, 1992), who applied these ideas to occupational therapy concepts. To summarise, the person (as an open system) takes in information and stimuli (referred to as input) from both its internal systems and external environment and converts or acts upon this information (a process referred to as throughput) to produce some sort of response, which may include observable behaviour (known as the person's output). The outcome of this behaviour in turn produces more information and stimuli and provides feedback as a cyclical process (for more information on open systems, see the section titled 'General Systems Theory and the Hierarchy of Living Systems' and Figure 11.1 in Chapter 11). The person repeats this cyclical process of *input* ⇒ *throughput* ⇒ *output* ⇒ *feedback* throughout life to meet the demands of a constantly changing external environment.

In this way, the repertoire of a person's actions develops throughout his life. People learn to associate stimuli (input) with action responses (for example, presentation of food with eating). Based upon this developed repertoire, the person has a limited number of responses (output) to a specific stimulus (input). The repertoire of an individual's acts develops throughout the life span as the result of interaction with its environment. The limitations of such a repertoire means that there are a limited number of responses (output) an individual can make to a given stimulus (input). Humans learn to associate stimulus and action responses, for example, presentation of food with eating. These associations form a conceptual framework of normal stimulus–response interactions. Observation of the demands of an individual's environment provides information about the nature of the information (input) received by that individual. Observation of the output produced in response to this environmental input gives the AHP an indication of the nature of the patient's internal organisation (throughput).

As AHPs, we have a conceptual framework of normal stimulus–response behaviours for the culture in which we live and work. When an AHP engages in observational assessment, they need to note the demands of the individual's environment to gain information about the nature of the information/stimuli (input) presented to the person. Observation of the person's behavioural responses (output), related to the observed input, gives the AHP an indication of the nature of the patient's internal organisation (throughput). As we have a repertoire of normal stimulus–response behaviours, we can predict what an acceptable behaviour response will be for a person of a particular age and background. Unusual output provides observational cues that prompt hypothesis generation. When an AHP observes an unpredicted output, they are alerted to the possibility of dysfunction. Unexpected output (which could take the form of an abnormal action, facial expression, or spoken word) prompts the diagnostic reasoning process, and the AHP begins a journey of questioning and hypothesising, which starts with a simple question such as: *Why did he do that? Why did he say that? Why did he react in that way?*

As an example, we will describe the diagnostic reasoning process used in the Structured Observational Test of Function (SOTOF; Laver and Powell 1995), a test developed as part of Alison's doctoral research (Laver 1994). The SOTOF is based on an error analysis assessment approach in which the AHP acts as a data processor who collects, sorts, selects, and then interprets assessment data obtained through both observation and interview. Cue acquisition is selective, based on the observer's expectations of the client's performance. The AHP observes the client's behavioural responses to defined stimuli and then selects any unexpected behavioural cues, or observed error, as the focus of the diagnostic reasoning process. Reasons for the observed errors are generated in the form of hypotheses, which are then tested against further observational cues, and theoretical and tacit knowledge.

All these hypotheses are related to performance component dysfunction (sensory, cognitive, and perceptual components). A further explanation could lie with the volitional subsystem. Dysfunction in a performance subsystem is only one explanation for unexpected responses; motivational factors, arising from the volitional subsystem, can have a profound effect on behaviour. From the example above, if the AHP were hypothesising about why the client did not name the cup when he was shown a cup and asked what it was, they would also need to consider that perhaps the person felt too depressed to answer or that they just could not be bothered to respond. Another explanation could be that he considered it was a trite question and was offended, or it was such an easy question they thought it was a trick question and, that a much more complicated response was required, and therefore they were too anxious to reply in case they made themselves look stupid.

An Example

If a person is presented with a cup and asked, 'What is the name of this object?' the expected response would be 'cup'. There are many reasons why the person may not have responded correctly, and the AHP is faced with a differential diagnosis.

A *differential diagnosis* (sometimes abbreviated DDx or $\Delta\Delta$ in therapy and medical notes) is the systematic method used by healthcare professionals to identify the causes of a person's problems and symptoms. If the client fails to respond correctly to a question or test item, the AHP would list the most likely causes and start to formulate a range of hypotheses which could explain the person's behaviour.

The AHP then asks questions and performs tests to eliminate possibilities until she is satisfied that the single most likely cause has been identified. When the person failed to identify the cup, the AHP might consider the most likely reason to be that he has reduced hearing acuity and did not hear the instruction. Otherwise, he might have heard, but had a language deficit, such as receptive aphasia, and did not understand the instruction.

A less common but possible cause, if receptive language and hearing are intact, is that the problem might still lie in the language domain, but be one of expressive aphasia. Alternatively, the AHP could hypothesise that if hearing and language are intact, the problem might have a visual origin, for example, visual acuity, visual attention, or visual field loss.

Further cues that would provide information about hearing, vision, and language would be sought and then used to evaluate each of these hypotheses. If hearing, vision, and language were all found to be intact, the AHP would need to generate further hypotheses to explain the original observed behaviour error (failure to name the cup). A further hypothesis could be visual object agnosia, which is the failure to recognise familiar objects although vision is intact.

The volitional subsystem should be considered to place observed behavioural cues into the context of the individual's internal, as well as, external environment. It is essential to engage the individual's motivation (Kuhl 2013). If judgements made from observational assessment are to be reliable and valid, then optimum performance needs to be elicited. The selection of an assessment domain must be made with reference to the interests, roles, and habits of the population on which the test is to be used. Motivation may be enhanced by allowing the individual some choice in the assessment activity to be performed. However, the benefits of individual choice have to be balanced against the requirements of standardisation.

PROBLEM-ORIENTATED CLINICAL REASONING PROCESS

Roberts (1996) states that 'in the process of clinical reasoning, there is usually a problem' and that 'the goal of the reasoning ... is to solve the problem' (p. 233). It should be remembered that in many instances in therapy, the product of a clinical reasoning process is not the definitive answer but a 'best guess'. Roberts acknowledges that [AHPs] cannot solve problems in the complete way that a mathematician solves a mathematical problem and acknowledges that 'there is not necessary a right answer to problems posed by humans who are ill' (p. 233). The problem-orientated clinical reasoning process is applied by AHPs to establish the *most likely cause* of the complex problems posed by their service users and to assist with the identification of the most appropriate intervention plan to attempt to address identified problems. Opacich (1991) has described six key steps, or stages, in a therapy *problem-orientated clinical reasoning process*:

1. problem setting (context)
2. framing the problem(s)
3. delineating the problem(s)
4. forming hypotheses
5. developing intervention plans
6. implementing treatment.

Diagnostic reasoning, as a component of clinical reasoning, primarily occurs during the first four stages of this process. These first four steps will now be described.

Problem Setting

Problem setting involves naming the phenomena/constructs that are to become the target of assessment. Defined problems are constructed from observed and reported problematic situations that are experienced by clients. Rarely in clinical practice do problems present themselves to the AHP as clear, obvious cause-and-effect relationships. These problematic situations can be puzzling, messy, and uncertain. The AHP needs to unravel the person's experience of a problematic situation in order to name the problem to be investigated. This involves selecting what will be perceived as the 'items' of the situation. The AHP then sets boundaries to focus the remit of the assessment and imposes upon it coherence that enables the statement of what is 'wrong' and how the problematic situation needs to be changed (Schon 1983).

Framing the Problem

This stage of framing the problem is where theory and conceptual frameworks play a key role. Framing the problem involves illuminating the problem(s) within a context (Opacich 1991). The process of framing involves the selection of an initial frame of reference to guide the AHP's reasoning. This is followed by the critique (see the section titled 'Step 3: Critical Appraisal of Assessment and Outcome Measures (Test Critique)' in Table 10.1 in Chapter 10) and selection of assessment tools designed to address the named constructs. The assessment tools selected should be consistent with the chosen theoretical framework (Rogers and Holm 1991). Assessment should be carefully structured in order to identify specific deficits/constructs. Constructs often are complicated, and it can be hard to discern whether dysfunction can be attributed to one or more constructs. This is why the AHP needs to select a frame of reference to structure the assessment and use sensitive, valid, and reliable measures in order to develop and test hypotheses about the relationships between dysfunction and underlying deficits/constructs. This process of beginning with a theory, or conceptual framework or a frame of reference, then proceeding to the formation of hypotheses, then selecting methods of assessment to collect data required to test the hypothesis is a deductive reasoning process (see earlier section and Figure 6.1).

Delineating the Problem

The stage of delineating a problem involves the implementation of the AHP's chosen assessment methods and strategies. AHPs often use multiple measures of performance and a range of data collection tools (see Chapter 2). Once data is collected, it is organised and categorised for interpretation. Standardised assessment should provide clear guidelines for the scoring and interpretation of data. With non-standardised assessments, the AHP should provide clear details and rationale for how data has been analysed.

Forming Hypotheses: Pattern Recognition, Hypotheses, and Heuristics

Earlier in this chapter, we drew your attention to the work of Fleming (1994), who found that the AHPs she studied utilised the three problem-solving methods that had been previously described by Newel and Simon (1972, as cited by Fleming 1994): 'recognition, generate and test and heuristic search' (p. 121). Recognition occurs to some degree when the AHP frames the problem. It occurs further when the AHP observes and selects cues related to the problem to help generate and test hypotheses. Payton (1985), who undertook research on clinical reasoning processes in a sample of 10 peer-designated expert physiotherapists, found they used a hypothetico-deductive model. Rivett and Higgs (1997), who undertook a comparative study with a small sample of 11 expert AHPs and 8 non-experts AHPs, reported that all AHPs in their sample generated hypotheses consistent with the use of hypothetico-deductive reasoning process.

Social perception is the process by which someone infers other people's motives and intentions from observing their behaviour and deciding whether the causes of the behaviour are internal or situational. Social perception helps people make sense of the world, organise their thoughts quickly, and maintain a sense of control over the environment. It helps people feel competent, masterful, and balanced as it helps people predict similar events in the future (Molden and Dweck 2006). AHPs will already have acquired skills in social perception before they even train to become therapists. During their training and subsequent clinical practice, AHPs draw upon and refine social perception processes to aid their assessment. AHPs need to develop a more refined process for identifying the likely causes of a client's observed behaviour or reported problems. This process involves hypothesis generation, testing, and the application of heuristics.

AHPs use hypotheses and heuristics to reduce the complex task of identifying the underlying causes of a client's problems to a simpler task. AHPs need to simplify the task because of the limits of working memory; 'working memory is the memory system component where active processing of information occurs ... several cognitive activities take place in working memory. These include encoding, rehearsal, recording/chunking and transfer of information to and from long term memory' (Carnevali et al. 1993, p. 18).

Encoding

Carnevali et al. (1993) state that 'accuracy and precision in encoding stimuli associated with one's professional practice is one dimension of clinical expertise and a necessary element of diagnostic reasoning and decision making' (p. 20). They describe how 'encoded bits of mental information coming in from sensory memory are further processed by assigning more precise meaning or interpretation to them' (p. 18). The AHP will be receiving multiple data into her working memory from all her sensory systems: vision, touch, smell, and hearing.

For example, suppose an AHP moves a client's arms through a passive range of movement and senses resistance in the client's muscle as they reach the outer range. AHPs use language to encode and they also link newly acquired data into systematic relations with previous knowledge. In the example above, the AHP might label the sensory data from the passive movements in terms of 'normal tone', 'stiffness', 'spasticity', or 'flaccidity'. AHPs can undertake encoding consciously when the sensory data received is unfamiliar and complex, but as they become more experienced, more and more encoding will become more automatic. So 'encoding expertise in [working memory] involves recognition of information from sensory memory and adequate professional language or imagery to further encode them' (p. 20).

Rehearsal

Rehearsal has been described as 'a mental recycling activity serving to retain stimuli in' working memory (Carnevali et al. 1993, p. 20). *Maintenance rehearsal* requires repeating information a number of times in order to help keep the information in working memory for a bit longer. For example, the AHP might rehearse a client's response to a test question, or goniometric measurements taken to assess range of movement. A second type of rehearsal is *Elaborative rehearsal*, which 'is a process reorganising new information using the information's meaning to help store and remember it' (p. 20). This is achieved by drawing on knowledge the AHP already has in their long-term memory and forming relationships with this previous knowledge and the current information in the working memory.

Recoding and chunking: The working memory only has a limited capacity. Most people can remember only between five to nine pieces of information at a time. These pieces of information are referred to as chunks. A chunk can comprise one item of information/data, or it can be formed of many related items of information. AHPs recode separate pieces of data by grouping them together and then remember this group of information as one chunk. Often, AHPs do this by grouping cues together linked to a recognised pattern. Pattern recognition is the AHP's ability to:

1. 'Observe a phenomenon
2. Identify significant characteristics (cues)
3. Perceive a relationship among cues (a configuration)
4. Compare a present configuration to a previously learned category or type (template)' (Fleming 1994, p. 145).

The recognition of patterns assists AHPs with the generation of hypotheses. There are two types of hypotheses generated by AHPs: familiar hypotheses retrieved from long-term memory that have been used before and proved successful in identifying a client's problem that was linked to the same pattern of cues; and new hypotheses generated when the AHP perceives this to be a novel situation. Fleming (1994) states that AHPs especially use heuristic search when new hypotheses are required or when they need to invent a particular solution for a client. She found that AHPs 'often use heuristic search method in the problem resolution phase of problem solving' (p. 147).

A *hypothesis* has been defined as a tentative explanation of the cause(s) of observed dysfunction (Rogers and Holm 1991). The delineation of the problem as a hypothesis involves the acquisition and interpretation of cues drawn from the assessment data.

A *heuristic* is a mental shortcut used in judgement and decision making. Heuristics have been defined as:

> *Involving or serving as an aid to learning, discovery, or problem-solving by experimental and especially trial-and-error methods. Also: of or relating to exploratory problem-solving techniques that utilize self-educating techniques (such as the evaluation of feedback) to improve performance.*

> https://www.merriam-webster.com/dictionary/heuristic)

Heuristics is a problem-solving technique in which the most appropriate solution is selected using rules. Usually, these are simplified rules used for processing information on a rule-of-thumb, trial-and-error basis. Heuristics help us to access information and make decisions more quickly because they reduce the amount of data to be processed, reduce processing time, move us beyond the presenting cue, and enrich the information accessed in the AHP's memory by inference. AHPs use heuristics as a problem-solving method by drawing upon what they have heard and seen in their past clinical practice to develop their own rules of thumb from how people with a particular diagnosis or problem have presented in the past and from what the underlying causes and solutions proved (Muoni 2012). Reoccurring patterns become embedded as rules of thumb, which are then accessed to help formulate hypotheses about the current client. The AHP reflects on the cues acquired and searches previous theoretical and experiential knowledge for rules of thumb, recognisable patterns, and metaphors to direct the formation of hypotheses.

Although heuristics can be very helpful, AHPs need to be aware that they can lead to suboptimal decision making, faulty beliefs, and systematic errors (Baron 2014). First, the formation of oversimplified categories can lead to stereotypes. Second, if a faulty belief underlies a rule of thumb used by an AHP, then significant and persistent biases will occur in the hypotheses you are likely to generate for particular client scenarios. One faulty belief relates to how common or frequent we perceive a particular client presentation, which we have formed as a category, to be.

The *availability heuristic* is a rule of thumb which occurs when people estimate the probability of an outcome based on how easy that outcome is to imagine (Searl et al. 2010). As such, vividly described, emotionally charged possibilities will be perceived as being more likely than those that are harder to picture or are difficult to understand, resulting in a corresponding cognitive bias. In clinical practice, a group of clients whose presenting features are readily available to the AHP's memory might appear to be more numerous than they really are. The events that easily come to mind might be judged more likely than they are. For example, a client falling at home and having to be readmitted after being assessed as fit for discharge by an AHP might lead to this AHP being overly cautious about the readiness of future clients for discharge because her perceived risk of falling in this client group is higher owing to this clearly remembered negative outcome. The availability of certain information may be biased because the AHP has had limited exposure to clients/interventions of a certain kind, or because the clients/outcomes are more remarkable and attract more attention, or because the AHP has stored the information in her memory in a particular fashion. The availability heuristic is of significance for AHPs and something we should be mindful of. When we are presented with a new client, we are more likely to match him to clients we have worked with recently because these cases are in our recent memory and easier to recall than clients treated a long time ago. Therefore, we will suppose his problems and related outcome will be similar to these easily recalled clients.

In addition, suppose a particular past client made a significant impression on us, for example, because the case was perplexing, or the outcome achieved was very positive or characteristics about the client resonated with us (they had the same hobby, liked the same television programme, looked like your Dad, etc.). This client will be more vivid in our long-term memory and will be easier to recall than less memorable clients.

We all have particular clients who *stick in our minds*, some because we really enjoyed working with them, others because they really challenged us and we struggled with their therapy. Because these clients are *memorable* and are easier to recall, the danger is that we will perceive the features of their presentation as being more common/frequent (Toft and Reynolds 2016). When we perceive the presentation of these cases to be more frequent, we are more likely to use them to generate rules of thumb, which then drive the development and analysis of clinical hypotheses. So if a new client has a couple of features that fit the heuristic generated by more recent and/or memorable clients, we will match the client in this category, and might ignore another set of features which would lead us to a category group that have a much rarer presentation. This is where standardised tests can help us, because a useful measure should address the full range of behaviours or presenting features under the domain of concern in equal measure, and such tests will prompt us to consider deficits that we might have only rarely seen or even never seen, such as ideational apraxia or colour agnosia.

Following the formation of a hypothesis, the AHP should conduct further assessment to test their hypothesis. This is the process of validating the hypothesis. Testing hypotheses helps to reduce the impact of bias. Care must be taken to be very objective during the hypothesis-testing process because a person is more likely to see what they expect to see (because they perceive it as more common and, therefore, more likely) and ignore data that refutes their beliefs. Cue interpretation and acquisition is often focused on the identification of confirmatory cues. AHPs also need to consider what behaviour would be observed if the hypothesis was false and then plan their further assessment to collect evidence to help confirm or refute the hypothesis, as well as considering what behaviour would be observed if the hypothesis was true. So when validating a hypothesis, you need to see if there are symptoms and signs that cannot be explained by your hypothesis and also think about whether your hypothesis would lead to the presence of any symptoms or signs that are not present in this case. The more discrete and targeted the tools and strategies used in the assessment, the easier it is for the AHP to test out their hypotheses and to make valid and reliable clinical decisions.

Standardised tests results can be used to help confirm or refute a hypothesis. For example, a standardised test might be selected to assist the evaluation of a hypotheses generated during an initial interview and/or from a review of presenting information such as a referral letter and medical notes. Standardised test results can also provide the cues that lead to further hypothesis generation. It is critical that standardised test results are used within the context of the whole assessment process and are not used for decision making in isolation. The AHP's clinical reasoning skills helps to both examine the test results in terms of the context in which they were obtained and apply them to the wider context of the client's presentation and situation. The test results need to be examined in the context of this particular client, tested in a particular test environment and at a particular time. A number of variables (fatigue, medication, test anxiety, motivation, time of day, distractions, etc.) could have influenced the obtained results. The results should also be examined alongside other client information, such as the client's self-report, informal observations, and proxy report. Consistencies or discrepancies that show up once data from different sources is triangulated are given particular attention during the diagnostic reasoning process. Some standardised assessments offer guidance to AHPs on how the test results should be interpreted and applied. For example, Abidin (1995) author of the Parenting Stress Index (PSI), provides interpretative guidelines in the PSI manual based on a combination of qualitative data drawn from clinical judgements and clinical literature (what he refers to as interpretations drawing upon the art of therapy) and quantitative data drawn from research conducted on the PSI and upon the relationship of individual PSI items to research outcomes reported in the child development literature (drawing upon science-based therapy). Abidin states that 'the interpretations suggested [for PSI scores] should be viewed as working hypotheses, the validity of which will need to be established by further inquiry with a particular parent' (p. 5).

Diagnostic reasoning produces a therapy diagnosis that reflects not just the pathology but also the observed performance deficit and the postulated causes of that deficit. A diagnosis (such as ideomotor apraxia resulting from stroke) formulated from formal neuropsychological testing tells neither the patient's exact pattern of functional deficit, nor his or her motivation and potential for independence. The flexibility provided by observational assessment allows the AHP to use judgement and improvisation in moving from theory to the requirements of a patient's unique experience. This produces a unique therapy diagnosis for each person.

Therapy Diagnosis

A diagnosis can be viewed in terms of both a process and a product (Rogers and Holm 1991) which moves forward 'from problem sensing to problem definition' (p. 1050), and the product of that reasoning. An occupational therapy diagnostic reasoning process refers to both the cognitive processes used by the practitioner to formulate a statement summarising the client's occupational status, and the outcome of that process, the diagnostic statement.

The therapy diagnosis can be presented as a *diagnostic statement*. This statement consists of four components: descriptive (functional problem) + explanatory (aetiology of the problem) + cue (signs and symptoms) + pathological (medical or psychiatric) (Rogers 1982, 2004).

Descriptive component: It should describe the specific deficits identified at each level of function that are impacting the person's ability to engage successfully in their chosen roles and activities. It articulates the identified problems that are addressed by either occupational therapy and/or physiotherapy. The descriptive component should name 'task disabilities, such as difficulty dressing, or social role dysfunctions, such as difficulty working as a seamstress'. Rogers (2004) clarifies that 'a task disability occurs at the level of individual tasks, while a social role dysfunction occurs at the level of social role, which is comprised of many tasks' (p. 18). (Note: For more information on assessment at different levels, refer to Chapter 11).

Explanatory component: The diagnosis should contain an explanatory component that indicates the AHP's hypothesis or hypotheses about the possible and most likely cause(s) of the defined problem described in the descriptive component. This is a very important aspect of the diagnostic statement because the cause of the problem may require a specific solution, and different therapy interventions will be selected for different causes of the same problem. A person's problem can be the result of an interaction between a number of impairments or hindrances, and so the AHP may need to list several causes in the explanatory component. Rogers (2004) provides a useful example: she explains how a dressing disability might be caused by (p. 18):

a. sensory impairment (e.g. low vision, paraesthesia);

b. physical impairment (e.g. limited movement or strength);

c. cognitive impairment e.g. apraxia, amnesia);

d. affective impairment (e.g. lack of motivation, fear of injury);

e. physical contextual hindrance (e.g. architectural barrier); or

f. social contextual hindrance (e.g. restrictive attitude of caregiver).

Cue Component: This identifies the observed and reported signs and symptoms that led the AHP to (a) conclude that there is a problem requiring therapy intervention and (b) hypothesise the nature and cause of the identified problem. A symptom is a condition that results from the problem. Data on *symptoms* is usually obtained through self-report and proxy data collection methods. For example, the client may tell the AHP, 'I can't reach to put on my socks and shoes' or a carer may explain, 'He gets in a muddle in the garden, he gets out the wrong tools for the job and I caught him pulling out well established plants the other day instead of the weeds'. Some clients or carers may be able to provide the AHP with a further explanation of why they have this problem: 'I can't put on my shoes as I'm too stiff and because it's too painful to stretch down' or 'He had such a good knowledge of plants and was such an avid gardener it must be because of his memory problems now he has dementia'.

In some cases, the AHP will wish to verify this explanation with an observation assessment method, and where the cause is unclear they will definitely need to undertake further assessment to elicit the underlying causes. This may include the use of standardised measures or setting up a task the client/carer has described as problematic and undertaking an informal observation to analyse the difficulty with performance. Data collected by the AHP using observational methods are referred to as *signs* (Rogers 2004). (Note: For more information on different methods of data collection, refer to Chapter 2.)

Pathologic component: This provides the pathological cause, if any, of the functional deficit (this part of the diagnosis often relates to, or is drawn from, the medical diagnosis). This is useful for AHPs because 'the nature of the pathology, the prognosis and pathology related contraindications establish parameters for ... therapy interventions' (Rogers 2004, p. 19). Interventions will be tailored not just to the underlying cause of the problem (as identified in the explanatory component of the diagnostic statement) but also by factors such as whether the person is terminally ill (diagnosis of cancer), has a long-term irreversible condition (diagnosis of dementia), or has curable illness (diagnosis of anxiety).

To illustrate the components of the diagnostic statement, two examples are provided below (Box 6.1). These two examples show how the same deficit and pathology can arise from different causes; both examples have the same descriptive and pathologic components (the client has had a stroke leading to dependence in dressing), but the cues leading to the explanatory component of the diagnosis are quite different and will lead on to different therapy interventions.

Rogers (2004) also provides an example of a diagnostic statement:

Mrs B ... is unable to prepare meals for herself (description) related to a memory deficit (explanatory) as evidenced by: her repeated requests for instructions; inability to remember salting the soup; failure to remove the soup when boiled; and burning the corner of the potholder (cues); caused by dementia of the Alzheimer's type (pathological). (p. 19)

In formulating the diagnosis, the AHP also considers the person's strengths, interests, and resources, and notes those physical and verbal prompts and cues that appear to facilitate function. Therefore, a therapy diagnosis is elaborate and is broader than the medical diagnosis as it also encompasses the person's physical and social environment, motives, and values. In addition to a diagnosis, the AHP formulates a prognosis in terms of projecting both the person's likely response to treatment and future functional ability.

Box 6.1   Examples of Diagnostic Statements

Therapy Diagnostic Statement Example 1: Mr A

Descriptive component:
Unable to get dressed independently.

Explanatory component:
Related to:

- reduced sensation in left upper limb
- reduced active range of motion in left upper limb
- spasticity in left upper limb

Cue component:
As evidenced by the following symptoms described by Mr A:

- 'My arm feels numb and heavy. If I concentrate really hard I can move it a little bit, but I can't feel things properly and I can't pick up fiddly things'.

As evidenced by the following signs identified through observational assessment:

- inability to identify objects through touch in left hand with eyes closed
- inability to report temperature or pinprick on left hand and arm on testing
- inability to move left elbow, wrist, and fingers through full range of motion on command
- inability to pick up and manipulate objects in left hand
- when left arm is moved through a passive range of movement, full range is present but resistance and increased tone are felt

Pathologic component:
Owing to a right Cerebral Vascular Accident (CVA)

Therapy Diagnostic Statement Example 2: Mrs B

Descriptive component:
Unable to get dressed independently.

Explanatory component:
Related to:

- left unilateral neglect

Cue component:
As evidenced by the following symptoms described by Mrs B:

- 'The nurse came along and said "Eat up Doris, you need a good meal" and I was annoyed because I had finished it all up and I said "What do you mean eat up – I've eaten it all up today" and she laughed and said "We're having a joke today are we? Have you finished then?" and then I felt really cross because I wasn't joking around and I said again "I've eaten it all up!" So then the nurse looked thoughtful and she said very seriously, "I'm not joking Doris so bear with me. Before I take your plate away can you take another look and tell me whether you see any food left on your plate?" I felt confused and annoyed because it seemed such a stupid question, but she's a nice girl you know and she was so serious, so I thought I'd humour her. I took another look and when I replied "Of course not!" she said "Oh" and then moved my plate a bit and told me to look again, and do you know what? I'd left some food after all – I think I'm going mad!'

As evidenced by the following signs identified through observational assessment:

- ignores objects to the left of the midline
- does not attempt to dress left side of the body
- puts both sleeves on right arm

Pathologic component:
Owing to a right CVA

The formation of a working diagnosis is just the beginning of the therapeutic journey with a client. As the AHP implements the chosen interventions and management strategies, they review their original therapy diagnosis in light of the client's response to the intervention. If the chosen interventions do not remedy the problem, they may decide to revisit the hypothesis and double-check that they had discovered all the relevant signs and symptoms during their initial diagnostic reasoning process. They may generate and test alternative hypotheses to explain the client's problem and try interventions linked to these alternative hypotheses to see if these deliver the desired outcome. In complex cases, the AHP may need to revisit the diagnostic reasoning process several times before they are convinced that they have identified the correct cause(s) of the client's problem *and* have selected the best intervention to address this underlying cause.

OTHER FORMS OF REASONING

As part of the assessment process, AHPs need to learn about people's individual experiences of their illness or disability. In the underlying philosophies of allied health professions, every individual is perceived as a unique person. This philosophy needs to be borne out in practice. Therefore, AHPs need to take a person-centred approach to understand the unique way in which diagnoses impact the lives of the people who receive therapy. Two people may be of the same age, sex, socio-economic background and have the same diagnosis, but their experiences of, and responses to, that diagnosis may be completely different. Consequently, AHPs need to engage in assessment and intervention in a phenomenological way. With a phenomenological approach, a person's experience of his body is inseparable from his experience of the whole world, and disability is viewed as an interruption or injury to a whole life (Mattingly and Fleming 1994). Therefore, the AHP needs to assess a person in the context of how he did, does, and hopes to live his life. Assessment is used to provide an understanding of a person in terms of his daily practices, life history, social relationships, and long term-goals and plans, that give him meaning in his life and his self-identity (Mattingly and Fleming 1994). In order to obtain this complex image of a person, and understand the impact of the diagnosis on his functioning, AHPs need to engage in several types of clinical reasoning during the assessment process. Mattingly and Fleming (1994) found that 'AHPs shift rapidly from one type of reasoning to another' (p. 18). They explain how:

> *The reasoning style employed changes as the AHP's attention is drawn from one aspect of the problem to another. AHPs process or analyse different aspects of the problem, almost simultaneously, using different thinking styles but do not lose track of their thoughts about other aspects of a problem as those components are temporarily shifted to the background and another aspect is dealt with immediately in the foreground (p. 18).*

Fleming (Mattingly and Fleming 1994) described this ability to utilise multiple modes of reasoning as 'the [AHP] with the three-track mind' (p. 119). She identified three distinct forms of reasoning which she labelled as procedural reasoning (this has been described briefly earlier in this chapter), interactive reasoning, and conditional reasoning. Other types of reasoning of particular relevance to assessment processes described by other authors include narrative reasoning (Mattingly and Fleming 1994), pragmatic reasoning (Schell and Schell 2008), and ethical reasoning. Although the forms of reasoning identified in the literature have some distinct strategies or components, there is some overlap between different types of reasoning as described by these different authors, and the following types of clinical reasoning are not mutually exclusive.

INTERACTIVE REASONING

AHPs require very interactive and collaborative relationships between the AHP and the client. Interactive reasoning occurs during the AHP's face-to-face interactions with clients and is used to create the collaborative therapeutic relationship. Other types of reasoning, such as procedural reasoning are usually factually based; by contrast, interactive reasoning is often intuitive (Unsworth 1999). Creating an effective collaborative relationship is a very skilled process that requires an AHP to evaluate a wide range of cues to understand the client's motives, meanings, and what he wants from therapy (Mattingly and Fleming 1994). Therapy involves an active 'doing with' process, as opposed to a passive 'doing to' process. This 'doing with' clients means that AHPs encourage and allow the person to do as much as he can for himself. The AHP creates a relationship that empowers the client to stretch himself; this is achieved by staying near to the client, coaching, encouraging, prompting, and cueing and only offering physical assistance when required. During assessment, the AHP needs to assess both what the client is capable of doing and what the client is willing to do. At times, the AHP may appear to be sitting back 'doing nothing' during an observational assessment, but much negotiation may have led to this point, and active observation and clinical reasoning will be underway as the AHP sits back while the client attempts the agreed activity or task. Mattingly and Fleming (1994) explain:

> *They often do not seem to be actually doing something themselves but are 'doing with' the client to help them in the transition from dependent patient to (as they say) 'independent living'. Doing with the patient also means having patients practice exercises in the hospital during times when they are not being seen by the AHP. Clients are asked to take an active role in their treatment. (p. 179)*

CONDITIONAL REASONING

Mattingly and Fleming (1994) perceive conditional reasoning as 'a complex form of social reasoning' that is used by AHPs 'to help the patient in the difficult process of reconstructing a life that is now permanently changed by injury or disease' (p. 17). In their studies of AHPs' reasoning, they saw how this 'reasoning style moves beyond specific concerns about the person and the physical problems and places them in broader social and temporal contexts' (p. 18). They selected the term 'conditional' because they perceived AHPs were thinking about 'the whole condition, including the person, the illness, the meanings the illness has for the person, the family, and the social and physical contexts in which the person lives' (p. 18). Unsworth (1999) noticed that Mattingly and Fleming (1994) utilise the term *conditional* in three different ways when discussing the AHP's reasoning:

1. Conditional reasoning involves the AHP reflecting on the whole condition; this includes the client's illness or problem, the meaning the client and his family attach to this illness, and the client's whole context.

2. The AHP imagines how the condition could change, both positively and negatively, and thinks about what this might mean for the client. These imagined outcomes are conditional to other factors and may or may not be achieved.

3. The AHP considers about whether or not the imagined outcomes can be achieved and understands 'that this is conditional on both the client's participation in the therapy program and the shared construction of the future image' (Unsworth 1999, p. 61).

Conditional reasoning has some overlap with both narrative reasoning (Mattingly and Fleming 1994) and pragmatic reasoning (Schell and Schell 2008), both of which will be briefly discussed below.

NARRATIVE REASONING

Narrative reasoning is used by AHPs to help them make sense of the illness experience of their clients, and is so named because it involves thinking in story form (Schell and Schell 2008). Through narrative reasoning, the AHP 'uses story making and story telling to assist ... in understanding the meaning of disability or disease to the client' (Unsworth 1999, p. 48). Narrative thinking is orientated to making sense of human experience in terms of understanding motives (Duncan 2011). Therefore, the AHP is very much interested in the person's struggle to engage in his everyday activities and roles as an arthritic person. In order to help solve the problems faced by this person with arthritis in his unique physical and social environment, the AHP must not only understand the condition of arthritis but must also seek to understand the particular situation of the individual. People's personal narratives are a key part of their identity (Smith 2006) and are of critical importance to an AHP trying to undertake a comprehensive, client-centred assessment. AHPs are encouraged to seek narratives from their clients because the person's construction of his situation enriches the AHP's understanding of:

- how the client experiences the condition;
- how the lived experience of the condition is shaping and constraining the client's day-to-day experiences;
- how other key people, such as family members, have reacted to the person since he developed this condition;
- how experiencing the condition has changed the person's priorities; and
- what solutions are desired by the client.

Client Stories

Through narrative reasoning, the AHP is empowering the person as the expert in his own story. Smith (2006) recommends: 'If we listen from the not-knowing position, people's stories will emerge as they begin to trust us. Through this transformative process, their stories lead us as AHPs to what is important to the individual. It is a process in opposition to the process of labelling, which leads to us seeing people in terms of only one or two categories'. He goes on to suggest that when the client's 'story has emerged, we have to let the person pick it up and make the process of doing and becoming his or her own. We do not create our clients' future lives, but we make space within which they can create their lives for themselves ... good therapy is not about observation but about negotiation, leading to interaction, shared memories and co-creation' (Smith 2006, p. 307). This is how AHPs use narrative reasoning beyond the assessment process to help clients engage in the therapeutic process. Hammell (2004) suggests that we often work with individuals whose life stories are so severely disrupted that they cannot imagine what their lives will look like. For many clients who experience disability as the result of an accident or the sudden onset of an illness, such as a heart attack or stroke, this unexpected onset/accident can make them feel like their life to all intents and purposes has ended. The AHP works to help the person see that this is not the end to his life, but rather the marking of the end of a chapter in his life story. The process of rehabilitation can be like turning to a fresh page to start a new chapter. The plot has taken a dramatic and often unexpected turn, but the story still goes on, and the unexpected can lead to positive as well as negative changes if the person can be helped to face the future with optimism and creativity. AHPs interweave treatment goals and interventions based on activities that have meaning for their clients to assist their clients to start to imagine what their lives could be in the future. Mattingly and Fleming (1994) describes how AHPs 'reason about how to guide their therapy with particular patients by using images of where the patient is now, and where this patient might be at some future time when the patient will be discharged' (p. 240).

To move the person through a therapeutic process from his current ability to a position of greater ability, the AHP needs more than the 'know-how to do a set of tasks'. The AHP rather needs to able to conceptualise a 'temporal whole' that captures the continuum from seeing the person as he functions at the beginning of the therapeutic story to the desired outcome, by imaginatively anticipating what the person could be in the future. Mattingly refers to this as a *prospective treatment story* (p. 241). This prospective treatment story helps the AHP to organise the tasks and activities that will form the intervention and to sell these tasks and activities to the client as worthy of engagement. In her research examining the clinical reasoning of AHPs, Mattingly and Fleming (1994) found that these prospective stories 'were useful not because they were completely accurate predictions of what would happen, but because they were plausible enough to give AHPs a starting point' (p. 242). Mattingly notes:

> *The clinical stories AHPs projected onto new situations often ran into trouble because the new situation was often resistant to the mould. Clinical practice is idiosyncratic enough and illness experiences are contextually specific enough that stories created from other times and for other patients often fall short in providing ideal guides to new situations. While clinical stories are rarely ever applied wholesale – the AHP is always tinkering, always improvising to make the fit appropriate ... (pp. 242–243)*

As the AHP engages with the client through interventions, they engage in informal assessment of the client's responses to their treatment approach. They may also undertake formal evaluation of progress. During this re-assessment, the AHP may find that their prospective treatment story does not fully fit the actual unfolding therapeutic story with this particular client. When AHPs experience a misfit between their original prospective story and the unfolding story, Mattingly found that 'they would revise the story accordingly, redirecting therapeutic interventions so that they were more in line with what was actually unfolding' (p. 242). However, this readjustment of the story is not always sufficient to achieve the desired outcome. In these cases, Mattingly found that 'AHPs experience the anxiety and frustration of falling out of the story, of losing their way' (p. 242). When this happens, AHPs find that their prospective story for this client 'no longer makes sense', and they start to 'lose faith in their strategies and plans for the patient because the outcomes are too far afield from the ones they consider desirable' (p. 243).

Not all therapeutic stories have 'happy endings'; as an AHP we have 'success stories' we like to share with our colleagues and students, but we also have our 'failures' – the clients where we failed to build rapport, or where the problem remained elusive, or the chosen interventions did not deliver the desired outcomes. These are the cases where our attempts to revise the prospective story, to mould it to this client, did not work out. In such cases, Mattingly and Fleming (1994) discovered:

> *If AHPs were … never able to locate and enact a story they considered clinically meaningful, the stories they told retrospectively were often explorations or justifications for who was to blame. When things go wrong in therapy… AHPs are no longer narrators with their images of the ending well in tow. Through difficult and unexpected turns in the therapeutic process, AHPs become readers of the story … they struggle to understand what has gone wrong and, sometimes, what another story might be that could substitute for the one they have had to abandon. (p. 243)*

These problematic clinical stories are the ones from which we have much to learn. These are the stories we should pay particular attention to and reflect upon and puzzle over. The clinical stories where we felt muddled and frustrated are useful to share with our peers and supervisors. So we can learn as much from what does not work as from what does, and also learn from the experience of others so that when faced with a similar client we do not construct the same unsuccessful prospective story as our starting point. Later in this chapter, we discuss the importance of reflective practice, and Box 6.4 provides a *Clinical Story Analysis Format* that may help you to write down and reflect upon a problematic clinical story of your own.

AHPs Sharing Stories

Another aspect of narrative reasoning relates not to how the AHP and client share stories, but to how AHPs share stories with each other. Health professionals often exchange stories about patients to assist in learning (Greenhalgh 2006). This sharing of stories among AHPs, in departments and staff rooms, has two important functions, the first being the method used by AHPs to puzzle out a problem. The problem might relate to how to engage a patient in therapy, the intervention to select, or figuring out the nature of underlying deficits that are impacting observed functional problems. AHPs will informally discuss cases over coffee or lunch as a way of figuring out things in their own mind, but also to seek help in an informal manner; 'I saw a patient this morning and …' Their colleagues often respond through storytelling: 'I had a patient like that and what I did was' or 'When I had a patient with … what worked was …'. Through these stories, AHPs offer each other suggestions, strategies, and solutions.

Second, sharing stories is a way to enlarge each AHP's fund of practical knowledge by vicariously sharing other AHPs' experience … these stories form a bond between AHPs and also teach them much more than they could learn in a classroom or through their own personal experience.

PRAGMATIC REASONING

Pragmatic reasoning relates to the AHP's clinical practice setting and personal context. Pragmatic reasoning is how the AHP obtains an understanding about how the personal context and the practice setting impact the assessment and treatment processes are implemented. It takes into account organisational, political, and economic constraints and opportunities that place boundaries around the assessment and treatment that an AHP may undertake in a particular practice environment (Unsworth 1999). The content of an AHP's pragmatic reasoning related to their practice setting may include:

- the availability of assessment and treatment resources;
- time limitations owing to their caseload and the priorities placed by other clients on their current caseload;
- the culture of the organisation within which they work;
- power relationships with their supervisor, manager, other AHPs, and across members of the multidisciplinary team;
- trends in clinical practice within their profession; and
- financial issues and constraints, for example, to pay for equipment, adaptations, placements, or services that may benefit the client.

The personal context which an AHP brings to their practice also plays a part in their pragmatic reasoning; this might include thinking related to their:

- clinical competence and confidence undertaking particular assessment procedures or interventions;
- preferences; these can include preferences for working with particular types of clients, or for working in particular environments (such as the therapy department versus the client's own home) or for working with particular colleagues (for example, having a very collaborative and mutually respectful relationship with nursing staff but feeling undermined by the physician in charge);
- level of commitment to the job and profession; and
- work life versus home life balance and the demands faced outside of work (for example, a child is sick and partner was unhappy about missing work to take care of their child).

Higgs et al. (2008) discuss how personal issues can drive clinical decisions on a daily basis, and call this 'the problem space' – 'Practitioners bring their personal and professional selves to the task of clinical decision making; these selves frame their problem space' (p. 13). Schell (2013) explained how personal issues can drive clinical decisions on a daily basis:

For instance, if a practitioner does not feel safe in helping a client stand or transfer to a bed, he or she is more likely to use table-top based activities. (p. 391)

So, in an assessment process, this AHP might opt for a bottom-up approach using a standardised battery of tests that can be administered at a table to explore performance component functioning, as opposed to a top-down approach that might involve observing the person undertake the activities that were of most importance to him, such as mobilising from his bed to the bathroom, transferring on and off the toilet, and toileting independently. Schell (2013) suggests that:

A [] practitioner may feel uncomfortable interacting with individuals who have depression and, therefore, might be quick to suggest that such clients are not motivated for therapy. (p. 391)

In this example, we see how the hypothesis selected by the AHP to explain the client's presentation is one related to motivation as opposed to a hypothesis related to low mood as the causal factor. In examining this hypothesis, the AHP's pragmatic reasoning is likely to guide them subconsciously towards cues that support their hypothesis related to the client's lack of volition and ignore cues that would point to a problem with depression. Finally, Schell (2013) offers the example of an AHP who:

has a young family to go home to might opt not to schedule clients late in the day so as to get home as early as possible. (p. 391)

In this example, we might find the AHP who phones a community-based client for monitoring and discovers the situation has worsened deciding that a home visit is not necessary that day and can be delayed until tomorrow. Alternatively, if they decide a face-to-face assessment is required today and perceives that this might involve complicated factors and a time-consuming visit, they may decide to refer to an out-of-hours crisis intervention team, even though that team are not familiar with their client. Another example is a hospital AHP who on undertaking an initial assessment towards the end of the working day decides to administer a brief screening test rather than lengthier standardised test battery even though the presenting information and initial interview point towards the more rigorous battery being necessary.

It is challenging to be consciously aware of how pragmatic reasoning shapes our decisions. However, if we truly want to act in the best interests of our clients, as opposed to the best interests of ourselves and/or our employing organisations, then we need to practice the art of reflection and look critically at the underlying reasoning behind our clinical decisions. However, although pragmatic reasoning may lead to actions that are not in the best interests of the client, it can be very useful in helping us to answer practical questions that shape our therapy positively; these include:

- Who referred this client for therapy and, why was this referral made?
- Who is paying for this treatment, and what are their expectations of the outcome of therapy?
- What family/carer support does the client have, what are these people's expectations and abilities, and can they provide resources (practical support, physical help, encouragement, finances) to assist with the client's intervention?
- How much time will I have to work with this client?
- What clinical and client-based environments are available for therapy and what standardised tests, equipment, and adaptations can I access to support the therapeutic process?
- What are the expectations of my manager, supervisor, and multidisciplinary colleagues?
- What are my clinical competencies, and will these be sufficient to provide the client with the therapy they need?

Source: Adapted from Schell 2013, Table 30.1, p. 389: Aspects of Reasoning in Occupational Therapy.

ETHICAL REASONING/MORAL REASONING

Bushby et al. (2015) highlighted a breadth of ethical tensions that have implications for practice, education, policy, and research, such as resource and systemic issues; upholding ethical principles and values; client safety; working with vulnerable clients; interpersonal conflicts; upholding professional standards; and practice management. Barnitt (1993) noted that ethics, morals, ethical reasoning, and moral reasoning are used interchangeably in the literature, and she offered some helpful definitions (p. 402):

> ***Ethics*** refers to identifiable statements about norms and values, used to guide professional practice. Codes of conduct, ethical guides, and guides to standards in professional practice are examples of this. Professional ethics are the rules and recommendations about appropriate behaviour in clinical work.
>
> ***Moral reasoning*** refers to a more philosophical enquiry about norms and values, about ideas of right and wrong, and about how AHPs make moral decisions in professional work. Moral issues have to be resolved through reflective thinking and problem solving because guideline to ethics cannot cope with specific instances.

Schell uses the term *ethical reasoning* and describes this as thinking that is concerned with the question of 'what should be done?' (Schell 2013, p. 391). Schell perceives that AHPs engage in ethical reasoning to help them to select morally defensible course of action, especially when faced with competing interests. Examples of the types of value-laden questions which AHPs try to address through ethical reasoning are the following:

- What are the benefits and risks to the person related to service provision, and do the benefits warrant the risks?
- In the face of limited time and resources, what is the fairest way to prioritize care?
- How can I balance the goals of the person receiving services with those of the caregiver, when they don't agree?
- What should I do when other members of the treatment team are operating in a way that I feel conflict with the goals of the person receiving services?

In this chapter, we have explored various types of clinical reasoning. We have seen how different modes of reasoning are undertaken for different purposes or in response to particular features of a problem or interaction with the client (Mattingly and Fleming 1994). These different types of reasoning are not undertaken in a sequential manner, but are interwoven during the complex thinking that the AHP engages in as they engage with a client during assessment and re-assessment. The AHP must draw together the thinking that results from these various modes of reasoning to form a coherent understanding of the patient and of what the therapy will be (Kielhofner 2009, pp. 284–287). The ability to pull together, synthesise, and make sense of the myriad pieces of information (from the referral, the client, the carer, and other colleagues) and marry these with standardised test results and informal observations is what AHPs learn through 'doing' therapy over time; expertise comes with practice.

This is why clinical placements form such a critical part of any AHP's education, and why ongoing reflection on practice is so important for any qualified AHP who wants to develop and improve their clinical skills. To reflect upon clinical reasoning involves metacognitive analysis – that is, engagement in 'thinking about thinking' (Schell 2013, p. 384). Finding a language to explain and un-package your clinical reasoning helps you to become a more insightful AHP and helps your students and colleagues to learn from your experience and expertise.

REFLECTIVE PRACTICE

All AHPs need to engage in reflective practice to ensure that what they are doing, and why they have made decisions to do this, is supported as far as possible by the evidence base and that this leads to safe and effective practice. Schon (1983, 1987) considered reflection to be a critical part of developing expertise in clinical practice and clinical decision making. His work has been drawn upon by both occupational therapy writers (such as Kielhofner 2009; Mattingly and Fleming 1994; Unsworth 1999) and physiotherapy writers (such as Larin et al. 2005; White 2004). Schon (1983) differentiated between 'reflection *in* action', which occurs while the AHP is engaged in an encounter with a client – this is thinking on one's feet (White 2004) – and 'reflection *on* action', which is a retrospective process that occurs after the therapeutic encounter when the AHP pauses to interpret and analyse what has occurred.

An AHP needs to draw from the evidence base as well as from theory and relate both to her practice. Swain (2004) defines reflective practice as 'the capacity of [an AHP] to think, talk or write about a piece of practice with the intention to review or research a piece of practice with clients for new meanings or perspectives on the situation' (p. 217). Taylor (2010) defines reflective practice from a number of health professionals' perspectives and use in practice, describing that it is not just about thinking individually, but also communicated and shared with others through conversation and written documents. Tate (2004) provides a simple figure for the reflective learning cycle (see Figure 6.3).

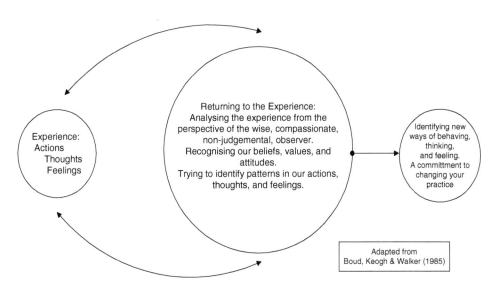

FIGURE 6.3   The Reflective Learning Cycle. *Source*: Tate and Sills (2004). © 2004, Westminster Research.

Tate adapted Figure 6.3 from work by Boud et al. (1985, e-book 2013). Boud and colleagues noted that experience alone is not sufficient for learning and posed the following questions:

- What is it that turns experience into learning?
- What specifically enables people to gain the maximum benefit from the situations they find themselves in?
- How can people apply their experience in new contexts?

They suggested that structured reflection is the key to learning from experience. They were particularly interested in the application of reflection during training. They linked the timing of reflective activities to the three stages in experience-based learning: preparation, engagement, and processing and highlighted the importance of including reflective activity at each stage. During the preparatory phase, students are prompted to examine what is required of them and consider the demands of their clinical placement site. During their experiences on placement, students are encouraged to process a variety of inputs arising from their clinical practice. Finally, once back in the academic setting, students are given time to consider and consolidate what they have experienced on placement (Boud et al. 1985).

Reflection, in both students and qualified AHPs, is undertaken all the time during interactions with clients as they make adjustments to their assessment approach and treatments based on feedback from the client and the clinical reasoning that draws upon their tacit knowledge and skills. Sometimes, this tacit reflection is made explicit when students/AHPs have to discuss decision making about a client, for example, with their supervisor, their student, or another member of the multidisciplinary team. However, the speed of decision making required during interactions with clients does not provide the 'time out' required for an AHP or student to reflect deeply on what they are doing. This is why students and AHPs need time outside of their day-to-day practice to think more deeply about what they are doing and why they are doing it. Reflection on action, therefore, requires a student/clinician to make time to step back from a particular client–AHP interaction, case, or experience in order to reflect upon and question their decisions, feelings, and actions. Being a reflective practitioner should make the AHP take a long hard look at the why, what, and how of a particular aspect of their practice, the way they handled a specific case or a significant incident, because in order to be most beneficial, reflection requires exploring taken-for-granted assumptions (Taylor 2010, p. 69).

Thomas et al. (2014) introduce how social constructivism, in very simple terms, is a viewpoint in which knowledge is not purely objective, but is at least partly socially constructed, and where the learner is an active participant. Social constructivism 'focuses on how individuals come to construct and apply knowledge in socially mediated contexts …, and supports the acquisition of cognitive processing strategies, self-regulation, and problem solving through socially constructed learning opportunities all of which are critical skills for evidence-based knowledge uptake and implementation in clinical practice' (p. 3). When AHPs use social constructivism to support reflection at a personal level, it can help to examine the beliefs and values they bring to their practice for signs of stereotypical thinking or prejudice. At a professional level, it can provide a framework for evaluating theories and models of practice in terms of their potential to oppress or marginalise people.

Reflective Practice as a Component of Continuing Professional Development

The requirement for undertaking and documenting continuing professional development (CPD) for registration to practice as AHPs has existed for some time (Westcott and Whitcombe 2012). In the United Kingdom, the Health and Care Professions Council (HCPC) guidelines on standards for Continuing Professional Development list reflective practice as an example of a work-based learning CPD activity (https://www.hcpc-uk.org/standards/standards-of-continuing-professional-development).

There are a number of ways in which reflection can be documented; these include diary entries, reflective journals, significant incident analyses, case analyses, clinical stories, and notes from supervision, mentorship, or peer reflection sessions. A good place to keep such reflections is in your portfolio of continuing development. Reflective journals are used across a number of health professions. Nursing, occupational therapy, and physiotherapy educators all use reflective journals to encourage their students to think about past experiences, current situations, and expected outcomes of their actions in order to assist students to find a language for explaining what they do in the clinical setting and why. Guidelines for structuring a reflective journal entry or for undertaking a significant incident analysis, either alone or in a group setting, are provided below.

As an AHP, you can be extremely busy and may not have time to stop and reflect immediately after a significant incident; unless you have an excellent memory, it can be very useful to jot a few key facts and feelings down in your diary as soon as possible and then complete a significant incident analysis later. Bassot (2016, p. 28) suggests a structure for reflecting writing.

Stage 1 Reflection
- Write freely and spontaneously to capture your thoughts.

Stage 2 Analysis – Ask yourself:
- What is happening here?
- What assumptions am I making?
- What does show about my underlying beliefs about my practice and myself?
- What are some of the alternative ways of looking at this?

Stage 3 Action
- What action can I take?
- How can I learn from what has happened?
- How would I respond if this situation occurred again?
- What does this experience tell me about my beliefs about my practice and myself?

Similar questions are posed by Larin et al. (2005) in their guidelines for physiotherapy students writing a weekly reflective journal entry while on clinical placement. These are provided in Box 6.2.

The reflective diary entry headings provide a useful process for teams or groups of people who have shared a significant experience or incident to follow to guide reflection and help the team/group to identify lessons and any actions or changes that they should make (see Box 6.3).

Box 6.2 Guidelines for Writing a Reflective Journal

1. Describe the learning event, issue, or situation. Describe prior knowledge, feelings, or attitudes with new knowledge, feelings, or attitudes.

What happened?

2. Analyse the learning event, issue, or situation in relation to prior knowledge, feelings, or attitudes.

What was your reaction to the learning event, issue, or situation? Your response may include cognitive and emotional reactions. Why did it happen?

3. Verify the learning event, issue, or situation in relation to prior knowledge, feelings, or attitudes.

What is the value of the learning event, issue, or situation that has occurred? Is the new knowledge, feeling, or attitude about the learning event, issue, or situation correct?

4. Gain a new understanding of the learning event, issue, or situation.

What is your new understanding of the learning event, issue, or situation?

5. Indicate how the new learning event, issue, or situation will affect future behaviour. Determine the clarification of an issue, the development of a skill, or the resolution of a problem.

How will you approach the same or similar event, issue, or situation in the future?

Source: Adapted from Larin et al. (2005).

Box 6.3 After Action Review Process

Step 1: Fix a time for the review – allow at least 20–30 minutes
Step 2: At the start of the review, propose some ground rules, for example:

- Everyone's experience is valid, irrespective of status in the organisation.
- Don't hold back, share what you saw, heard, and experienced.
- No 'thin skins' – don't take anything personally, focus on the impact of the experience on the team/group.
- Propose changes – what could be done differently or better?

Step3: Work through the basic questions of the After Action Review. Ask each person to make brief notes on:

- What was supposed to happen?
- What actually happened?
- What accounts for the difference?

Step 4: Taking each question in turn, ask each person present to comment, and note down the points on which most people agree on a flip chart.
Step 5: When all the questions have been dealt with, ask:

- 'What could we do differently next time?'

Note any ideas and actions which are feasible and which you agree could improve practice.

Step Six: Close the meeting, thank everyone for their input, and give all participants in the process a copy of the results.

Writing and analysing case studies and clinical stories can be very useful for helping you to undertake reflection *on* action. Mattingly and Fleming (1994) provide a number of case examples and clinical stories throughout the text; they also provide an 'Appendix of Clinical Stories' (pp. 343–359) which have been written by different AHPs. Each clinical story is followed by some discussion questions to prompt reflection. Unsworth (1999) also structures much of her text around case studies, through which AHPs' reasoning related to the evaluation and intervention of a range of cognitive and perceptual dysfunctions is explored. Box 6.4 provides a Clinical Story Analysis Format to help you write and reflect on a clinical story of your own.

There are advantages and disadvantages to undertaking reflective activities individually or with colleagues in pairs or groups and between unsupervised and supervised reflection (Tate 2004). These advantages and disadvantages are presented in Table 6.1.

Reflective practice has been seen as an individual or small group activity undertaken by professionals. In a healthcare environment in which systematic and embedded service user and carer involvement is being increasingly highlighted as essential to good practice, the involvement of service users in your reflective activities should be implemented.

Box 6.4   Clinical Story Analysis Format

1. **Identification of Themes**
    (a) Develop a descriptive title for the client's point of view.
    (b) Develop a descriptive title for the AHP's point of view.
    (c) Who is constructing the plot? What are they doing to emplot (make the story 'come true')?
    (d) Describe the motives and morals, desires and passions reflected in the story.
    (e) Discuss the following:
        (i.) Does the story explain and/or blame or not explain and blame?
        (ii.) Does the story take credit or not take credit?
    (f) Does revision take place? If so, describe the process.

2. **Action and Inquiry**
    - What are the puzzles/questions being worked upon?
    - What actions make a pivotal point – insights/inferences promoted by the AHP or client?
    - Describe action and reaction clusters, together with reciprocity of action on the part of each.
    - Describe the revisions made in the therapeutic process as a result of inquiry.
    - Describe the inquiry which resulted from action, and vice versa.

This story analysis format has been taken from a handout used with occupational therapy students at in the Occupational Therapy Program at Washington University School of Medicine, St. Louis, United States. The handout was developed by colleagues Karen Barney and Christine Berg in 1991.

TABLE 6.1   Advantages and disadvantages of different methods of critical reflection.

Method	Advantages	Disadvantages
Unsupervised		
Individual	• Not threatening • Can be undertaken according to individual needs • May enable greater honesty • Concentrates on personal issues	• More difficult to challenge self • Have only one world perspective • May become negative • May deceive oneself
Pairs	• More than one world perspective • Can feel supported • Can provide a more objective view of the experience	• May collude rather than challenge • Need to consider another person when engaging in the process
Group	• Many world perspectives • Have a support group when initiating action • Can learn from the experiences of others	• Need to adhere to ground rules • May be scapegoated • 'Cliques' may develop
Supervised		
Individual	• Can be undertaken according to individual needs • May enable greater honesty • Concentrates on personal issues • Can be undertaken according to individual needs • Benefit from the experience of a facilitator (see pp. 7 and 8) • May be more motivating for supervisee	• May respond to please the facilitator • Need to find a personal facilitator • Need to trust and respect the facilitator • May be costly
Pairs	• More than one world perspective • Can feel supported • Can provide a more objective view of the experience • Benefit from the experience of a facilitator • May be more motivating for supervisee	• Need to consider another person when engaging in the process • May respond to please the facilitator • Need to find a personal facilitator • Need to trust and respect the facilitator • May be costly
Group	• Many world perspectives • Have a support group when initiating action • Can learn from the experiences of others • Benefit from the experience of a facilitator • Less costly than individual supervision • May be more motivating for supervisee	• Need to adhere to ground rules • May be scapegoated • 'Cliques' may develop • Need to consider another when engaging in the process • May respond to please the facilitator • Need to find a personal facilitator • Need to trust and respect the facilitator • Participants may be at different developmental stages • Personal needs may not be the priority for the group

Source: Tate and Sills (2004). © 2004, Westminster Research.

COGNITIVE DISSONANCE

Finally, in this discussion about reasoning, reflection, and decision making, it is important to draw your attention to cognitive dissonance (Thomas et al. 2014). We do not like to have inconsistencies between our attitudes/beliefs and our behaviours. When this happens, we experience an uncomfortable feeling known as cognitive dissonance. Cognitive dissonance is a psychological phenomenon first identified by Leon Festinger (1962). It occurs when there is a discrepancy between what a person believes knows and values and persuasive information that calls these into question. The discrepancy causes psychological discomfort, and the mind adjusts to reduce the discrepancy. This leads some people who feel dissonance to seek information that will reduce dissonance and avoid information that will increase dissonance. People who are involuntarily exposed to information that increases dissonance are likely to discount that information, by either ignoring it, misinterpreting it, or denying it. Cognitive dissonance can affect our judgement and decision making (Toft and Reynolds 2016). One way of dealing with dissonance is to change our viewpoint. However, changing our views to agree with another persons can be very problematic in clinical situations and can work to the disadvantage of the client.

For example, an AHP may find that their views, beliefs, or assessment results in conflict with those of other members of the department or multidisciplinary team. Cognitive dissonance is likely to occur under these circumstances, particularly if they are less experienced or less qualified than their colleagues. Changing their views/beliefs/conclusions by deferring to the superiority of senior colleagues, such as a consultant or senior AHP, will help to reduce the feeling of dissonance. To justify such a change, they may rationalise that the senior colleague has more experience, greater qualifications, is wiser, and/or is further up the organisational hierarchy and responsible for their supervision/management. This type of reasoning is known as *argument from authority*, and it is a type of inductive reasoning. An argument from authority draws a conclusion about the truth of a statement based on the proportion of true propositions provided by that same source. It has the same form as a prediction. Therefore, if the AHP has found 99% of the claims of authority by their senior colleague to have been true, then they infer that there is a 99% probability that this claim of authority from the same colleague is also true. However, this situation may the 1% occasion when the senior colleague is wrong. Toft (2001), in an external enquiry into an adverse incident, found cognitive dissonance to be one of the factors leading to the death of a patient. Toft's report provides a stark example of the consequences of junior staff not questioning senior colleagues; in this case, a senior doctor passed a junior doctor a drug to administer through lumbar puncture. The drug administered in this way proved fatal. When interviewed, the junior doctor admitted that he had responded to being handed the drug by repeating the drug's name in a questioning manner, he received an affirmative response and repeated the drug's name with the method of administration in a questioning manner, but then proceeded after receiving a further affirmative response from the senior doctor. The junior doctor felt his limited experience of the type of treatment and his junior status meant that he was not in a position to challenge a senior colleague. Had he followed his initial convictions and refused to administer the drug as a spinal administration, the patient would not have died in his hands.

Although it can be uncomfortable to challenge senior colleagues, our responsibility as AHPs to act in the best interest of our clients mandates that we handle our dissonance and make challenges if needed.

Analysing your approach to conflict can be useful. The *Thomas-Kilmann Conflict Mode Instrument* (Thomas and Kilmann [1974] 2009) is an interesting self-report instrument which is designed to assess a person's behaviour in conflict situations. The test taker choses from a series of paired statements related to her most likely response in a series of conflict situations. The test results provide a profile for how often the person is likely to use each of five responses to conflict; these are labelled as the competing, collaborating, compromising, avoiding, and accommodating modes. These modes fall into two behavioural dimensions, that of assertiveness and cooperativeness. Therapy is a very collaborative process, and client-centred therapy involves a great deal of cooperativeness, negotiation, and accommodation on the part of the AHP. A competing stance, where the AHP has to be assertive and uncompromising, may not come naturally, and AHPs may need to work on developing skills in assertiveness in order to become effective advocates for clients receiving health or social care in a disempowering system.

As the use of self is so important as a therapeutic tool for building a therapeutic relationship (Mosey 1981) and for how you handle yourself as a member of a multidisciplinary team, a reflective activity called 'Analysis of therapeutic self' can be very valuable. The purpose of this activity is to help you to become more aware of the personal resources you can bring to your therapeutic relationships. Box 6.5 provides a format for describing your personal style as an AHP.

Box 6.5   Analysis of Therapeutic Self

1. Describe your personal style in terms of the qualities listed below. In your descriptions, try to include examples of behaviours you have demonstrated in clinical helping relationships. The following qualities are listed in alphabetical order – but you do not have to follow this order. You may wish to undertake this activity over time, reflecting on one or two qualities at a time. Comments, in brackets, are provided after each quality to give you some ideas and/or clarify concepts.

   (a) Affect, emotional tone (for example, are you enthusiastic, energetic, serious, low key)

   (b) Attending and listening (including your ability to reflect back and/or add to what the speaker has said)

   (c) Cognitive style (detail or gestalt orientated, abstract or concrete, ability to understand diverse points of view)

   (d) Confidence (not only what you feel, but what you show to others)

   (e) Confrontation (can you do it and with whom)

   (f) Empathy (for what emotions, in what situations)

   (g) Humour (do you use it, and if so, how)

   (h) Leadership style (directive, facilitative, follower)

   (i) Non-verbal communication (facial expressiveness, eye contact, voice tone and volume, gestures)

   (j) Power sharing (need to control or comfortable with chaos)

   (k) Probing (when you are comfortable doing it, with whom, and about what)

   (l) Touch (do you use it automatically or consciously, when, where, and with whom)

   (m) Verbal communication (vocabulary, use of vernacular, ease of speaking)

2. Write a summary of what you see as your strengths and weaknesses relative to establishing therapeutic relationships.

3. Review your reflections on your personal style, your strengths, and weaknesses:

   (a) Which areas or skills would you like to improve?

   (b) Prioritise these and suggest strategies for improving your top two priorities.

   (c) Draw up an action plan for implementing these strategies for improvement.

This activity has been based on a handout provided to ALF when visiting colleagues engaged in clinical reasoning research at Tufts University, Boston (April 1992). The handout does not acknowledge an author or date. It was developed as an activity for occupational therapy students. Colleagues involved with the Institute on Clinical Reasoning for Occupational Therapy Educators at Tufts in the 1990s were Maureen Fleming, Cheryl Mattingly, Ellen Cohn, Janice Burke, Maureen Neistadt, and Sharan Schwartzberg.

Novice to Expert Continuum

'Professional expertise is a goal of health care professionals and an expectation of health care consumers' (Higgs and Bithell 2001). Expertise is hard to measure (Case et al. 2000) and is often measured in terms of an AHP's length of clinical experience, seniority, and academic qualifications rather than in terms of knowledge, skills, and qualities. The quality of an AHP's advanced clinical reasoning skills can be a factor in separating an expert from a competent practitioner, and clinical expertise should be considered as a continuum along multiple dimensions (Higgs et al. 2008).

A number of writers have drawn upon the work of Dreyfus and Dreyfus (1986) to understand the journey taken as clinicians move from novice to expert practitioners. This novice to expert continuum comprises five stages and is outlined in Figure 6.4.

Schell and Schell (2008) drew on the work of a number of authors, including Mattingly and Fleming 1994 and Benner 1984, to apply the novice to expert continuum proposed by Dreyfus and Dreyfus (1986) to clinical reasoning in occupational therapy practice. The *novice* is perceived as someone with no experience who has to be dependent on theory to guide their practice. A novice uses rule-based procedural reasoning to guide their clinical decisions, and is not yet able to recognise contextual cues. At this stage, narrative reasoning is apparent when forming social relationships but is not being used to inform clinical practice (Schell and Schell 2008). A novice will recognise overt ethical issues, and will 'judge their actions by how well they adhered to the rules' (Mitchell and Unsworth 2005).

An *advanced beginner* is likely to have less than one 'year of reflective practice' (Schell and Schell 2008). At this stage, the AHP starts to 'incorporate contextual information into rule-based thinking' and is able to start recognising the differences between expectations from theory and real clinical problems. A lack of experience means that the AHP has yet to form patterns/heuristics to help prioritise her competing hypotheses. An advanced beginner is developing skills in both pragmatic and narrative reasoning.

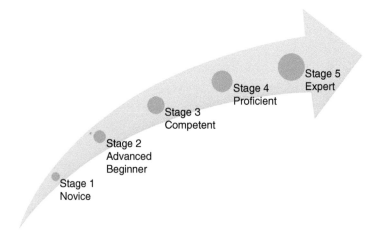

FIGURE 6.4   The Novice to Expert Continuum. Source: Based on Dreyfus and Dreyfus (1986).

The *competent* AHP will have been engaged in reflective practice for about three years. An AHP at this stage is able to apply more skills automatically and so can focus attention on more issues. They are more efficient at sorting data and at setting priorities. Planning becomes 'deliberate, efficient and responsive to contextual issues' (p. 250), and a competent AHP can use conditional reasoning to shift treatment during sessions and to anticipate needs. At this stage, Schell and Schell (2008) state that the AHP can recognise 'ethical dilemmas posed by [their] practice setting, but may be less sensitive to justifiably different ethical responses' (p. 250).

The *proficient* AHP is likely to have engaged in reflective practice for around five years. This AHP will have developed a wealth of experience, which enables them to be more targeted in their assessment approach, efficient in diagnostic reasoning, and flexible in alternating between different treatment options. These AHPs are able to 'creatively combine different diagnostic and procedural approaches'; they also have more refined narrative reasoning skills and become 'more attentive to occupational stories and the relevance [of these stories] for treatment' (p. 250). In terms of pragmatic reasoning, a proficient AHP becomes better at accessing and negotiating resources to meet her clients' needs. At this stage, Schell and Schell (2008) state that the AHP has become sophisticated in her ability to recognise the 'situational nature of ethical reasoning' (p. 250).

Finally, an *expert* AHP will have undertaken 10 or more years of reflective practice. Schell and Schell state that for an expert, 'clinical reasoning becomes a quick an intuitive process which is deeply internalized and imbedded in an extensive store of case experiences', and that this 'permits practice with less routine analysis, except when [the AHP is] confronted with situations where [her] approach is not working' (p. 251). An expert AHP will have become highly skilful in her use of stories and will have refined narrative reasoning skills, which they apply to their assessment and intervention.

REFLECTION QUESTIONS

1. Where are you on this novice to expert continuum?
2. Are you a first-year AHP student who is working at a novice level, or a third-year student who is moving towards the stage of advanced beginner?

3. Have you recently graduated into the profession and although capable can see that you have much to learn still?

4. Have you come to this text as a postgraduate student with a wealth of clinical experience, or as an educator or practice supervisor and perceive yourself to be proficient or expert in your practice?

5. Try to place yourself on this novice to expert continuum and then reflect on some goals to help you move your skills to the next stage.

Case Study: Mrs Ellis' Initial Assessment Process

by **Karen Innes** and **Alison Laver-Fawcett**

This case study has been written to illustrate the AHP's (an occupational therapist) clinical reasoning related to the initial assessment of a client with whom she is likely to work with over many months. The case is provided to illustrate several of the different types of reasoning outlined earlier in this chapter. It is a detailed study, so that students and novice AHPs can see an example of how an AHP frames and explains her assessment approach. The AHP's thinking is given in italics and is mostly provided in boxes to separate the reasoning from the description of what happened during the assessment process for this case.

Introduction to the AHP: The AHP undertaking the following referral has worked as a qualified occupational therapist for five years. Prior to that she has had 12 years' experience as a technical instructor (TI) working with people with learning disabilities, working-age adults with mental health problems, and older adults with mental health problems; she worked across inpatient, outpatient, and community settings. Presently the AHP is a Community Mental Health Team (CMHT) member, together with a consultant psychiatrist, AHP, community psychiatric nurse, social worker, and healthcare assistants, based in a rural location.

Models and Approaches that Guide the AHP's Practice

The two main models used by this AHP are:

- The *Model of Human Occupation* (*MOHO*; Kielhofner 1985; Kielhofner and Burke 1980). 'MOHO seeks to explain how occupation is motivated, patterned, and performed. By offering explanations of such diverse phenomena, MOHO offers a broad and integrative view of human occupation. Within MOHO, humans are conceptualised as being made up of three interrelated components: volition, habituation, and performance capacity. Volition refers to the motivation for occupation, habituation refers to the process by which occupation is organised into patterns or routines, and performance capacity refers to the physical and mental abilities that underlie skilled occupational performance. MOHO also emphasises that to understand human occupation, we must understand the physical and social environments in which it takes place. Therefore, this model aims to understand occupation and problems of occupation that occur in terms of its primary concepts of volition, habituation, performance capacity, and environmental context. These concepts have been consistent throughout the nearly three decades of development of this model. Theoretical refinement has taken place over the years to achieve a clearer and more accurate explanation of how these four factors interact to influence what people do in their everyday, occupational lives and to explain why problems can arise in the face of chronic illness and impairments and when environmental factors interrupt occupation'. (Taken from the MOHO website Introduction to MOHO found at: https://www.moho.uic.edu/resources/about.aspx)

• The *Canadian Model of Occupational Performance* was developed by a group of AHPs associated with the Canadian Association of Occupational Therapists in 1991 (History of the COPM | COPM. The Occupational Performance Model promotes working in a client-centred way respecting the client's choice and autonomy and advocating for the client's needs and wishes. This model focuses on the dynamic relationship between people, their environment, and their occupations (activities related to self-care, productivity, and leisure). It provides a framework for enabling occupation in all people, and can be applied across age groups, diagnoses, and clinical settings. Using this model, client-centred practice is based on a collaborative assessment of occupational needs of the person within his specific physical and social environment (accessed from the COPM resource website at: http://www.thecopm.ca).

The process of change that the AHP hopes to elicit with the clients are through the use of:

Rehabilitation (although not applied as frequently with people with a terminal illness such as dementia);

Education, which is mainly undertaken with the carers;

Adaptation and Facilitation of the environment and/or the task and

Risk Management especially risk related to the environment and the activities that the client is engaged with.

Often, the treatment process is a combination of most of these models, approaches, and processes, as the needs of the client are considered and changes occur.

In relation to the models and approaches used by the AHP in this case study, the main standardised tests used by the AHP are as follows:

Assessment of Motor and Process Skills (AMPS): The AMPS (Fisher 2003) is a specialised assessment of function that requires the occupational therapist to attend a one-week intensive training course. The course costs approximately £900 (which in this case was funded by raising money through the local training consortium and sponsor money through a drug company.) The test assesses motor and process skills deficits which impact a person's quality of performing tasks. It can be administered in the person's own environment.

COTA Safer Tool for environmental Assessment (SAFER Tool) (Community Occupational Therapists and Associates, COTA 1991). The AHP found the SAFER tool an excellent tool to use, as it provides a comprehensive environmental prompt list, and it gives some good pointers to help the AHP with solutions to environmental risk factors. However, it can be time consuming and can lead people to stray from the purpose of the assessment; therefore, the AHP has to remain focused upon the purpose of using the assessment and guide the client through it.

Canadian Occupational Performance Measure (COPM) (Law et al. 1991). This is a self-report tool used to evaluate a client's self-perception of occupational performance. However, for clients with organic impairment, depending on what stage the client is at with the dementia, this tool may not be appropriate owing to a client being unable to think through a situation in an abstract manner. This tool is used alongside the Canadian Model of Occupational Performance (CAOT 1991).

Mini Mental State Examination (MMSE) (Folstein et al. 1975). This assessment is a short test that is easy to use, and it provides an indication of the level of cognitive function and is good for test/retest purposes.

The Activity Card Sort (Baum et al. 2000) gives visual prompts which help a person with cognitive impairment, and it can be easier for the person to identify levels of activity with this test compared to checklist formats.

Bradford Wellbeing Profile (Bruce 2000). This is an observational assessment that subtly identifies small changes in a person's well-being, and cognitive decline level at the moderate to moderately severe and onwards). It is a relevant assessment for the AHP as it assesses the person's well-being.

Zarit Caregiver Burden Survey (Zarit et al. 1986) is a proxy measure that the AHP uses as a prompt to encourage conversation with the carer to assess for carer burden and to find out where they are having difficulties in caring for the client.

Memory and Behavioural Problems Checklist (MBPC; Zarit et al. 1986) is a proxy report checklist used to identify memory and behaviour problems observed by carers of people with cognitive impairment. The checklist collects data on the presence and frequency of problems/behaviours.

Interest Checklist (Katz 1988;) and *Role Checklist* (Oakley et al. 1986) were tools the AHP used in a previous clinical setting and are measures that fit with the MOHO (Kielhofner 1985).

These standardised tools, together with the structured and semi-structured interviewing techniques and informal observations, are the assessment tools used by the AHP in this case.

From the initial assessment information gathered, the AHP then forms some hypotheses around the underlying causes of the stated problems. She then switches to a 'bottom-up approach' and engages in diagnostic reasoning to test her working hypotheses. This may involve searching for further cues, which are obtained by conducting appropriate standardised assessments and undertaking further interviews with the client and carer to gain a more detailed history of symptoms. At the end of the diagnostic reasoning process, she has developed an idea as to why, how, and where the client's problems are occurring. She then engages in conditional reasoning to develop treatment goals linked to her prognosis and then build a treatment plan to deliver these goals.

Case History: Mr and Mrs Ellis

Referral Information Received and Further Information Gathering

A very brief written referral was received from the general practitioner (*GP*) by the CMHT requesting support for a gentleman struggling with his wife's care during her three-year history of an Alzheimer's type dementia. During a Multidisciplinary Team (*MDT*) meeting, it was decided that it was important to determine level of difficulty being experienced. This information could come from two sources, the GP and the husband of the lady with the illness. On receiving the referral, the AHP's reasoning moved towards her prior experience of working with people with Alzheimer's disease. She was able to consider the types of problems that the lady and her husband might be experiencing and hypothesised that given the lady had been diagnosed three years ago she was likely to be at a moderate stage of dementia. The Community Occupational Therapist decided to start the information-gathering process by investigating the referral further, to establish a more in-depth history to get a flavour of where the difficulties lie. This information would initiate a procedural reasoning process to understand the person's problems and to consider ways to alleviate, or reduce the impact of, these problems. She also wanted to phone the GP to clarify the GP's expectations of what role the CMHT might play in the care of this couple; this approach is linked to pragmatic reasoning and attempts to address the questions of 'Who referred this client for therapy and why was this referral made?'

A telephone call was made to the GP to acknowledge the referral and request further information about the situation and what had triggered the referral to be made. It transpired that the family had been known to the practice for approximately 30 years. Mrs Ellis' recent illness had been treated by a consultant privately after relations had broken down with the local hospital at the start of the illness. The GP also reported that the family were willing to accept help from the team because they wanted to be in closer proximity to their care providers. The GP said that the family were well respected within the community, having been very actively involved with local groups in the past. This involvement had reduced over recent years. It was also established that the main problems reported to the GP were around the patient's disturbed sleep pattern, and some sleeping tablets had been prescribed.

Pragmatic reasoning: *The AHP's immediate impression was one of caution; it was going to be very important to start off on the correct footing to establish a trusting therapeutic relationship in order to be able to engage effectively with this couple to meet the care needs of the client and her family. The AHP wondered what 'relations had broken down with the hospital' meant? She wondered whether this implied some sort of formal complaint had been made and decided that she should be very thorough with all her documentation pertaining to this case.*

The next step was to contact the client's husband over the telephone to make an introduction and to set up a mutually appropriate appointment to meet him and his wife. This phone call was made. Mr Ellis was polite and appeared to be expecting a call from the team; he seemed pleased she had phoned promptly, and a date was agreed. The AHP followed this up with a letter of confirmation.

Pragmatic reasoning: *The AHP was very conscious of the importance of following a correct and thorough procedure to build up an efficient and effective client-centred first impression, and to provide information of the role of the AHP and the CMHT. She was relieved that Mr Ellis had been expecting her contact and appeared pleased to be receiving a home visit. Some of her initial anxieties about building an effective therapeutic relationship were reduced after she had spoken to Mr E and had a positive first interaction.*

First Home Visit and Initial Assessment

Procedural reasoning: *It is important that each client's circumstances are considered as a unique case, therefore, prior to the home visit the AHP had to determine what the objectives of the initial assessment are and the information to be gathered. In this scenario, these included*

- *Establishing a trusting therapeutic relationship*
- *Gaining a history about the couple and finding out how the family are coping*
- *Establishing where both Mrs and Mr Ellis see their difficulties*

- *Informally assessing Mrs Ellis' orientation and perception of her difficulties*
- *Determining what the action plan formulation is to be for future care needs.*

Problem-orientated clinical reasoning process: *The AHP decided that an observational assessment approach would be used to gather information about physical and social environmental factors – this assessment would be informal, but her observations would be framed in terms of SAFER tool items (COTA 1991). She also planned to observe how the couple communicated with each other with her, and she planned to seek cues related to the quality of the couple's relationship. The Interest Checklist (Katz 1988) and a Role Check list (Oakley et al. 1986) can be used during the initial interview to help gather client-centred information; this information can help inform narrative reasoning and is useful for both assessment and treatment planning processes. The AHP decided to take these checklists with her and then see once she was there whether their use in the first interaction would be appropriate.*

Pragmatic reasoning: *As with any home visit, it is important to set a realistic time scale to conduct the visit, allowing enough travelling and interview time. For an initial home visit, the occupational therapist (OT) usually allows two hours (it can take a while for the client/OT to settle down to the assessment); one hour is normally allowed for subsequent visits unless complex assessments are conducted. Care was taken by the OT to create the right impression of the service offered, particularly in the light that the relationship had broken down on a previous contact.*

The couple's home was a large luxury bungalow. They said they had lived there for over 45 years. Access to it was via a long drive, and there were five steps up to entrance. Mr and Mrs Ellis appeared at the door at the same time and greeted the AHP with polite formality, inviting her into their home. The AHP waited for the couple to decide where it was convenient for the interview to take place. Mr Ellis allowed Mrs Ellis to determine this and whether she wanted him present throughout the visit also. Both of them were very well dressed. Mrs Ellis was well groomed, her hair looked like it had been professionally set, and she wore under-stated, but expensive-looking jewellery. *(The AHP noted that there were no obvious signs of self-neglect but wondered how much support her husband offered to maintain this standard of presentation and whether a special effort had been made for her visit.)* The bungalow was immaculately presented in terms of décor, tidiness, and cleanliness. *(The AHP wondered who undertook domestic chores in this household.)* There were photos of them in exotic locations (what appeared to be on safari in Africa, by Ayres Rock, in front of a pyramid, and on some tropical looking island) and items of interest collected from their travels as well as many family photographs around the room. A grand piano stood in one part of the room.

Narrative reasoning: *The AHP started to construct a story around this couple's past life experience. The photos of their travels appeared to have been taken since their fifties, and they were clearly well travelled. She postulated that the couple had a very active life together. She hypothesised that the onset of dementia had reduced their trips abroad and wondered how they were coping with the changes in their lifestyle. She also wondered if anyone played the piano. The AHP observed that this was a couple that considered each other's needs and made decisions jointly. They took pride in their surroundings, and appeared to have a large family and a range of personal interests. She decided to proceed with a semi-structured interview to start building rapport and initiate a working relationship and to seek some insight into the difficulties being experienced.*

During the interview, it was revealed that Mrs Ellis was 81 years old, and she and Mr Ellis had been married for 62 years after being childhood sweethearts. Mrs Ellis lost her mother at a very young age. The couple had 4 children and 15 grandchildren. Mrs and Mr Ellis had been very accomplished in their respective professional careers, as headmistress and doctor of engineering, respectively. Both individuals had continued with interests in music, travel, and languages once they had retired. Mrs Ellis was an accomplished pianist and continued to play the piano up to the present time; however, Mr Ellis had to prompt her to play now, and he said she was no longer interested in picking up new tunes but preferred to play old favourites from memory.

Procedural reasoning: *The AHP wondered how much prompting was required to initiate other activities. She wondered how much Mrs E's range of interests could be maintained through drawing on long-term memory, such as the years of practice that had led to her ability to read music and play a wide variety of tunes from memory.*

Diagnostic reasoning: *The AHP took cues from this initial conversation and began hypothesis generation. Her experience of working with other people with organic impairment was that when a client with dementia required prompting to initiate one task or activity, this impairment was generalised to other areas of functioning; so she hypothesised that Mrs E had impairments in the area of task initiation that would affect ADLs as well as leisure activities. She also hypothesised that Mrs Ellis showed little interest in learning new tunes because she experienced difficulties with attending to an unfamiliar piece music and that her ability to learn a new tune would be impacted by cognitive deficits, particularly problems with short-term memory and working memory, related to her Alzheimer's disease.*

The AHP continued with her interview, asking more specific questions to ascertain which interests had been relinquished or reduced since the diagnosis. The couple reported that up until four years ago they had lived very full lives with lots of time spent with their family and frequent visits from grandchildren as they had liked to babysit and to have their grandchildren who lived future away to stay. Mrs Ellis had been heavily involved with the local Girl Guides for many years. She had taught languages and after her retirement had become a member of a local interest group speaking French and Italian and enjoying exchange visits. The couple had enjoyed entertaining, going to the theatre and had frequent holidays abroad, both as a couple and with family. The AHP asked more about the onset of problems which had prompted them to seek medical help. Short-term memory problems (mainly with forgetting names) were reported to have started approximately four years ago. A diagnosis of Alzheimer's type dementia had been made. Cognitive functioning had been maintained for a couple of years with the help of drug therapy, following the couple seeking help through a consultant psychiatrist.

Diagnostic reasoning – cue acquisition: *The AHP noted that both Mr and Mrs Ellis were happy to talk and appeared confident in their views and their account of the history of her illness. Mrs Ellis had an extensive vocabulary, was articulate, and presented socially very well owing to her high intellectual ability. However, as the interview unfolded, it became evident that although Mrs Ellis could cover up the some of the difficulties she was experiencing in a brief conversation, when a conversation was continued over several minutes, repetition and confabulation became evident. Repetition of some information, such as her being a headmistress and having four children, occurred several times over the duration of the hour's interview. Mrs Ellis also appeared to become fatigued towards the end of the interview, allowing her husband to answer more of the questions and staring vacantly at times. The AHP hypothesised that Mrs Ellis' role of mother and teacher were very important to her sense of self, and she also felt that her initial hypotheses about problems with attention and short-term memory had been supported further.*

The AHP asked if Mrs Ellis was feeling tired and would prefer to end the visit for today. Mr Ellis suggested they leave her to rest for a moment while they went to the kitchen and made them all a cup of tea. Once he was alone with the AHP, he explained that his wife had been a very energetic person but that she did tire quickly these days. He reported that he often had to speak for his wife when she was in tired or appeared to have difficulty replying. He described how her speech had become very quiet, almost inaudible on occasions, and said that this coupled with her confabulation and repetition was extremely frustrating.

Procedural reasoning: *The AHP wondered about the causes of the reduced speech volume and decided to ask Mrs Ellis if she was aware of any communication problems. She did not have expertise in the area of communication and thought a referral to a speech and language AHP might be useful.*

Mrs Ellis was aware that she had problems but was unable to identify what they were specifically. She appreciated that her husband found it frustrating when he could not hear what she was saying. She agreed to have an assessment on her communication difficulties and said she would see a speech and language AHP if it might help the situation for her husband's sake.

As the interview unfolded further, some emotional distress was expressed by Mrs Ellis; this was in the form of fear and anxiety, relating to the delusional belief that when her husband left her for any length she believed that he would not come back. Mrs Ellis became quite tearful.

Pragmatic reasoning: *The AHP wondered about potential separation problems should day or respite care be required in the future for the couple. The AHP had to be particularly sensitive to these verbal and non-verbal communication signs, careful to achieve a balance between acknowledging the client's expressed fears and emotion but without turning the interview into a counselling situation.*

Physically, Mrs Ellis' mobility did not initially cause any concerns to the AHP, as she appeared to mobilise quite well. However, Mr Ellis reported that his wife had experienced a couple of minor falls lately, and was on occasion unsteady on her feet. He explained that she also had started to drop things. The AHP was informed that Mrs Ellis had experienced two heart attacks over the last three years and was unable to participate in any strenuous activity.

Diagnostic reasoning: *In terms of the reported falls, the AHP hypothesised about neurological changes occurring as a result of the disease and postulated about deficits in movement and balance. She also thought about person-occupation-environment fit and the possibility of environmental risk factors. She decided that a detailed home environment assessment to seek further cues around physical hazards would be useful.*

Pragmatic reasoning: *She did not consider herself a specialist in falls and felt she should suggest to the couple that an assessment around balance, strength, falls risk, and prevention with the team's physiotherapist would be helpful.*

Mr Ellis was very informative during the interview, reporting that his wife no longer participated in complex levels of decision making for ADL. He explained that he did try to involve her in making decisions where he could, for example, in meal choice, daily clothing, and where they should go if they went out for the day.

Conditional reasoning: *The AHP was aware of the insight and interest Mr Ellis had and took about his wife's abilities and the importance of retaining her independence as much as he could. However, her intuition questioned his emotional acceptance of the situation, how much he was actually doing around the house, and what degree of carer stress he was under.*

Procedural reasoning: *The AHP thought about the assessments that might be appropriate to use to gain some further insight into the abilities of Mrs Ellis so that some constructive interventions could be used to help Mr and Mrs Ellis perform some tasks together and maintain Mrs Ellis' role about the house in a safe and least restrictive way (retrieving past theoretical knowledge. She felt this course of action might also allow Mr Ellis to gradually come to terms with his wife's failing abilities. Tests that would help to provide valuable information for the AHP included MMSE (Folstein et al. 1975), which would give an indication of Mrs Ellis' cognitive function. The AHP was keen to observe Mrs Ellis directly in the performance of familiar tasks, so she chose the AMPS (Fisher 2003) as a measure that would help her to identify what the impact her cognitive function was having on functional abilities. The dilemma for the AHP was how not to insult the couple's intellectual integrity and highlight the deficiencies; she decided to focus the interview upon Mr Ellis and think about that later.*

As she talked to Mr Ellis about the couple's daily and weekly routines, it became apparent that all the ADL tasks were left to Mr Ellis to undertake. He reported his wife had difficulty following instructions and would often 'end up in a confused muddle with familiar things if she was left to her own devises'. Mr Ellis had initially presented with strong composure throughout the interview, but at this point his eyes filled up with tears, and it became apparent that he was struggling to come to terms with his wife's illness and difficulties. He explained how capable his wife had once been, his distress over the change that he was seeing his wife go through, and the helplessness he felt about the situation. Mr Ellis explained that he found it very difficult coping with the disrupted sleep pattern that his wife was experiencing and how the sleep deprivation was impacting him negatively. He said he had gone to his GP because he was suffering from severe headaches, which his GP felt were linked to sleep deprivation and stress. He explained that his GP had told him that it was quite common for partners of people with dementia to begin grieving even while their loved one was alive because you lose the person you knew and the roles between you change. He said his chat with the GP had 'been very validating' as he was distraught by his wife's loss of ability and was feeling increasingly fearful about his ability to care for her adequately and their future.

Reason for Intervention – Needs Identification

Narrative reasoning: *The lived experience of dementia was proving distressing for both the client and her husband. It was becoming apparent that it was not only a practical supporting role that may be required but also an emotional one, for both Mrs Ellis and her husband needed support to come to terms with the losses in function associated with her dementia. She started to construct a prospective treatment story, imaging what the intervention might look like and what the outcome could be. The AHP felt confident, owing to the candour with which the couple had described their situation, that the therapeutic relationship and trust had started to develop.*

The AHP then summarised her initial findings from the information given by the couple and her preliminary observations. She explained that from what they had told her today, it was clear that the memory problems that Mrs Ellis was experiencing were causing some reduction in her independence which, together with the recent falls, had affected her confidence. The AHP also expressed her concerns over how distressed Mrs Ellis sometimes became over her anxieties and how the change in role for Mr Ellis, coupled with impact of the disrupted sleep pattern, was affecting them both. The AHP stressed the value of continuing their involvement in social activities together and gave positive reinforcement for this. The AHP explained that she would use information provided at today's visit to identify further assessments required to formalise a treatment and intervention plan. She explained that this intervention plan would be developed in accordance with their priorities and agreement. The AHP followed the CMHT referral procedures and protocol for confidentiality and explained that the next step would be to discuss her findings with the consultant psychiatrist and the other members of the CMHT, which included a nurse, social worker, and a healthcare assistant. She gained their permission to make referrals to the physiotherapist and speech and language therapist. She told them that she would then set up another home visit to discuss her ideas for addressing identified problems and needs.

Pragmatic reasoning: *On this occasion, it was felt by the AHP that it was inappropriate to use either the Role or Interest Checklists as the time was at a premium. However, she felt they would provide useful data and be acceptable to Mr and Mrs Ellis. Therefore, she left the two checklists with the couple to complete as a self-report/ proxy assessment and to give them some control and involvement over the assessment. Using Mrs Ellis' roles and interests would help her to tailor the treatment process and ensure any activities selected as the basis for intervention were meaningful to the client.*

Identifying the Problems and Focusing the Assessment

The AHP now engaged in *problem setting;* this involved naming the phenomena/ constructs that were to become the target of assessment. Defined problems were constructed from the observed and reported problematic situations that were identified from the referral information, discussion with the GP, and the initial home visit interview. From the initial contact, a lot of information was gleaned without the use of standardised tests. From this information, the AHP developed a problem list around the difficulties that the couple were experiencing. She then selected appropriate assessments to provide the data required to explore these further and test related hypotheses.

Problem List

From the information given by Mr Ellis, the AHP identified that:

- *Mrs Ellis had short-term memory problems and presented some challenging behaviour towards her husband by being easily distracted, confused, disorientated in time, and presenting with disrupted sleep pattern.*
- *Mrs Ellis had become increasingly dependent for some personal activities of daily living (PADL) and most domestic activities of daily living (DADL).*
- *Mrs Ellis had communication difficulties, confabulation, and quietness of speech.*
- *There was some evidence of delusional beliefs and insightfulness exhibited by Mrs Ellis which made her feel tearful and anxious.*
- *The AHP hypothesised that perhaps perceptual and cognitive changes were occurring. Related cues were falls, and dropping items was the result.*
- *Physically, Mrs Ellis was quite frail as a result of a history of cardiac problems; related to this, her lack of regular exercise reduced her stamina and possibly muscle tone.*

  - *Mr Ellis was rational and realistic in the care for his wife; however, he was experiencing emotional difficulties in association with increased responsibility of being a carer, struggling to come to terms with the changes his wife was going through, and struggling with an increased loss of sleep he was enduring.*
  - *Mr Ellis was taking increased responsibility in all domestic ADLs.*
  - *The couple still enjoyed a social life, mainly focused around their family and long-standing friends; however, both Mr and Mrs Ellis were becoming more isolated from social involvement owing to the situation.*

Feedback to the Team

In the past, drug therapy had been the main focus of intervention; however, as there had been deterioration in the well-being of Mrs Ellis, a joint care approach was taken following discussion with the consultant psychiatrist and CMHT.

Delineating the Problems

The stage of delineating a problem involves the implementation of the AHP's chosen assessment methods and strategies. The AHP needed to apply multiple measures related to these various problems, such as:

Occupation: The AHP needed to assess Mrs Ellis' remaining abilities in personal care (washing, dressing), domestic involvement, and role activity. She wanted to understand the underlying causes of any dysfunction and to see how Mrs E tackled tasks and to assess whether any particular cues or prompts facilitated her function. Therefore, she decided to assess Mrs Ellis' functional ability through use of AMPS (Fisher 2003). From the assessment results, the AHP anticipated she would be able to identify ways of working with Mrs Ellis to maintain her capabilities.

Challenging Behaviour: Mrs Ellis was exhibiting a number of challenging behaviours. The AHP wanted to assess the frequency and intensity of these problems further. She thought she would ask Mr Ellis to complete an MBPC (Zarit et al. 1986). She anticipated that carer education would be valuable to explain to Mr Ellis why such behaviours may be occurring and ways of trying to minimise the displayed behaviours.

Communication: Communication appeared problematic particularly in social situations; therefore, investigation into support opportunities could be included in the treatment process of speech problems. A referral to *Speech and Language Therapy* was made.

Physical Function: Mrs Ellis was experiencing difficulties which were putting her at risk of falls and accidents and limiting her involvement in activity. It was felt that physiotherapy intervention would be valuable for the couple to maintain mobility and physical well-being. A referral to a *physiotherapist* was made.

Environment: An occupational therapy environmental risk assessment could be used to minimise further hazards around the home. The AHP planned to use the SAFER Tool (COTA 1991).

Carer Stress: Mr Ellis seemed to be experiencing carer stress, and the nature of his physical and emotional burden needed to be investigated to gain some insight into the extent of the burden, and offer appropriate support where necessary. The AHP decided to tell Mr Ellis about *The Alzheimer's Society* and *Carer's Resource*. She would encourage engagement with these services but give him the option of self-referral so that he could take control over the extent and timing of his engagement with these agencies. The AHP considered that a referral to a day care service would offer Mr Ellis some respite and Mrs Ellis socialisation, but she wondered whether this would be an acceptable option for the couple at this time.

Pragmatic reasoning: *The AHP was aware that this battery of assessments would be too much for Mr and Mrs Ellis to undertake all at once. She was also aware that the sudden involvement of healthcare colleagues (physiotherapist and speech and language therapist) and of workers from voluntary agencies (Carers Resource and Alzheimer's) may be too much straight away, as the couple seemed to like to make considered decisions about things that happened. It would, therefore, take a number of visits to follow the assessment and intervention process through with full approval and support of Mr and Mrs Ellis.*

A second home visit was planned by the occupational therapist with consent from the couple.

The objectives for the visit were as follows:

- Discuss the couple's thoughts about the previous meeting.
- To discuss the findings of the first contact and agree some prioritised goals with Mrs and Mr Ellis.
- Collect the Role and Interest Checklists, and use these as the basis for looking at some options of intervention.
- Conduct an environmental risk assessment.
- Conduct a MMSE (Folstein et al. 1975) to gain a baseline figure to monitor any cognitive changes later in treatment.

From the data gathered from the initial meeting with the client and the outcome of the team meeting, the next visit was primarily to discuss the proposed assessment, treatment, and management. The AHP felt that it was important to keep the couple informed of ideas and thoughts about CMHT intervention so that they did not become increasingly anxious in an already emotional situation.

The next visit was again conducted by the AHP alone; the couple were pleased to see her and happy to discuss their thoughts over the last visit. Mrs Ellis was very pleased at the thought of some help for her husband, and she recapped her concerns over how she felt a burden to him owing to her memory problems.

Mr Ellis again presented calm initially when discussing the care of his wife; however, the tears were evident again as the discussion progressed. The AHP wondered about the use of 'CRUSE' Counselling service to help with the loss/helplessness he was feeling, but felt that this was not the time to discuss this. She also wondered whether Mr Ellis might be suffering from a mild reactive depression and wondered whether it would be worth using a brief depression screen.

The AHP discussed some of her thoughts about the previous meeting and suggested that this meeting was about prioritising goals for the couple and the AHP to work together on. The AHP's approach was to look both at the couple's joint needs and also at their individual problems.

The AHP discussed the history of falls previously mentioned, and the couple were happy that a referral to Physiotherapy for a falls assessment had been made. In conjunction with this, the couple allowed the occupational therapist to make an assessment of the environmental factors in the couple's home; this would identify any potential risks that could be elevated prior to the physiotherapist's visit.

The tool that the OT used was the COTA Safety Assessment of Function and the Environment for Rehabilitation, known as the *SAFER Tool* (COTA 1991). This is a comprehensive checklist that addresses an individual's occupational performance tasks in their own home. The AHP found that all furniture was of a suitable height for safe transfers.

From the information received, a few problems were highlighted and addressed. For example, the AHP suggested removing the scatter rugs in the home. In the kitchen, Mr Ellis reported that his wife used to be a magnificent cook, but that now she found it difficult even to make a cup of tea or use the toaster. Mr Ellis reported that he felt that his wife would be unable to identify how to put together a nutritional meal. He also reported that he usually carried hot food and drinks for her, for fear of Mrs Ellis falling while transferring hot items to the table. The AHP suggested using a compensatory technique in the form of a kitchen trolley; this was gratefully accepted. Mr Ellis informed the AHP that he was considering getting an au pair to help with domestic tasks so that he could devote more time to the more pleasurable side of life with his wife. He felt that this might take the pressure off himself as he did not enjoy domestic tasks. In the area of personal ADL, Mr Ellis reported that his wife spent a lot of time in the bedroom 'fidgeting' and would often require help with dressing as she would get dressed inappropriately, selecting the wrong items of clothing, or mislaying items that she was looking for.

Procedural reasoning: *The AHP wondered what level Mrs Ellis was functioning at, where the difficulties were in performing tasks, and also how much of this was Mr Ellis protecting his wife's feelings over her reduced abilities. Again, the AHP had to be subtle in performing any assessments so that some positive outcomes could be developed from the results. She decided that she would like to undertake an AMPS (Fisher 2003) as soon as possible.*

Narrative reasoning: *During this visit, the AHP was aware that Mrs Ellis had said very little. She wanted to keep engaging with her lived experience of dementia and maintain rapport with her client, as well as with her husband, so the conversation was directed more towards her to try to identify what her priorities were. The AHP gave Mr Ellis the Memory Problems and Behaviours Checklist (MPBC; Zarit et al. 1986) and suggested he might want to do this at the kitchen table. She said that she would chat to Mrs Ellis in the living room while he was doing the checklist. The AHP used the completed Role Checklist and Interest Checklists as a focus for her conversation with Mrs Ellis, as she did not feel that the COPM (Law et al., 1991) would be a valuable tool in Mrs Ellis' case owing to her confabulation, which would affect the test requirements for subjective answers. She felt Mrs Ellis might struggle with the 10-point rating scale, and this could cause distress. She hoped that the Interest and Role checklists would help her engage Mrs Ellis in exploring her past life history and current life style and future wishes.*

The Role Check list indicated that Mrs Ellis had enjoyed being a mother and now loved being a grandmother, she was proud of her professional achievements and work in the various charities, and that she enjoyed participating in regular worship at church.

From the Interest Checklist, the AHP discovered that Mrs Ellis had enjoyed the arts, theatre, dance, and cookery. She continued to be involved with a local language group, which she got a lot of pleasure from as she attended with her husband. Mrs Ellis also reminisced about the camping holidays that the family used to take. Mrs Ellis stated that she would love to remain involved in many of these pleasurable activities for as long as possible as they gave her a sense of usefulness. The AHP explained that another questionnaire would provide an even more detailed picture of Mrs Ellis' quality of life and would help them monitor her participation in these important activities. She then administered the Mayers' Lifestyle Questionnaire (Mayers, 2003) as an interview. Mrs Ellis appeared to enjoy one-to-one conversation with the AHP and did not appear to tire. As they explored her lifestyle and quality of life, she became quite animated and was fully engaged in the conversation. The AHP wondered whether Mrs Ellis would enjoy formally working on recording her life story and might benefit from reminiscence work.

Narrative reasoning: *The AHP noted that Mrs Ellis had a strong sense of herself and when speaking about these roles she had good self-esteem, feeling as if she had and does contribute well within the family but not so much with the community now.*

Priority Areas for Goals Identified by Mrs Ellis

- To maintain her personal care skills
- To assist her husband with some light household tasks
- To continue to be involved with her family
- To continue to engage in the language group
- To enable her to be a companion for her husband

Conditional reasoning: *The AHP felt that this had been a valuable visit as it had opened up some possible areas of occupational therapy intervention. It appeared that although there were difficulties with domestic activities, outside help in the form of an au pair help would support Mr Ellis with these. The couple identified that the most important areas for them to enjoy were around pleasurable pursuits. The AHP felt that given the degenerative nature of the disease, this was a sensible and philosophical way of moving forward once the safety issues were tackled.*

Action Plan

- Arrange a visit to introduce the physiotherapist.
- Conduct a baseline assessment for cognitive function using the MMSE (Folstein et al. 1975). This will give an indication of any cognitive changes that may affect drug therapy decisions (she planned to do this last time, but had chosen to undertake the Mayers' Life Style questionnaire and thought it had been too much to do this afterwards).
- Conduct an AMPS (Fisher 2003) to investigate the quality of occupational performance to identify areas that can be modified and enable the couple to do activities together or to enable Mrs Ellis to perform her own personal care independently.
- Speak with Mr Ellis privately about carer stress and possible support available.

During the next week, she took the physiotherapist to visit the couple. He conducted assessments which took the form of gaining a verbal history from the client and her husband about physical functioning, environment, habit, and ADL in conjunction with measuring intact balance through two measures; the *Berg Balance Scale* (Berg et al. 1992), and the *Get up and Go Test* (Mathias et al. 1986), which identify people with poor balance, either sedentary or dynamic, who are at risk of falling. The outcome from these assessments indicated that Mrs Ellis had relatively good dynamic balance, but on rising from a sedentary position she would occasionally feel unsteady. Advice was given on this, and some general Tai Chi–based exercises were prescribed for the couple so that Mr Ellis could support his wife in performing exercises routinely. It was also suggested that a six-week attendance to a local day hospital for older people with mental health problems would enable monitoring of progress and allow further physiotherapy assessment and treatment to be conducted. Mrs Ellis would also be able to join a group exercise class at the day hospital. Mrs Ellis was happy to consider this option. The AHPs also felt this short-term intervention would provide Mr Ellis with some much-needed respite.

Prior to the next occupational therapy home visit, there was a telephone call from Mr Ellis requesting some help with night-time wandering. He sounded quite exasperated by the experience of his wife wandering around the house and even trying to leave the house at night. The AHP suggested that he call into the team's office after dropping his wife at the day hospital for her preliminary visit, so that they could talk without Mrs Ellis being there and she could give him the time that he needed to discuss his worries without feeling that he had to protect his wife's feelings. In the meantime, the AHP sent out some information about wandering and sleep problems related to dementia and reinforced the availability of the Carer's Resource team and Alzheimer's worker for advice. This was the start of the educative role that the AHP would play, and it was also an indication of the trust that had been built up between carer and AHP. The AHP noted that the skill would be to keep the relationship a positive therapeutic one that supported Mr Ellis but prevented dependence.

During the visit to the day hospital, Mrs Ellis met the rest of the team and participated in some of the activities that were conducted; she was particularly good in quizzes and enjoyed the baking, requiring verbal prompts throughout. Mrs Ellis was slightly anxious when her husband left her to speak with the AHP but became distracted by the rest of the group enough to alleviate her separation anxiety. During her visit, the nurse administered the MMSE and agreed to share the results with the AHP. Mr Ellis took the opportunity to speak frankly about the strain he was under through lack of sleep and how sad and frustrated he was feeling about being helpless in respect of being unable to help his wife.

Procedural reasoning: *The AHP had a few thoughts about what was going on and what may help. She decided to encourage setting up a life story book about their life together, as it may help to consolidate some of their feelings, and celebrate their life together as well as giving the couple a joint activity to perform. It may also involve other family members to support Mr Ellis. Also, it refocused the AHP's role in this person's treatment; as the occupational therapist was aware that although she was a generic CMHT member, her professional expertise was with occupational performance, role engagements, and activity analysis. The need to assess the quality of functional performance by using AMPS could determine the level of involvement that Mrs Ellis can function at and provide one way of allowing Mrs and Mr Ellis to achieve some level of satisfaction in occupation, as this has been a major theme* *throughout the couple's life. Mr Ellis was partly grieving at the diminished functional performance that his wife was now subject to after a life of high achievement.*

The AHP requested that she conduct the Zarit Caregiver Burden Survey and undertook this as an interview. She found that although Mr Ellis wanted to do the best he could to help his wife, he was finding it increasingly tiring. He understood that it was important to maintain her independence and sense of individuality, but had concerns over her safety and felt that this was a huge worry to him. The AHP acknowledged his concerns and discussed her thoughts about the life story book and undertaking an AMPS assessment with a view to providing advice on cues and prompts to maximise functional ability. Both suggestions were accepted by Mr Ellis, but the AHP felt that there was a lack of confidence in the suggestions. It was also explained that once a treatment plan was set up, support could be initially offered to the couple from the AHP but ongoing support from the CMHT would be provided by the healthcare assistant. The assistant would follow through with some of the treatment plan, for example, supporting Mrs Ellis to prepare a drink and snack, so that Mr Ellis did not feel that it was another thing to overwhelm him in caring for his wife.

Focusing the Treatment

The next home visit was conducted early in the morning so that options for selecting AMPS tasks for assessment could be broadened. One of the priorities identified by Mrs Ellis had been personal care activities, and the AHP agreed she would arrive before Mrs Ellis had got dressed. On arriving, the AHP was greeted at the door by an unfamiliar lady, who introduced herself as the new au pair who had been employed by the family to help with domestic tasks and meals. The impact upon Mr Ellis was obvious; he looked much more relaxed as he now felt he could devote time to spending productive and quality time with his wife. Mrs Ellis was pleased that as a result of her husband having more free time they had initiated a life story book which had brought back some lovely memories, and the AHP observed lots of photographs scattered on the coffee table.

The AHP explained the process of the AMPS and sought consent from Mrs Ellis to conduct the assessment. Mrs Ellis grasped most of what was being asked of her and agreed to participate; however, the AHP sensed that Mr Ellis still had reservations about assessing his wife's ability to undertake tasks and the possibility that her inabilities would be highlighted. The AHP explained that she only assesses activities that the individual wants to do and that the assessment looked at the quality of the performance so that the process can be modified to maintain success and indicate possible risk. The AHP was aware of the tentative beginnings and how these had developed into a positive relationship, so it was important that a full explanation was given to this couple at every stage of assessment and intervention to ensure fully informed consent and maintain trust and rapport.

Based upon the priorities identified by Mrs Ellis on the Mayers' Lifestyle Questionnaire, the tasks offered for assessment where limited to those of an average complexity to provide a reasonable challenge to Mrs Ellis. The AMPS tasks identified were Upper and Lower body dressing, and preparing a cold cereal and beverage.

Interpreting the Results

The results of the AMPS assessment indicated that in the grooming task Mrs Ellis found difficulty locating appropriate clothing and required some prompts to help her choose her clothing and struggled on occasion with fine finger dexterity and grip. She was slow in conducting the process of the task and had difficulties with starting the various parts of the task; for example, she would stop in between putting on her blouse and then her cardigan, requiring assistance to select the garment. Mrs Ellis asked questions frequently. The preparation of cold cereal and drink indicated difficulties finding items and returning them to their original positions, and she had problems gauging the distance and speed of pouring the liquid. Again, prompts were required to assist Mrs Ellis through the process, but she completed the tasks successfully.

Procedural reasoning: *The AHP determined from the results that Mrs Ellis was inefficient in performing tasks graded by the assessment as being of average difficulty; however, when given verbal prompts and only items that she required to complete the tasks, she could succeed. The physical difficulties with her motor control meant that activities required grading so that she could achieve desired levels of performance. For example, the AHP decided she should educate Mr and Mrs Ellis not fill jugs too full so that she could pour without spilling fluid. The repeated deficits seen across both tasks of being unable to find items and with sequencing problems meant that only items required should be in view so that Mrs Ellis could respond to verbal cues in an uncluttered and confusing environment. Mrs Ellis did not compensate for her actions, and there was potential to create a risk situation.*

Negotiated Goal Setting

The AHP discussed her findings with the couple, and they agreed to the following treatment goals:

- Education for Mr Ellis regarding setting up the environment so Mrs Ellis can perform personal care tasks and simple domestic tasks safely and with minimal verbal prompting. Mr Ellis was to assist by choosing items and tools to be used in a task and setting them up in view for Mrs Ellis to use.
- Mr Ellis will use simple verbal cues to help Mrs Ellis complete the tasks.
- The AHP undertook some environmental modifications required to help Mrs Ellis to perform ADL.

After the assessment, the AHP explored the environmental changes required to assist in Mrs Ellis' independence. These included de-cluttering surfaces and cupboards to cut down inappropriate stimuli, setting out tools required for the task, and the modelling of an activity with Mrs Ellis to show Mr Ellis how to reinforce task processes and cut down on the need for prompts.

The AHP also discussed the use of orientation prompts to help address the sleep problems, for example, using notices to prompt Mrs. Ellis to return to bed, going to bed later in the evening, bladder management to minimise the need to go to the toilet, etc.

Summary of the Assessment Process

The AHP had gathered her information to explore the referral from various sources, discussed the proposed visit formally over the telephone with the carer, started initial assessment procedures during the first home visit, and worked on building up the therapeutic relationship from initial telephone contact and during home visits. The AHP was aware of the limits of her own expertise and attempted to provide treatment boundaries with the couple by involving appropriate other professionals and focusing her support upon both the client and the carer's needs.

Although the occupational therapist had a list of assessments she wanted to use and a preferred order of administration, in a complex condition like dementia where contact with the client and family is likely to be long term, the assessment process rarely follows a linear route. Instead, what often happens is that the assessment pathway can be one of exploring and revisiting options time after time in a client-centred way even though the AHP's experience may already include a certain predicted path of treatment options – the prospective story. The client's unique treatment process comes from the priorities set from the initial assessments, and these will change over time as an illness develops or circumstances alter. Sometimes an AHP may feel that the treatment is on a designated route, but then things happen to make the treatment route change; there is a constant reviewing of the situation, and a flexible approach needs to be adopted.

In this case, the AHP administered her chosen assessments over a number of visits with Mr and Mrs Ellis, trying to work in a client-centred way to engage in problem solving and risk assessments. Her assessment process included professional expertise from other team members to gain a holistic view of the individual's perceived and observed difficulties. The selection of assessments provided a combination of observational, self-, and proxy-reported data. Initially, the focus was upon gaining verbal information through a semi-structured interview with both client and carer. Standardised measures, such as Memory and Behaviour Problems Checklist and Carer Burden Scale, helped to build interview data with more specific proxy and self-report data. These helped to identify the client's and carer's perceived priorities and negotiate what they wanted to work upon. The next step was to conduct some observational standardised assessments in the form of AMPS and the physiotherapy balance scales. This enabled baseline measurements of function and movement to be taken, so that treatment could be discussed with the couple together, and a joint working approach could be adopted in the planning stage.

This case provides an example of the complexity of assessment and of the various reasoning forms that the AHP undertakes to make sense of the presenting condition and move towards negotiated goals and treatment plans.

Worksheets

The following worksheet is designed to assist you in applying clinical reasoning to your own practice. See Worksheet 6.1 on p. 224. The worksheet takes you through a series of headings to guide you to write a therapy diagnostic statement. Use the worksheet to develop a therapy diagnostic statement for one of your clients. If you are a student, write a therapy diagnostic statement for a person you have worked with on placement. Refer to diagnostic statement examples earlier in this chapter.

REVIEW QUESTIONS

6.1   What is clinical reasoning?

6.2   What type of questions do AHPs attempt to answer through pragmatic reasoning?

6.3   What are the four components of diagnostic reasoning?

6.4   How could you document your reflections on your practice?

You will find brief answers to these questions at the back of this book on p. 445.

WORKSHEET 6.1 Clinical Reasoning – Writing a Therapy Diagnostic Statement

Client's name	
Descriptive component:	
Explanatory component:	
Cue component: As evidenced by the following symptoms described by service user and/or proxy	
Cue component: As evidenced by the following signs identified through observational assessment:	
Pathologic component:	

REFERENCES

Abidin, R.R. (1995). *Manual for the Parenting Stress Index*. Odessa, FL: Psychological Assessment Resources.

Allport, G.W. (1968). The historical background of modern social psychology. In: *The Handbook of Social Psychology*, 2e (eds. G. Lindzey and E. Aronson), 1–80. Addison-Wesley.

Barnitt, R.E. (1993). 'Deeply troubling questions': the teaching of ethics in undergraduate courses. *British Journal of Occupational Therapy* 56 (11): 401–406. https://doi.org/10.1177/030802269305601104.

Baron, J. (2014). Heuristics and biases. In: *The Oxford Handbook of Behavioral Economics and the Law* (eds. E. Zamir and D. Teichman), 3–27. Oxford University Press, USA.

Bassot, B. (2016). *The Reflective Journal*. Macmillan International Higher Education.

Baum, C.M., Perlmutter, M., and Edwards, D.F. (2000). Measuring function in Alzheimer's disease. *Alzheimer's Care Today* 1 (3): 44–61.

Benner, P. (1984). *From Novice to Expert*. Menlo Park.

Berg, K.O., Wood-Dauphinee, S.L., Williams, J.I., and Maki, B. (1992). Measuring balance in the elderly: validation of an instrument. *Canadian journal of public health= Revue canadienne de sante publique* 83: S7–S11.

Boud, D., Keogh, R., and Walker, D. (1985, e-book 2013)). *Reflection: Turning Experience into Learning*. Routledge.

Bruce, E. (2000). Looking after well-being: a tool for evaluation Residents' emotional needs can be easily neglected in a busy care home environment. *Journal of Dementia Care* 8 (6): 25–27.

Bushby, K., Chan, J., Druif, S. et al. (2015). Ethical tensions in occupational therapy practice: a scoping review. *British Journal of Occupational Therapy* 78 (4): 212–221. https://doi.org/10.1177/0308022614564770.

Carnevali, D. L., Thomas, M. D., Godson, L. T., & Waterloo, I. A. (1993). *Diagnostic reasoning and treatment decision making in nursing*. Philadelphia, PA.

Case, K., Harrison, K., and Roskell, C. (2000). Differences in the clinical reasoning process of expert and novice cardiorespiratory physiotherapists. *Physiotherapy* 86 (1): 14–21. https://doi.org/10.1016/S0031-9406(05)61321-1.

Cohn, E. S., & Czycholl, C. (1991). *Facilitating a foundation for clinical reasoning. Self-paced instruction for clinical education and supervision: An instructional guide, 159–182*.

Donaghy, M.E. and Morss, K. (2000). Guided reflection: a framework to facilitate and assess reflective practice within the discipline of physiotherapy. *Physiotherapy Theory and Practice* 16 (1): 3–14. https://doi.org/10.1080/095939800307566.

Dreyfus, H. and Dreyfus, S. (1986). *Mind Officer Machine: The Power of Human Intuition and Expertise in the Era of the Computer*. New York: Free Press.

Duncan, E.A. (ed.) (2011). *Foundations for Practice in Occupational Therapy-E-BOOK*. Elsevier Health Sciences.

Festinger, L. (1962). *A Theory of Cognitive Dissonance*, vol. 2. Stanford University Press.

Fisher, A.G. (2003). *AMPS: Assessment of Motor and Process Skills Volume 1: Development, Standardisation, and Administration Manual*, 378–382. Ft Collins, CO: Three Star Press Inc.

Fleming, M.H. (1991). Clinical reasoning in medicine compared with clinical reasoning in occupational therapy. *American Journal of Occupational Therapy* 45 (11): 988–996. https://doi.org/10.5014/ajot.45.11.988.

Fleming, M.H. (1994). Procedural reasoning: addressing functional limitations. In: *Clinical Reasoning: Forms of Inquiry in a Therapeutic Practice* (eds. C. Mattingly and M.H. Fleming), 37. Philadelphia: FA Davis.

Folstein, M.F., Folstein, S.E., and McHugh, P.R. (1975). "Mini-mental state": a practical method for grading the cognitive state of patients for the clinician. *Journal of Psychiatric Research* 12 (3): 189–198.

Greenhalgh, T. (2006). *What Seems to Be the Trouble?: Stories in Illness and Healthcare*. Oxford: Radcliffe.

Hammell, K.W. (2004). Dimensions of meaning in the occupations of daily life. *Canadian Journal of Occupational Therapy* 71 (5): 296–305. https://doi.org/10.1177/000841740407100509.

Higgs, J. and Bithell, C. (2001). Professional expertise. In: *Practice Knowledge and Expertise in the Health Professions* (eds. J. Higgs and A. Titchen), 59–68. Butterworth-Heinemann.

Higgs, J., Jones, M.A., Loftus, S., and Christensen, N. (eds.) (2008). *Clinical Reasoning in the Health Professions E-Book*. Elsevier Health Sciences.

Johns, C. (ed.) (2017). *Becoming a Reflective Practitioner*. Wiley.

Jones, M.A., Jensen, G., and Edwards, I. (2008). Clinical reasoning in physiotherapy. In: *Clinical Reasoning in the Health Professions* (eds. J. Higgs and M. Jones), 245–256. Oxford Boston Melbourne: Butterworth Heinemann.

Katz, N. (1988). Interest checklist: a factor analytical study. *Occupational Therapy in Mental Health* 8 (1): 45–55.

Kielhofner, G. (1978). General systems theory: implications for theory and action in occupational therapy. *American Journal of Occupational Therapy* 32 (10): 637–645.

Kielhofner, G. (1985). *A Model of Human Occupation: Theory and Application*. Baltimore: Williams & Wilkins.

Kielhofner, G. (1992). *Conceptual Foundations of Occupational Therapy Practice*. FA Davis.

Kielhofner, G. and Burke, J.P. (1980). A model of human occupation, part 1. Conceptual framework and content. *American Journal of Occupational Therapy* 34 (9): 572–581.

Kielhofner, G. (2009). *Conceptual Foundations of Occupational Therapy Practice*. FA Davis.

Kilmann, R.H. and Thomas, K.W. (2009). *Conflict Mode Instrument*. CPP.

Kuhl, J. (2013). Motivation and volition. *International Perspectives on Psychological Science* 2: 311–340.

Larin, H., Wessel, J., and Al-Shamlan, A. (2005). Reflections of physiotherapy students in the United Arab Emirates during their clinical placements: a qualitative study. *BMC Medical Education* 5 (1): 3. https://doi.org/10.1186/1472-6920-5-3.

Laver, A. J. (1994). *The development of the Structured Observational Test of Function (SOTOF) (Doctoral dissertation, University of Surrey)*. https://ethos.bl.uk/OrderDetails.do?uin=uk.bl.ethos.259917

Laver, A.J. and Powell, G.E. (1995). *The Structured Observational Test of Function (SOTOF)*. NFER Nelson.

Law, M., Baptiste, S., Carswell-Opzoomer, A. et al. (1991). *Manuel de la Mesure canadienne du rendement occupationnel*. Toronto: Publications de l'ACE.

Line, J. (1969). Case method as a scientific form of clinical thinking. *The American Journal of Occupational Therapy* 23 (4): 308–313.

MacKay, D. M. (1969). *The informational analysis of questions and commands*. https://ieeexplore.ieee.org/abstract/document/6290206

Mathias, S., Nayak, U.S.L., and Isaacs, B. (1986). The "Get up and Go" test: a simple clinical test of balance in old people. *Archives of Physical Medicine and Rehabilitation* 67: 387–389.

Mattingly, C. (1991). What is clinical reasoning? *American Journal of Occupational Therapy* 45 (11): 979–986. https://doi.org/10.5014/ajot.45.11.979.

Mattingly, C. and Fleming, M.H. (1994). *Clinical Reasoning: Forms of Inquiry in a Therapeutic Practice*, 37. Philadelphia: FA Davis.

Mayers, C.A. (2003). The development and evaluation of the Mayers' Lifestyle Questionnaire (2). *British Journal of Occupational Therapy* 66 (9): 388–395.

Mitchell, R. and Unsworth, C.A. (2005). Clinical reasoning during community health home visits: expert and novice differences. *British Journal of Occupational Therapy* 68 (5): 215–223. https://doi.org/10.1177/030802260506800505.

Molden, D.C. and Dweck, C.S. (2006). Finding "meaning" in psychology: a lay theories approach to self-regulation, social perception, and social development. *American Psychologist* 61 (3): 192. https://doi.org/10.1037/0003-066X.61.3.192.

Mosey, A.C. (1981). *Occupational Therapy: Configuration of a Profession*, vol. 63, 67–69. New York: Raven Press.

Muoni, T. (2012). Decision-making, intuition, and the midwife: understanding heuristics. *British Journal of Midwifery* 20 (1): 52–56. https://doi.org/10.12968/bjom.2012.20.1.52.

Newel, A. and Simon, H.A. (1972). Human problem solving. In: *Clinical Reasoning: Forms of Inquiry in a Therapeutic Practice* (eds. C. Mattingly and M.H. Fleming), 37. Philadelphia: FA Davis.

Oakley, F., Kielhofner, G., Barris, R., and Reichler, R.K. (1986). The role checklist: development and empirical assessment of reliability. *The Occupational Therapy Journal of Research* 6 (3): 157–170.

Opacich, K. J. (1991). *Assessment and informed decision-making. Occupational therapy: Overcoming human performance deficits*, 354–372. Slack Thorofare, NJ

Payton, O.D. (1985). Clinical reasoning process in physical therapy. *Physical Therapy* 65 (6): 924–928. https://doi.org/10.1093/ptj/65.6.924.

Rivett, D.A. and Higgs, J. (1997). Hypothesis generation in the clinical reasoning behavior of manual therapists. *Journal, Physical Therapy Education* 11 (1): 40–45. https://journals.lww.com/jopte/Abstract/1997/01000/Hypothesis_Generation_in_the_Clinical_Reasoning.8.aspx.

Roberts, A.E. (1996). Approaches to reasoning in occupational therapy: a critical exploration. *British Journal of Occupational Therapy* 59 (5): 233–236. https://doi.org/10.1177/030802269605900513.

Rogers, J.C. (1982). Order and disorder in medicine and occupational therapy. *American Journal of Occupational Therapy* 36 (1): 29–35.

Rogers, J.C. (1983). Eleanor Clarke Slagle lectureship—1983; clinical reasoning: the ethics, science, and art. *American Journal of Occupational Therapy* 37 (9): 601–616. https://doi.org/10.5014/ajot.37.9.601.

Rogers, J.C. (2004). Occupational diagnosis. In: *Occupation for Occupational Therapists* (ed. M. Molineux), 17–31. Blackwell Science Oxford, UK.

Rogers, J.C. and Holm, M.B. (1991). Occupational therapy diagnostic reasoning: a component of clinical reasoning. *American Journal of Occupational Therapy* 45 (11): 1045–1053. https://doi.org/10.5014/ajot.45.11.1045.

Sackett, D. L., Rosenberg, W. M., Gray, J. M., Haynes, R. B., & Richardson, W. S. (1996). *Evidence based medicine: what it is and what it isn't*. https://doi.org/10.1136/bmj.312.7023.71

Schell, B.A.B. (2013). Professional reasoning in practice. In: *Willard and Spackman's Occupational Therapy* (eds. B.A. Schell, G. Gillen, M. Scaffa and E.S. Cohn), 384–397. Lippincott Williams & Wilkins.

Schell, B.A.B. and Schell, J.W. (eds.) (2008). *Clinical and Professional Reasoning in Occupational Therapy*. Lippincott Williams & Wilkins.

Schon, D.A. (1983). *The Reflective Practitioner: How Professionals Think in Action*. New York: Basic Books.

Schön, D.A. (1987). *Educating the Reflective Practitioner: Toward a New Design for Teaching and Learning in the Professions*. Jossey-Bass.

Searl, M.M., Borgi, L., and Chemali, Z. (2010). It is time to talk about people: a human-centered healthcare system. *Health Research Policy and Systems* 8 (1): 35. https://health-policy-systems.biomedcentral.com/articles/10.118/1478-4505-8-35.

Smith, G. (2006). The Casson memorial lecture 2006: telling tales — how stories and narratives co-create change (sagepub.com). *British Journal of Occupational Therapy* 69 (7): 304–311. https://doi.org/10.1177/030802260606900702.

Stewart, S. (1999). The use of standardised and non-standardised assessments in a social services setting: implications for practice. *British Journal of Occupational Therapy* 62 (9): 417–423. https://doi.org/10.1177/030802269906200907.

Swain, J. (2004). Interpersonal communication. In: *Physiotherapy: A psychosocial approach* (eds. J. Sim, M. Smith and S. French). Oxford: Butterworth Heinmann.

Tate, S (2004) *Using critical reflection as a teaching tool. In Tate S., Sills M (2004) The Development of Critical Reflection in the Health Professions. Learning and Teaching Support Network (LTSN) at the Centre for Health Sciences and Practice (HSAP). https://westminsterresearch.westminster.ac.uk/item/93476/the-development-of-critical--reflection-in-the-health-professions* check

Taylor, B. (2010). *Reflective Practice for Healthcare Professionals: A Practical Guide*. McGraw-Hill Education (UK).

Thomas, A., Menon, A., Boruff, J. et al. (2014). Applications of social constructivist learning theories in knowledge translation for healthcare professionals: a scoping review. *Implementation Science* 9 (1): 54. https://doi.org/10.1186/1748-5908-9-54.

Toft, B. (2001). *External Inquiry into the Adverse Incident that Occurred at Queen's Medical Centre, Nottingham, 4th January 2001*. London: Department of Health https://www.who.int/patientsafety/news/Queens%20Medical%20Centre%20report%20(Toft).pdf.

Toft, B. and Reynolds, S. (2016). *Learning from Disasters*. Springer.

Tomlin, G.S. (2008). Scientific reasoning. In: *Clinical and Professional Reasoning in Occupational Therapy* (eds. B.A.B. Schell and J.W. Schell), 91–124. Lippincott Williams & Wilkins.

Unsworth, C. (1999). *Cognitive and Perceptual Dysfunction: A Clinical Reasoning Approach to Evaluation and Intervention*. FA Davis.

Von Bertalanffy, L. (1951). General system theory, a new approach to unity of science. 5. Conclusion. *Human Biology* 23 (4): 337. https://www.ncbi.nlm.nih.gov/pubmed/14907030.

Westcott, L., & Whitcombe, S. (2012). *Continuing professional development: The personal and public interface*. https://doi.org/10.4276/030802212X13548955545378

White, P. (2004). *Using reflective practice in the physiotherapy curriculum. The development of critical reflection in the health professions*, 24–31. London: Health Sciences and Practice Subject Centre.

Zarit, S.H., Todd, P.A., and Zarit, J.M. (1986). Subjective burden of husbands and wives as caregivers: a longitudinal study. *The Gerontologist* 26 (3): 260–266.

SECTION 2

CONCEPTS FOR ASSESSMENT AND MEASUREMENT

CHAPTER 7

Standardisation

OVERVIEW

This chapter discusses what is meant by standardisation and a standardised test. The chapter also explores the definitions of key terms, including the normal distribution, percentile ranks, standard deviation, and mean.

See Chapter 1 to review terminology. The process for developing an assessment for use in practice is described in Chapter 14.

QUESTIONS TO CONSIDER

1. What is standardisation?
2. What are the benefits of standardisation versus non-standardisation?
3. What is a normal distribution curve? Why is this important in standardisation?
4. What is standard deviation?

STANDARDISATION

Standardisation (see Chapter 1, p. 22) is the process of taking an assessment and developing a fixed protocol for its administration and scoring, and then conducting psychometric studies (see Chapter 15) to evaluate whether the resulting assessment has acceptable levels of validity and reliability. There are two ways in which assessments can be standardised: either in terms of procedures, materials, and scoring or in

Principles of Assessment and Outcome Measurement for Allied Health Professionals:
Practice, Research and Development, Second Edition. Alison J. Laver-Fawcett and Diane L. Cox.
© 2021 John Wiley & Sons Ltd. Published 2021 by John Wiley & Sons Ltd.

terms of normative standardisation (de Clive-Lowe 1996). The first method of standardisation involves the provision of detailed descriptions and directions for the test materials; method of administration; instructions for administration; scoring; and interpretation of scores (Jones 1991; see Chapter 14). Standardisation 'extends to the exact materials employed, time limits, oral instructions, preliminary demonstrations, ways of handling queries from test takers, and every other detail of the testing situation' (Anastasi 1988, p. 25). This information should be provided in the *test manual* or, if a test is published in its entirety in a professional journal, should be included in the description of the test.

To standardise the *test materials*, the exact test materials should be listed or included. Some tests provide materials as part of a standardised test battery. If the allied health professional (*AHP*) has to collect the materials together for the test, then the precise details of how to construct the test (with exact sizes, colours, fabric of materials, etc.) are required (see Chapter 14 for more information on test development).

To standardise the *method of administration*, the test conditions should be described in detail. The number of people tested at any one time should be specified (i.e. individual or group assessment, size of the group). Information about the time required for administration should be given. In order to produce standardised instructions for administration, detailed written instructions for the AHP should be provided. Exact wording for any instructions to be given to the test taker is required. To maintain standardisation, AHPs should be told to follow all instructions exactly.

To standardise the *scoring system*, clear guidelines need to be provided for scoring. The person's performance on the test should be evaluated on the basis of empirical data. Scoring methods vary from test to test and may include the use of raw scores, which may then be converted to another type of score. If scores are being added, subtracted, divided, or multiplied, then make sure the level of measurement allows the numbers to be handled in that way (see Chapter 4 for more information).

Information should be included in a standardised test to guide the AHP in the interpretation of scores. AHPs should be aware that a number of factors may influence the person's performance on the test, including test anxiety, fatigue, interruptions, and distractions. In addition to basic administration details, other subtle factors might affect a person's test performance. For example, when giving oral instructions, 'rate of speaking, tone of voice, inflection, pauses, and facial expression' all may influence how a person responds (Anastasi 1998, pp. 25–26).

STANDARDISED ASSESSMENTS

AHPs need reliable, valid, and sensitive outcome measures in order to obtain an accurate baseline for intervention and to examine whether that intervention has been effective. Quantifiable data is required in order to undertake the statistical analyses required to demonstrate that results obtained from an intervention are significant and not just owing to chance factors (de Clive-Lowe 1996). As discussed in Chapter 1, the requirement to demonstrate the effectiveness of therapy interventions has led to an increase in the development and use of standardised assessments within AHPs.

WHY SHOULD AHPs USE STANDARDISED TESTS?

Most testing errors occur when the AHP has done one or more of the following (Vitale and Nugent 1996):

- collected insufficient data
- collected inaccurate data
- used unsystematic data collection methods
- obtained irrelevant data
- failed to verify data collected
- obtained data that has been contaminated by bias or prejudice (e.g. either by the person completing the self-report or proxy survey or by the AHP)
- not accurately communicated data collected.

The use of standardised tests can help reduce the chances of errors resulting from such practices. A rigorously developed and psychometrically robust test will:

- involve the collection of sufficient data for the purpose of the test (e.g. to screen for a specific impairment);
- will have established reliability, so that data is collected accurately;
- will use a systematic data collection method;
- will have established validity, so that data obtained is related to the stated purpose and focus of the test;
- will provide information about confidence intervals, so that the AHP can judge how likely it is that this test result has provided a true picture of the person's ability and / or deficits;
- will reduce the influence of bias or prejudice on test results; and
- will have a record form for recording, analysing, and communicating scores.

The AHP must establish that the assessment they plan to use will accurately provide the information needed for the purpose required (see Chapter 3). Using standardised tests can facilitate objectivity, and this is very important because when assessing human functioning it is virtually impossible to obtain complete accuracy and objectivity. Bartram (1990) stated that 'the major advantage of a statistically-based assessment – and it is crucial to professional effectiveness and quality of decision making – is that it provides an objective source of data, unbiased by subjective feeling' (p. 3).

Subjective
'is based on personal opinions, interpretations, points of view, emotions and judgment'

Objective
'is fact-based, measurable and observable'
https://www.diffen.com/difference/Objective_vs_Subjective

WHAT IS A STANDARDISED TEST?

AHPs may refer to a published tool used for data collection as a standardised test, standardised assessment, standardised evaluation, standardised measure/outcome measure, standardised instrument, or a standardised scale. (Note: Definitions of assessment, outcome measure, scale, and instrument and discussions about the use of these terms in therapy have been provided in the chapter titled 'Introduction').

So What Do We Mean by *Standardised in AHP Practice?*

The word *standard* has been defined as 'a level of quality or achievement, especially a level that is thought to be acceptable' or 'something that you use in order to judge the quality of something else' or 'an accepted or approved example of something against which others are judged or measured' (https://www.collinsdictionary.com/dictionary/english/standard). Pentland et al. (2018) define standardised measurements as designed to capture outcomes in each of the different categories [], with the majority of different tools being used to evaluate changes in body function, symptomology, and functional performance (p. 38). Standardisation, therefore, 'implies uniformity of procedure in administering and scoring [a] test' (Anastasi 1988, p. 25).

Cole et al. (1995) described a standardised test as a measurement tool that is published and has been designed for a specific purpose for use with a particular population. They state that a standardised test should have detailed instructions explaining how and when it should be administered and scored and how to interpret scores. It should also present the results of investigations to evaluate the measure's psychometric properties. These instructions are usually contained in a *test protocol* that describes the specific procedures that must be followed when assessing a patient (Christiansen et al. 2005). Details of any investigations of reliability and validity should also be given. In order to maintain standardisation, the assessment must be administered according to the testing protocol. The conditions under which standardised tests are administered have to be the same if the results recorded from different service users by different AHPs, or from the same person by the same AHP on different occasions, are to be comparable.

Being standardised does not necessarily mean that the test is an objective measure of externally observable data. AHPs also develop standardised tools that enable clinicians to record internal, unobservable constructs, for example, a person's self-report of feelings, such as pain, sadness, or anxiety. However, any standardised test, whether of observable behaviours or psychological constructs, should be structured so that the method of data collection will yield the same responses for a person at a specific moment in time and the same responses for the person being tested regardless of which AHP is administering the test. Some standardised tests are referred to as a *'battery'*; this is an assessment approach or instrument with several parts. For example, the Rivermead Perceptual Assessment Battery (*RPAB*; Lincoln et al. 1985) comprises 16 subtests covering several domains of perception: form constancy, colour constancy, sequencing, object completion, figure-ground discrimination, body image, inattention, and spatial awareness.

What Is an Un-standardised Assessment in AHP Practice?

The terms *non-standardised* and *un-standardised* are used interchangeably in the literature. These are assessments that provide the AHP with information but have no precise comparison to a norm or a criterion. Some un-standardised tests are structured assessments that are constructed and organised to provide guidelines for the content and process of the assessment, but their psychometric properties have not been researched and documented. (see Chapters 8, 9, and 15).

NORMATIVE DATA

Normative data (often referred to as norms) provide a numerical description of the test performance of a defined and well-described sample group (known as the normative group, normative sample, or reference group) that then serves as a reference from which AHPs can evaluate the performance of the other people who take the test. Most norms tables provide, in descending order, the range of test scores and the percentage of people in the normative sample who scored below each score level.

By obtaining a client's score, the AHP can then determine how he compares with the normative group. Statistical analyses are undertaken to give technical information about the distribution of the normative group's test scores, such as the average score. These statistics may be presented as a labelled normal curve with specified values attached to standard deviations above and below the mean (Anastasi 1988). AHPs should understand statistical concepts such as mean, standard deviation, and normal distribution. The definitions presented below have been developed following an examination of some measurement literature, for example, Anastasi (1988) and Crocker and Algina (1986).

Terminology Related to Non-referenced Tests

Obtained Score

The score achieved by a person taking a test.

Raw Score

A raw score is the original numerical score that has not been transformed. In therapy measurement, the raw score is the original result obtained by a client on a test (e.g. the number of correctly answered items) as opposed to that score after transformation to a standard score or percentile rank.

Frequency Distribution

A frequency distribution is a table of scores (either presented from high to low, or low to high scores) providing the number of people who obtain each score or whose scores fall in each score interval. Frequency distributions are used to determine tables of percentile ranks.

Mean

The mean (μ) is a measure of central tendency. It is the arithmetic average: the sum divided by the number of cases. Therefore, in testing, the mean score is the average score obtained by a group of people on a test. The mean score is calculated by adding the scores obtained by all people taking the test and then dividing this total by the number of obtained scores. For normal distributions, the mean is the most efficient and, therefore, the least subject to sample fluctuations of all measures of central tendency (Manikandan 2011). The mean can be affected by a few extremely high or low values.

Median

The median is the value above and below which half the cases fall. If there is an even number of cases, the median is the average of the two middle cases when they are sorted in ascending or descending order. With test scores, the median is the score below which 50% of people's scores fall. Like the mean, the median is a measure of central tendency. But unlike the mean, the median is not sensitive to

(*continued*)

(continued)

outlying scores. Therefore, if the distribution of scores is distorted by a few atypical scores (that are considered to have little clinical relevance), then the median may be a better summary description of the group's performance than the mean. If the distribution is symmetric, then the median and mean will be almost identical. The median is also by definition the 50th percentile (Manikandan 2011).

Normal Distribution

The normal distribution is a theoretical frequency distribution for a set of variable data, usually represented by a bell-shaped curve symmetrical about the mean. The normal distribution is also known as the *Gaussian distribution* (after the nineteenth-century German mathematician Karl Friedrich Gauss). It is used to represent a normal or statistically probable outcome. Normal distributions are symmetric with scores more concentrated in the middle than in the tails. They are defined by two parameters: the mean (μ) and the standard deviation (σ). The normal distribution curve is symmetrical and bell shaped, showing that scores will usually fall near the mean value, but will occasionally deviate by large amounts. The normal distribution curve has a line representing its mean at the centre (see Figure 7.1 below).

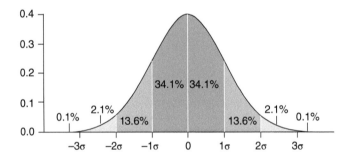

FIGURE 7.1   A normal curve showing standard deviations above and below the mean. *Source:* Toews (2007).

Test developers frequently discover that the results for a group of people who have taken their test match a normal distribution curve (bell curve; see Figure 7.1). This means that they find a large number of people perform moderately well on their test; i.e. their results fall in the middle of the bell. Some people do worse than average, and some do better than average on the test; i.e. their results fall in the sloping sides of the bell, and a very small number of people achieve very high or very low scores (i.e. their results fall in the rim of the bell) (Streiner et al. 2015).

The normal distribution is important to AHPs because many psychological and behavioural constructs are distributed approximately normally. Although the distributions are only approximately normal, they are usually quite close. The normal distribution is also important for test developers and for AHPs undertaking research, because many statistical tests can be applied to normally distributed data. If the mean and standard deviation of a normal distribution are known, it is easy to convert back and forth from raw scores to percentiles (Streiner et al. 2015).

Some tests use standard deviations to provide a cut-off point at which a person's performance is said to be dysfunctional or at which a specific deficit is considered to be present. For example, the RPAB (Lincoln et al. 1985) provides a graph that profiles scores in relation to expected levels for people of average intelligence and sets a cut-off level of 3 standard deviations below the mean to indicate a level below which perceptual deficit is presumed.

Standard Deviation

The standard deviation (σ) is a measure of the spread or extent of variability of a set of scores around their mean. It is the average amount a score varies from the average score in a series of scores. The standard deviation reflects the degree of homogeneity of the group with respect to the test item in question. That is, the less the scores are spread across the range of possible scores, the smaller will be the standard deviation. Therefore, a large standard deviation indicates that the scores obtained are scattered far from the mean, whereas a small standard deviation indicates that the obtained scores are clustered closely around the mean. The standard deviation is defined as the square root of the variance. This means it is the root mean square (*RMS*) deviation from the average. The standard deviation is always a positive number (or zero) and is always measured in the same units as the original data (Streiner et al. 2015).

The standard deviation is the most commonly used measure of spread. An important attribute of the standard deviation as a measure of spread is that if the mean and standard deviation of a normal distribution are known, it is possible to compute the percentile rank associated with any given score. In a normal distribution, about 68% of the scores are within one standard deviation of the mean, and about 95% of the scores are within two standard deviations of the mean.

The standard deviations from the mean indicate the degree to which a person's performance on the test is above or below average. It is helpful to think about these as 'deviations from assumptions of normality' in order to emphasise that the concept of both norm and deviance are constructed either by society and/or the application of statistics (Hammell 2004, p. 409).

- One standard deviation either side of the mean represents 34.13% of the population (decimal points are often not used, and this is represented as 34% of scores, or is given with only one decimal point as 34.1% – see Figure 7.2). So, a score falling between minus one or plus one standard deviation from the mean represents a score obtained by 68.26% (or roughly 68%) of the population (Anastasi 1988).

- The percentage population that falls between one and two standard deviation above the mean is 13.59%, and as the curve is symmetrical, the percentage population that falls between one and two standard deviation below the mean is also 13.59%. So, scores falling between minus two or plus two standard deviations above the mean represent those of 95.44% of the population (Anastasi 1988).

- The percentage population that falls between two and three standard deviations above the mean is 2.14%, and as the curve is symmetrical, the percentage population that falls between two and three standard deviations below the mean is also 2.14%. So, scores falling between minus two or plus three standard deviations above the mean represent those of 99.72% of the population (Anastasi 1988).

Percentile Rank

Percentile values are values of a quantitative variable (e.g. numerical test scores) that divide the ordered data into groups so that a certain percentage is above and another percentage is below. Quartiles (the 25th, 50th, and 75th percentiles) are used to divide the obtained scores into four groups of equal size.

Percentile Values

It is the percentage of people in the norm group scoring below a particular raw score. It indicates a person's relative position in the group for the ability/characteristic tested. Percentile rank is widely used (e.g. for infant growth charts) and is quite easily understood. With a percentile rank, the remaining scores are at the same level (equal scores) or are higher/greater scores. For instance, if a physiotherapy student received a score of 95 on a test and this score were greater than or equal to the scores of 88% of the other physiotherapy students taking the test on that course, then the student's percentile rank would be 88, and they would be in the 88th percentile. Percentiles provide a useful way of comparing people and identifying when a person's attributes (such as height, weight, and head circumference) or performance is significantly below a level expected for his age and background.

For many tests of dysfunction, the cut-off point for identifying a deficit falls 1 standard deviation below the mean.

A norm-referenced test, therefore, determines a person's placement on a normal distribution curve. It is used often in education and students/pupils compete against each other on this type test; this is sometimes referred to as 'grading on a curve'. In therapy, it is a test that is used to evaluate performance of a person against the scores of a peer group whose performance has been described using a normative sample. Types of scoring on normative tests can include developmental norms, within group norms (standard scores, percentiles), and fixed reference group norms.

A good example of a norm-referenced test, whose test manual clearly explains the application of the normal curve, is provided by (Dunn and Daniels 2002) in the Infant and Toddler Sensory Profile Manual. In Figure 7.2 below, the normal curve is shown and indicates that typical performance of infants from birth to six months is found to fall in the range of minus 1 standard deviation (sd) to plus 1 sd from the

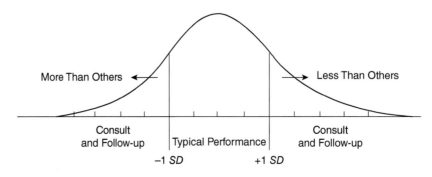

FIGURE 7.2   The normal curve and the Infant/Toddler Sensory Profile Classification System for children ages birth to six months. Infant/Toddler Sensory Profile. *Source:* Dunn (2002). © 2002, Pearson.

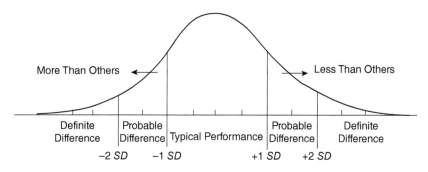

FIGURE 7.3   The normal curve and the Infant/Toddler Sensory Profile Classification System for children ages 7–36 months. Infant/Toddler Sensory Profile. *Source:* Dunn (2002). © 2002, Pearson.

mean. Scores falling outside this range are either more or less than the majority of other infants of this age, and the AHP is recommended to follow up these babies. As the Infant/Toddler Sensory Profile assesses responsiveness to sensory stimuli, scores representing both under-responsiveness and over-responsiveness are of concern to an AHP. In many other normative assessments, the AHP would focus on scores below the mean, which equated with a dysfunction, and would not concern herself with people who showed a greater than average ability on the test.

The next Figure 7.3 shows how the normal curve is used to identify children exhibiting typical performance for their age from children with a probable difference (whose scores fall within the 1–2 sd range) and a definite difference (whose scores fall ±2 sd from the mean).

The standard against which a person is assessed should be what is typically seen for a person of the same age, and the process through which the person accomplishes the assessment task must be evaluated against the process for that age and cultural background. It is, therefore, critical for AHPs to understand normal human development, from birth to old age, and to understand the impact of cultural and environmental factors upon performance. In order to be sure that the data from the normative sample can be generalised to their service users, AHPs should review the representativeness and sample sizes of the normative data upon which assessments have been standardised. To do this, the AHP must consider the characteristics of their service users (such as age, sex, education, sociocultural background) and compare these to the characteristics of the normative sample. The importance of these factors will vary depending on the construct measured.

The AHP should consider which characteristics are likely to be relevant to the skills or constructs that the test is designed to measure (de Clive-Lowe 1996). For example, with a paediatric developmental assessment, a child's age will have a profound effect on the motor, language, cognitive, and perceptual skills that an AHP would expect a child to have mastered. With an older client group assessed on an Instrumental Activities of Living (*IADL*) scale, the sex and sociocultural background of the client and normative sample might have an effect on people's prior experience and performance of specific IADL items. For example, an older woman might not have dealt with the family's finances, and an older man might not have dealt with laundry.

Norms are not 'universal truths' but are based upon 'cultural judgements' (Hammell 2004, p. 409). Therefore, norms in any society can be fluid and may change in response to changes in other aspects of society, such as value systems. Therefore, depending on the construct being tested, some normative data should be updated at regular intervals.

TRAINING AND INTERPRETING STANDARDISED TEST SCORES

It is important to check whether you as the AHP administering the test have the appropriate knowledge and skill to administer, score, and interpret the results of the test correctly. Most published tests require that the person administering the test has obtained certain qualifications and expertise. Some tests require that the test administrator has undertaken specific training on the administration and scoring of the test (de Clive-Lowe 1996). For example, to be calibrated to administer the Assessment of Motor and Process Skills (*AMPS*; Fisher 2003, Fisher and Merritt 2012), AHPs have to attend a one-week training course.

Most standardised assessments provide raw or standard scores. These scores are not sufficient alone and must be interpreted within the wider context of the specific testing situation and influences of the test environment and the client's current situation and personal idiosyncrasies (de Clive-Lowe 1996). For more information on interpreting test scores, see Chapter 5.

REVIEW QUESTIONS

7.1   What makes a test standardised?

7.2   What is a norm-referenced test?

7.3   What is standard deviation, and how is it used in measurement?

You will find brief answers to these questions at the back of this book on p. 445 .

Worksheet 7.1 takes you through a series of questions to help you establish whether a test has been standardised.

Please complete this for the test you are using, mark whether Yes or No, and add your comments on the test.

Name of the test:
Full reference:

	Yes	No
Is there a test manual?		
Does the test manual describe the test development process?		
Does the test manual describe the purpose of the test and the client group for whom the test has been developed?		
Does the test manual provide details of psychometric studies undertaken to establish reliability and validity?		
Does the test manual describe the materials needed for test administration or are these included as part of the test package?		
Does the test manual describe the environment that should be used for testing?		
Is there a protocol for test administration that provides all the instructions required to administer the test?		
Is there guidance on how to score each test item?		
Is there a scoring form for recording scores?		
Is there guidance for interpreting scores?		
If it is a norm-referenced test, is the normative sample well described?		
Are there norm-tables from which you can compare a client's score with the distribution of scores obtained by the normative group?		

Comments:

REFERENCES

Anastasi, A. (1988). *Psychological Testing*, 5e. New York. NY: Macmillan.

Bartram, D. (1990). Reliability and validity. Chapter 3. In: *Testing People. A Practical Guide to Psychometrics* (eds. J.R. Beech and L. Harding). Windsor, Berks: NFER-Nelson.

Christiansen, C., Baum, C.M., and Bass-Haugen, J. (eds.) (2005). *Occupational Therapy: Performance, Participation, and Well-Being*, 2–22. Thorofare, NJ: Slack.

de Clive-Lowe, S. (1996). Outcome measurement, cost-effectiveness and clinical audit: the importance of standardised assessment to occupational therapists in meeting these new demands. *British Journal of Occupational Therapy* 59 (8): 357–362. https://doi.org/10.1177/030802269605900803.

Cole, B., Finch, E., Gowland, C., and Mayo, N. (1995). *Physical Rehabilitation Outcome Measures*, 24–78. Toronto, Ont.: Canadian Physiotherapy Association.

Crocker, L. and Algina, J. (1986). *Introduction to Classical and Modern Test Theory*. Harbor Drive, Orlando, FL: Holt, Rinehart and Winston.

Dunn W (2002) *Infant/Toddler Sensory Profile*. Harcourt Assessment. Pearson

Dunn, W. and Daniels, D.B. (2002). Initial development of the infant/toddler sensory profile. *Journal of Early Intervention* 25 (1): 27–41. https://doi.org/10.1177/105381510202500104.

Fisher, A. G. (2003). *Assessment of motor and process skills. Administration and Scoring Manual*. AMPS Overview | Center for Innovative OT Solutions

Fisher, A. G., & Merritt, B. K. (2012). *Conceptualizing and developing the AMPS within a framework of modern objective measurement*. Assessment of Motor and Process Skills, 1, 14-11

Hammell, K.W. (2004). Deviating from the norm: a sceptical interrogation of the classificatory practices of the ICF. *British Journal of Occupational Therapy* 67 (9): 408–411. https://doi.org/10.1177/030802260406700906.

Jones, L. (1991). The standardised test. *Clinical Rehabilitation* 5 (3): 177–180. https://doi.org/10.1177/026921559100500301.

Lincoln, N.B., Whiting, S.E., Cockburn, J., and Bhavnani, G. (1985). An evaluation of perceptual retraining. *International Rehabilitation Medicine* 7 (3): 99–101. https://doi.org/10.3109/03790798509166132.

Manikandan, S. (2011). Measures of central tendency: median and mode. *Journal of Pharmacology and Pharmacotherapeutics* 2 (3): 214. https://doi.org/10.4103/0976-500X.83300.

Pentland, D., Kantartzis, S., Clausen, M.G., and Witemyre, K. (2018). *Occupational Therapy and Complexity: Defining and Describing Practice*. London: Royal College of Occupational Therapists www.rcot.co.uk/sites/default/files/OT%20and%20complexity.pdf.

Streiner, D.L., Norman, G.R., and Cairney, J. (2015). *Health Measurement Scales: A Practical Guide to their Development and Use*. USA: Oxford University Press.

M. W. Toews, 2007. *File Standard deviation diagram*. File:Standard deviation diagram.svg - Wikimedia Commons

Vitale, B.A. and Nugent, P.M. (1996). *Test Success: Test-Taking Techniques for the Healthcare Student*. FA Davis Company.

CHAPTER 8

Validity and Clinical Utility

This chapter will define the main types of validity of relevance to allied health professionals (AHPs). This will include definitions of content validity, construct validity, and criterion-related validity as well as descriptions of subtypes of these three main validation studies, such as predictive validity, discriminative validity, and concurrent validity. External validity and face validity are also discussed. The chapter ends by considering the concept of clinical utility.

1. How do I ensure that my measurements are valid?
2. How do I evaluate whether the measures I use are acceptable to my clients?
3. How do I identify whether an assessment will be clinically useful in my practice setting?

In order for any measurement to be clinically useful, it should meet two essential requirements:

1. It should measure what it intends or is supposed to measure.
2. It should make this measurement with a minimum of error (Pynsent et al. 2004).

The first type of requirement is called *validity* and is explained in this chapter. The second type of requirement is known as *reliability* and will be explored in the next chapter (Chapter 9). A test is considered valid when research demonstrates that it succeeds in measuring what it purports to measure. When a test is developed, the researcher needs to define the domain to be assessed in order to construct relevant test items. This definition of the domain specifies what the test is supposed to measure, but is no guarantee that the resultant test will actually assess this intended domain (Bartram 1990). AHPs need to know whether the items contained in a measure, both individually and as a whole, adequately represent the performance domains and/or constructs they are supposed to measure, and whether the assessment items address these domains and/or constructs in the correct proportions (Asher 1996). Therefore, AHPs need some evidence that the test is an indicator of what it was designed to measure. This is known as validity.

Definition of Validity

Validity relates to the appropriateness and justifiability of the things supposed about the person's scores on a test and the rationale AHPs have for making inferences from such scores to wider areas of functioning (Bartram 1990).

Validation is undertaken by a test developer to collect evidence to support the types of inferences that are to be drawn from the results of an assessment (Crocker and Algina 1986). Bartram (1990) stated that the evidence used to establish validity, and justify inferences made from test scores, ranges from 'appeals to common sense at one extreme to quantifiable empirical evidence at the other' (p. 76). There are several types of validity, which AHPs should be able to understand in order to critically review test manuals to identify whether psychometric studies have shown the test has appropriate levels of validity. Three types of validation studies, known as *content validity*, *construct validity*, and *criterion-related validity*, are traditionally performed during test development (Crocker and Algina 1986).

These areas of validation can be further subdivided into specific validity study areas exploring aspects such as *predictive validity*, *discriminative validity*, *factorial validity*, and *concurrent (also referred to as congruent or convergent) validity*. *External validity* is relevant when we want to generalise findings. *Face validity* is also considered by some researchers and has a strong link to clinical utility. Examination of validity should be built into a test development process from the outset, and the development of a valid test will involve several sequential processes undertaken throughout test development. This is particularly true for content and construct validity, whereas criterion-related validity studies are more often conducted towards the end of test development (Anastasi 1988).

CONTENT VALIDITY

Content validity (also sometimes called content relevance or content coverage) refers to the degree to which an assessment measures what it is supposed to measure judged on the appropriateness of its content. Also see Table 8.1, pp. 260 later in this chapter.

Definitions of Content Validity

Content validity consists 'of a judgement whether the instrument [assessment] samples all the relevant content or domains' . (Streiner et al. 2015, p. 8)

The ability of the selected items to reflect the features of the construct in the measure. This type of validity addresses the degree to which items of an instrument sufficiently represent the content domain. It also answers the question that to what extent the selected sample in an instrument or instrument items is a comprehensive sample of the content. (Zamanzadeh et al. 2014, p. 164)

Content validation examines the components of a test and examines each test item as to its representativeness of the entire sample of potential items representing the domain to be measured. Content validity, therefore, relates to the rigour with which items for a test have been gathered, examined, and selected. Content validation is needed when the AHP wants to draw inferences from the test scores about the person's ability on a larger domain of activities similar to those used on the test itself (Crocker and Algina 1986). For example, if you want to measure balance and have 10 different items related to aspects of balance, you would need to examine each item separately to see if it really did relate to the domain of balance (Lewis and Bottomley 2008). Content validity relates to the relevance of the person's individual responses to the assessment items, rather than to the apparent relevance of the assessment item content. Asher (1996) noted that content validity is descriptive rather than statistically determined. Therefore, it is sometimes considered a weaker form of validity, compared to other types of validity, such as predictive or discriminative validity.

Crocker and Algina (1986) state that a content validation study should as a minimum involve:

1. a definition of the performance domain being measured; in achievement tests this is often defined by a list of instructional objectives;
2. the use of a panel of qualified experts in the content domain;
3. the development of a structured framework for the process of matching test items to the overall performance domain; and
4. the collection and summarising of data collected by the expert panel when undertaking this matching process.

Test developers can make a dichotomous decision when matching test items to the performance domain to be measured; for example, the item either is or is not an aspect of the performance to be assessed. Alternatively, rate the degree of match between the test item and the performance domain, for example, using a 5-point scale where 5 = an excellent match and 1 = no match.

One issue that should be considered during content validation is whether aspects of the performance domain to be measured should be weighted to reflect their importance. Sometimes all aspects of the performance domain are of equal value. However, in AHP assessments, sometimes some aspects of performance are more critical than others. For instance, when undertaking an assessment of the person's functioning to assess readiness for discharge home, the AHP may decide that the assessment of items related to risk, such as the ability to manage the gas, likelihood of falling or wandering, and ability to self-medicate, is more important than other areas which are more easily addressed, such as the inability to cook meals, which can be addressed by the provision of meals on wheels. In a content validation study where weighting importance is required, the researcher needs to provide the panel of experts with a definition of importance and may use a scale to identify the importance of different test items to the critical aspects of the performance domain.

Clemson et al. (1999) provide a good example of a content validity study which offers clear details of the methodology followed. They describe a series of studies that contributed to the content validity of the Westmead Home Safety Assessment (WeHSA), a test developed to identify fall hazards in a client's home environment. The first study they undertook to ensure content validity involved content analysis of the literature that studied falls and the home physical environment. They followed a process comprising four steps for this type of analysis:

1. Develop operational definitions of the key variables
2. Decide what to include in the analysis
3. Classify and record data
4. Analyse data.

Their literature search identified 26 relevant studies that were analysed during WeHSA test development. The test developers used their initial version of the WeHSA 'as an organising framework for the content analysis and the types of home environmental hazard reported in each study were tallied' (p. 173). If a new hazard was identified in the literature, this was added. Frequencies for each hazard cited across the 26 studies were calculated, and tables summarising this analysis included in the test manual.

Clemson et al. (1999), to construct test specifications for a criterion-referenced assessment, wrote of a 'descriptive scheme' (p. 173) that provided:

- A general description of the tool's purpose that gives a brief overview of what is being assessed and a description of the purpose of the test.
- A list of stimulus attributes to define the assessment's attributes (instrument specifications) that includes all the factors that influence the composition of test items, for example:
  - "the assessment needs to be in a form manageable on a home visit and able to be completed in a home situation, or soon afterwards.
  - items must identify features of the environment that may impact on the risk of falling" (p. 178), such as: 'design and condition of objects (for example, equipment, furniture, footwear' (p. 178).
- Specification of eligible content.

The expert review process used for the *WeHSA* study comprised 'assessment users, developers and beneficiaries, medical and interdisciplinary workers in falls speciality areas and care of older people, and those with expertise in the areas of geriatric home assessment, falls, older people and disability issues and architecture' (p. 174). The expert panel also include some laypeople to represent the views of clients and carers. The panel comprised 14 expert reviewers, of whom 13 completed stage 1, 12 completed stage 2, and 8 responded to the final review. Clemson et al. (1999) used a Delphi panel approach for their review that involved 'anonymous gathering of responses, feedback from respondents and the opportunity to alter responses based on their feedback' (p. 174). For stage one of the content validity study, an open-ended questionnaire was used to record the expert panel's examination of the stimulus attributes, coverage domain, and completeness.

For stage 2 of the expert review, the panel were asked to rate the degree of relevance of the WeHSA items using a 5-point scale 'relevance-taxonomy' (p. 174):

1. Essential: defined as 'item is essential and must be included in the home assessment for falls risk assessment. It would be a hazard for any elderly person who is at risk of falling'
2. Important
3. Acceptable
4. Marginally relevant
5. Not relevant: defined as 'This item would never be a hazard for falls'.

The test developers decided to quantify the level of content validity of the WeHSA by calculating the percentage agreement of experts using a content validity index (CVI). This CVI is calculated by dividing the proportion of items judged by an expert panel to have content validity by the total number of items in a test. They examined the content validity of each item on the test by calculating the proportion of expert judges who rated each item as valid. The article by Clemson and colleagues provides a clear summary of results for each part of their content validity study. The expert panel were asked to review 250 WeHSA items, and 98% of these (n = 245 items) were judged relevant. The test developers used an individual item cut-off of CVI > 0.78, which is the level recommended when using a panel of 10 or more judges. Comments from the expert panel also 'led to rewording or subsuming of some items, for example "Lighting and Dark/dim" were combined into "Poor illumination"' (p. 176). Clemson et al. cite an overall CVI of 0.80; this indicated that 'the proportion of items that was rated as having acceptable relevancy or higher by *all* the experts (that is, a CVI = 1.00) was 0.80' (p. 176).

COSMIN (COnsensus-based Standards for the selection of health Measurement Instruments) is an initiative of an international multidisciplinary team of researchers with a background in epidemiology, psychometrics, medicine, qualitative research, and healthcare, who have expertise in the development and evaluation of outcome measurement instruments https://www.cosmin.nl/about). Terwee et al. (2018a) completed a Delphi study considering the content validity of patient-reported outcome measures (PROMs). From this study, they produced a user manual on assessing content validity (2018b). The Table 8.1 is from the user manual.

For a detailed review of the definition, importance, conceptual basis, and functional nature of content validity, along with quantitative and qualitative methods of content validation, see Haynes et al. (1995).

CONSTRUCT VALIDITY

A construct can be described as idea or mental representation or conceptual structure that is generated from informed scientific imagination in order to categorise and describe behaviour and assist thinking about the factors underlying observed behaviour (Cronbach and Meehl 1955; Welk 2002). It is an abstract quality or phenomenon that is thought to account for behaviour. Construct validation is needed if the AHP wants to draw inferences from the person's performance on an assessment to performances that can be grouped under the labels of a particular construct (Crocker and Algina 1986), for example, generalising from the score on an item testing an aspect of short-term memory to the overall construct of short-term memory.

Definition of Construct Validity

Construct validity involves the extent to which an assessment can be said to measure a theoretical construct or constructs.

Construct validity has also been described as relating to the ability of an assessment to perform as hypothesised (Streiner et al. 2015). For example, individuals discharged to an independent living situation should score higher on a self-care assessment than individuals discharged to a long-term care living situation. Any assessment that uses observed behaviour as an indicator of functioning related to theoretical constructs about unobservable areas of function should clearly state the underlying assumptions regarding the relationships between observed behaviour and related concepts of function. Fitzpatrick (2004) regards construct validity as a more quantitative form of validity (as compared to content and face validity) and states that, as no single correlation provides sufficient support of construct validity, a test developer or AHP should look for a cumulative pattern of evidence. For example, the construct of disability 'is expected to have a set of quantitative relationships with other constructs such as age, disease status and recent use of healthcare facilities' (p. 55).

A four-step process for establishing construct validity has been described by Crocker and Algina (1986):

1. Formulate one or more hypotheses (based on an articulated theory) about how people who will vary on the construct are expected to differ on other variables, such as observable behaviours measured as performance criteria, demographic characteristics (e.g. age, sex, ethnicity, occupation, level of education), or performance on another measure of the same construct that has already been validated.
2. Select a test that has items covering behaviours that are considered manifestations of the construct.
3. Collect data related to the hypothesised relationship(s) to be tested.
4. Establish whether the data collected supports the hypothesis and determines the extent to which the data could be explained by alternative explanations or theories. If data could be explained by a rival hypothesis, try to eliminate these if possible; this might require more data collection.

A group of five occupational therapists (Letts et al. 1998) who examined the construct validity of the Safety Assessment of Function and the Environment (SAFER Tool) provides an example of a construct validity study for rehabilitation. They thought that clients 'who were more independent in completing self-care and instrumental activities would be less likely to have problems related to their ability to function safely in their homes' (p. 128). They also thought that for people 'with cognitive impairments, it would be expected that the number of safety concerns would be greater due to their impaired judgement' (p. 128). For the study, they set a hypothesis that stated: "lower scores on the SAFER Tool (meaning fewer problems) would be associated with:

1. Subjects who were more independent in activities of daily living (ADL) and instrumental activities of daily living (IADL)
2. Subjects who had mild to no cognitive impairment" (p. 128).

To examine these hypotheses, these AHPs administered a battery of tests to a sample of 38 subjects recruited from across five therapy sites in Ontario and British Columbia, Canada. All subjects were 65 years old or above, able to communicate in English, and living in the community. The sample, comprising 11 men and 27 women, had a mean age of 77.3 years and the standard deviation (sd) was 6.5 years. The tests used were:

- The SAFER Tool (Community Occupational therapists and Associates COTA; 1991)
- The Physical Self-maintenance Scale (PSMS, Lawton and Brody 1969)
- The IADL Scale (Lawton and Brody 1969)
- Standardised Mini-Mental State Examination (SMMSE, Molloy et al. 1991).

For the analysis, three hypotheses were explored, and three correlation coefficients (for more information about correlation coefficients, see Chapter 9) were calculated to examine these. The researchers set a level of Pearson correlation coefficients of 0.40 or greater as the acceptable level for construct validity, stating that 'this value is high enough to demonstrate a medium to large effect size' (Letts et al. 1998, p. 129). The first hypothesis looked at the relationship between the SAFER Tool and PSMS scores, and a negative correlation was expected in which people with fewer safety problems as measured by the SAFER Tool would be more independent in ADL and higher PSMS scores. However, the researchers report that 'the correlation was slightly positive and did not meet the criterion of 0.40' (p. 131). In discussing this result, they note that the range of scores on the PSMS for their sample was very small and the sample 'were quite independent in ADL', and wonder whether 'the lack of range of PSMS scores may have contributed to this finding' (p. 131). In terms of the second hypothesis, scores on the SAFER Tool were correlated with the IADL Scale. In this case, the correlation was negative, as hypothesised; the Pearson Correlation Coefficient was −0.2471 and did not meet their 0.40 criterion. The final hypothesis was supported by the results with a negative correlation of −0.41 found between SAFER scores and SMMSE scores. Although the construct validity of the SAFER Tool was partly supported through the demonstration of a relationship between cognitive impairment and safety functioning, further construct validity studies are required to examine the relationship between the SAFER Tool and other measures of ADL and IADL.

FACTORIAL VALIDITY

Asher (1996) reports that 'factorial validity may be considered with construct validity because it can identify the underlying structure and theoretical construct' (p xxxi).

Definition of Factorial Validity

Factorial validity relates to the factorial composition of a test. The correlation between a test and the identified major factors that determine the test scores (Anastasi 1988).

Test developers use factor analysis to explore this type of validity. Factor analysis is a statistical technique that is used for analysing the inter-relationships between data that records behaviours, and was developed to isolate psychological traits.

Anastasi (1988) considers it 'particularly relevant to construct validation' (p. 154). Through the process of factor analysis, a number of variables (which could be total scores from different tests or items from the same test) that describe some aspect of a person's performance/behaviour are reduced to a smaller number of common traits, which are labelled factors. Anastasi states 'a major purpose of factor analysis is to simplify the description of behaviour by reducing the number of categories from an initial multiplicity of test variables to a few common factors, or traits' (p. 155). For example, Baum and Edwards (1993) used factor analysis 'to explore the component structure of the variables' (p. 434) and 'identify common relationships among the variables' (p. 432) in their Kitchen Task Assessment (KTA).

The KTA was developed as a functional measure that assesses the level of cognitive support needed by a client with Senile Dementia of the Alzheimer's Type (SDAT) to undertake a cooking task successfully. The test looks at practical organisation, planning, and judgement skills. Baum and Edwards (1993) performed an analysis to 'determine the internal structure of the variables and to establish the KTA as a unidimensional instrument' (p. 434) using data from a sample of 106 people diagnosed with SDAT. They reported that only one major factor was identified and that this accounted for 84% of the variance.

Dunn and Daniels (2002), provide another example of a factor analysis study, used in test development. During the development of the Infant/Toddler Sensory Profile, the test developers conducted several principal components factor analyses to determine whether items clustered meaningfully into independent groupings. The first analysis was undertaken using data from a sample of 150 infants aged from birth to six months who did not have disabilities. They report that 'the initial factor analysis yielded 6 factors .... that accounted for 48.19% of the variance (i.e., 40% of the variation among the scores of the children could be accounted for by these factors)' (p. 19). The six factors identified were labelled as low threshold (self) = 9.29%; low registration = 9.18%; seeking = 9.06%; avoiding/high noticing = 8.37%; low threshold (regulation) = 7.79%; and context awareness = 5.11%. In a second study, the researchers undertook principal components factor analyses on a sample of 659 children aged seven to 36 months who did not have disabilities. In this study, the factor analysis yielded 10 factors accounting for 40.5% of the variance. Further analysis 'using a varimax rotation' found 'that a 6 factor solution was the most interpretable' and accounted for 44.3% of the variance (p. 22). Further factor analyses were conducted on samples of children with diagnoses disabilities. Dunn concluded that the results of all the factor analyses appeared to fit with constructs she had described in her Model of Sensory Processing and noted that items on the Infant/Toddler Sensory Profile had not loaded according to related sensory systems but according to their sensory-processing characteristic. Each analysis had included 'factors in which items cluster based on thresholds and behavioural responses (i.e. Low Registration and Sensation Seeking, which are the high threshold components of Dunn's Model of Sensory Processing, and Sensory Sensitivity and Sensation Avoiding, which reflect low threshold components)' of Dunn's model (p. 22). She found that, in general, the same constructs had emerged from these factor analyses as had emerged during the development of other versions of the Sensory Profile for adolescents/adults and for children aged 3 to 10 years.

DISCRIMINATIVE VALIDITY

A discriminative test is a measure that has been developed to 'distinguish between individuals or groups on an underlying dimension when no external criterion or gold standard is available for validating these measures' (Law 2004).

Definition of Discriminative Validity

Discriminative validity relates to whether a test provides a valid measure to distinguish between individuals or groups.

Discriminative validity is explored when a test is developed to measure a construct in order to distinguish between individuals or groups. For example, a test might be developed to measure the construct of memory in order to discriminate between people with dementia versus people with memory deficits associated with normal ageing processes, or between people exhibiting temporary memory problems associated with depression as opposed to people with permanent memory impairment related to organic problems, such as dementia. Test developers obtain samples of the groups of interest and then compare their scores on test items to see whether the clinical group, for example, people with dementia, do in fact obtain scores indicating higher levels of deficit on the construct of interest, such as showing a greater degree of memory deficit, than the group of matched norms. In this type of study, the clinical groups and normative samples should be comparable in terms of significant or potentially significant factors (confounding variables), such as age, sex, educational level, and socio-economic background.

DeGangi et al. (1995), who examined the discriminative validity of the Infant and Toddler Symptom Checklist by testing samples of infants assessed by other measures as either developing normally or as having regulatory problems, provide an example of a discriminative validity study. They then computed the mean scores for the norm and clinical groups for each item in their draft version of the checklist. They evaluated mean differences to provide a discrimination index and calculated t-test values to look at level of significance. They reported that only items with a medium (0.5–0.8 difference in means) to a large (>0.8 difference in means) were included in the final version of the Infant and Toddler Symptom Checklist. Because of their discriminative validity study, they discarded 14 items on the draft test version because they did not significantly discriminate between normally developing infants and infants known to have regulatory disorders.

CRITERION-RELATED VALIDITY

As discussed in Chapters 7 and 14, a criterion-referenced test is a test that examines performance against predefined criteria and produces raw scores that are intended to have a direct, interpretable meaning (Crocker and Algina 1986). Criterion-related validity 'can best be characterized as the practical validity of a test for a specified purpose' (Anastasi 1988, p. 151).

Definition of Criterion-Related Validity

Criterion-related validity looks at the effectiveness of a test in predicting an individual's performance in specific activities; this is measured by comparing performance on the test with a criterion which is a direct and independent measure of what the assessment is designed to predict.

Criterion-related validation is needed when AHPs want to draw an inference from the person's test score to other behaviours of practical relevance (Crocker and Algina 1986). Both *predictive* and *concurrent* measures can be used to determine criterion-related validity. The most frequent analysis used to explore criterion-related validity is the correlation coefficient. Crocker and Algina (1986, p. 224) describe a five-step process for undertaking a criterion-related validation study:

1. 'Identify a suitable criterion behaviour and a method for measuring it.
2. Identify an appropriate sample of examinees representative of those for whom the test will ultimately be used.
3. Administer the test and keep a record of each examinee's score.
4. When the criterion data are available, obtain a measure of performance on the criterion for each examinee.
5. Determine the strength of relationship between test scores and criterion performance.'

CONCURRENT VALIDITY

Concurrent validity studies enable researchers to correlate the test of interest with other test variables. Concurrent validity is also sometimes referred to as *congruent* or *convergent* validity or *diagnostic utility*.

Definition of Concurrent Validity

Concurrent validity is 'the extent to which the test results agree with other measures of the same or similar traits and behaviours' (Asher 1996, p. xxx).

Concurrent validation is undertaken by comparing two or more measures that have been designed to measure the same or similar content or constructs (Streiner et al. 2015). Lewis and Bottomley (2008) give the example of correlating a manual muscle test with mechanical tests, or correlating a balance assessment developed within their own department with a standardised and accepted balance measure used within the field of physiotherapy. Davis et al. (2008) provide a useful example of how 'to determine the concurrent validity of the 4 hamstring length measures, simple linear regression and Pearson's correlation coefficient were calculated' (p. 586).

With concurrent validity, the test developer is hoping to find sufficient correlation with an established and recognised measure of the same trait or behaviour to indicate that the same trait/behaviour is being measured by their new test. However, if their new test correlates too highly, and does not have the added advantage of improved clinical utility (for example, it is shorter or easier to administer), then it will be perceived as simply reinventing the wheel and having no extra clinical advantage over the already established measure (Anastasi 1988).

Concurrent validity studies are one of the most frequent types of validity study reported in therapy literature. Wright et al. (1998) correlated three sets of scores on the Rivermead Mobility Index (RMI) and the Barthel Index (BI) obtained by a physiotherapy patient sample. They reported that 'scores on the BI and RMI were highly correlated prior to admission, and at admission and discharge (Spearman's rank 0.74, 0.78, 0.87 respectively $p < 0.001$ for all comparisons)' (p. 219). Scudds et al. (2003) provide another good example of a concurrent validity study examining the concurrent validity of an Electronic Descriptive Pain Scale (EDPS), which they described as a pain scale built into a transcutaneous electrical nerve stimulation device, compared to three other recognised measures of pain in a sample of 100 physiotherapy outpatient clients. The three concurrent measures selected were a visual analogue scale (VAS), a numerical pain rating scale, and the McGill Pain Questionnaire's Present Pain Intensity (MPQ PPI; Melzack 1987). The authors used Spearman's rank correlation coefficients to test for concurrent validity, and statistics were calculated for the EDPS and the other three measures before and after physiotherapy treatment. They reported that 'correlation coefficients ranged from 0.76 to 0.80 before treatment and from 0.84 to 0.88 after treatment' (p. 207). They concluded that 'the EDPS has a reasonably high level of concurrent validity when compared with three scales that are routinely used in clinical practice' (p. 207).

In addition to using a concurrent validity study to show that a new test measures content or constructs as well as or better than some accepted gold standard of measurement, concurrent validity studies can also be used to show that a new test is offering measurement of some distinct content or construct compared to available measures. DeGangi et al. (1995) examined the discriminative validity of the Infant and Toddler Symptom Checklist by calculating inter-correlations among Symptom Checklist scores and test scores. They obtained samples of 157 normal and 67 regulatory-disordered infants on the Bayley Scales of Infant Development, Mental Scale (Bayley 1993), the Test of Sensory Functions in Infants (DeGangi and Greenspan 1989), and the Test of Attention in Infants (DeGangi 1995). They found that none of the inter-correlations were significant for the regulatory-disordered sample and that only a few correlations were significant for the normal sample. They concluded that the findings 'suggest that, for the most part, the Symptom Checklist provides information that is distinct from that obtained by other diagnostic measures (such as sensory processing, attention), particularly for 10 to 30 month olds' (p. 44).

PREDICTIVE VALIDITY

A critically important type of criterion-related validity is predictive validity. A predictive test is designed to classify individuals into a set of predefined measurement categories, concurrently or prospectively, to determine whether individuals have been classified correctly (Kirshner and Guyatt 1985).

Definition of Predictive Validity

Predictive validity is 'the accuracy with which a measurement predicts some future event, such as mortality' (McDowell 2006 p. 714).

Predictive validation refers broadly to the prediction from the test to any criterion performance, or specifically to prediction over a time interval (Anastasi 1988). Crocker and Algina (1986) define predictive validity as 'the degree to which test scores predict criterion measurements that will be made at some point in the future' (p. 224). Predictive validity is also sometimes referred to as *predictive utility* (Anastasi 1988). For example:

1. predicting meal preparation ability from a kitchen assessment undertaken in an occupational therapy department to how the client's should manage in his own kitchen when discharged home; or

2. predicting mobility from a mobility assessment undertaken on a flat, lino sur-
    face in a ward or therapy department to how the person should be able to
    mobilise in a home environment containing a range of flooring including
    carpet, rugs, laminate, and tiles.

Therefore, AHPs need to be careful that the predictions made from specific test
results to other areas of function really are valid. For example, Donnelly (2002)
explored whether the Rivermead Perceptual Assessment Battery (RPAB; Whiting
et al. 1985) could predict functional performance. The aims of her study were 'to
determine if a relationship exists between RPAB and functional performance and to
ascertain if the RPAB could predict discharge functional performance' (p. 71). She
assessed 46 adults with stroke on the RPAB and a functional measure, the Functional
Independence Measure (FIM), over an 18-month period. She found 'little relationship between the RPAB results and functional performance on admission to rehabilitation' and concluded: '... the RPAB results may not be useful to clinicians when
attempting to ascertain if the functional problems experienced by some people on
admission to rehabilitation are perceptually based. Also, if the prediction of functional
outcome is desired, the RPAB may be seen as far too time consuming and therefore
not cost-effective when age of the subject can be included into the predictive equation
with the same degree of confidence' (p. 79).

Duncan et al. (1992) provide a useful example of a study that demonstrated good
levels of predictive validity. They examined the predictive validity of the Functional
Reach in identifying elderly people at risk for falls. The functional reach measure is
the 'maximal distance one can reach forward beyond arm's length whilst maintaining a fixed base of support in the standing position' (p. M93). A sample of 217 older
men living in the community were given baseline screening, including a functional
reach test, and were then followed up for six months. One of the challenges of predictive studies is the follow-up of subjects, particularly where the construct of interest
cannot be measured directly by the researcher, as in the case of falls. These researchers
used a rigorous method for supporting subjects to accurately report falls. Each subject was given six calendars covering a 30-day period. They were asked to mark any
falls on the calendar and were given stamped addressed envelopes to encourage
return. The subjects were telephoned once a month by the researcher to ask about
any falls, and any changes in health or medication. They were also gave subjects
stamped, addressed post cards to post to the researchers as soon as they had a fall,
and any person sending in a post card were contacted straight away for a telephone
interview to record the details of the fall, including any injuries sustained. Two members of the research team, who were blinded to all other subject data, then reviewed
the falls records and classified the falls as either counting or not counting as a fall for
the purpose of this study, and if these two researchers did not agree, a third researcher
reviewed the falls record. Subjects were then classified as being either fallers or non-
fallers at the end of the six months, and any older person who had fallen two or more
times was classified as a recurrent faller. The authors undertook a logistic regression
and examined the relationship between the history of falls and functional reach baseline data, as well as exploring a number of other variables measured at baseline
(including mental state, mood, vision, and blood pressure). They reported 'the
association between functional reach and recurrent falls was not confounded by age,
depression, or cognition' and concluded 'that functional reach is a simple and easy
to use clinical measure that has predictive validity in identifying recurrent falls'
(p. M93). Note that this paper by Duncan et al. (1992) also provides a succinct table
comparing the established psychometric properties (inter-observer and test retest

reliability, criterion and construct validity, and sensitivity to change) of 14 measures of balance as part of their literature review.

Another example of a predictive validity study is found described in the manual for the Infant and Toddler Symptom Checklist (DeGangi et al. 1995), which is used with parents of 7-to-30-month-old babies to predict infants and toddlers 'who are at risk for sensory-integrative disorders, attentional deficits, and emotional and behavioural problems' (p. 1). In a study of 14 infants, from paediatric practices in the Washington DC area of the United States, 12 subjects were assessed on the Symptom Checklist as falling within the risk range. These 12 infants were then assessed on a number of standardised observational tests. The authors report that all 12 infants 'demonstrated regulatory problems when tested … nine had sensory-processing deficits as determined by the Test of Sensory Functions in Infants (DeGangi and Greenspan 1989), three had attentional deficits as determined by the Test of Attention in Infants (DeGangi 1995) and one child had both sensory and attentional problems' (p. 42).

One issue identified by Anastasi (1988) is that of sample size: 'samples available for test validation are generally too small to yield a stable estimate of the correlation between predictor and criterion … the obtained coefficients may be too low to reach statistical significance in the sample employed and may thus fail to provide evidence of the test's validity' (p. 152). AHPs, therefore, need to pay particular attention to sample sizes when examining validity data in journal articles or test manuals.

Validity is more than just the *matching* of what a test *actually measures* with that which it was *designed to measure*. Sometimes there can be uncertainty about what a test really measures, yet it may still be a good predictor of an outcome of concern because we have evidence that scores on the test are related to that outcome (Bartram 1990). Therefore, if AHPs need to make predictions about future performance (for example, safety at home alone), the predictive validity of a test could be more important than its content validity.

OTHER TYPES OF VALIDITY

There are some other types of validity of relevance to AHPs, but less frequently mentioned or addressed in therapy/rehabilitation literature and test manuals. These include ecological and external validity, which are very closely related.

Definition of Cross-Cultural Validity

The degree to which the performance of the items on a translated or culturally adapted measurement instrument is an adequate reflection of the performance of the items of the original version of the measurement instrument. (Prinsen et al. 2016, p. 6)

Definition of Ecological Validity

Ecological validity addresses the relevance of the test content, structure, and environment to the population with whom the test is used (Laver 1994).

Definition of External Validity

External validity is the extent to which findings can be generalised to other settings in the real world (Lewis and Bottomley 2008).

External validity is also sometimes referred to as *validity generalisation* and has been defined as follows.

External and ecological validity are relevant to AHPs for a few reasons. Individual therapy departments may develop criterion-related tests for a specific service; external validity explores the generalizability of test validity to different situations outside of the original service where the test was developed (Anastasi 1988). For example, Wolf (1997) reports that 'ADL scales often used in rehabilitation are not valid and reliable measures of outcome for clients of community services' (p. 364). Many tests are originally developed as research tools and are administered to research subjects in highly controlled formal testing environments. A patient's home environment, or the assessment space available in an outpatient department or on a ward, may have many more potential distractions. There are pros and cons to both situations. In a highly controlled testing environment removed from the client's home or hospital ward setting, the formality and unfamiliarity of the testing environment could lead to test anxiety, which could affect performance and hence the reliability of results. However, the background noises and possible interruptions that occur in home and therapy/ward environments can impact the client's concentration and may therefore also negatively impact performance.

CLINICAL UTILITY

Just because a test is well standardised, valid, and reliable does not mean it automatically will be useful in the clinical environment. Many an expensive test gathers dust in AHP departments for practical reasons, such as the AHPs discovering after purchase that it was too lengthy to administer or too cumbersome to move around. Therefore, it is critical to consider the clinical utility of potential assessments for your service to ensure that the selected assessment can be easily and economically administered (Jeffrey 1993).

Definition of Clinical Utility

Clinical utility is the overall usefulness of an assessment in a clinical situation and covers aspects of a test such as reasonable cost, acceptability, training requirements, administration time, and interpretation of scores, portability, and ease of use.

Tyson and Connell (2009) completed a systematic review to identify measures for balance in clinical practice by considering the psychometric properties and clinical feasibility.

COST AND CLINICAL UTILITY

When estimating the overall cost of a test for your service, there are a number of factors to consider. The most obvious cost is the initial financial outlay required to purchase the test (this might comprise a manual, forms, test materials, etc.). The cost of standardised tests varies considerably; some brief tests are published in professional journals and are freely available, others can be purchased cheaply, but some are very expensive. You will need to justify to the budget holder that the financial outlay will bring sufficient benefit for your service. In addition, you may need to purchase some of the equipment required for test administration if this is not provided with the test. This is more common with tests described in journal articles, where the equipment required is described. The expertise required of the rater is another cost factor. Some tests specify that the rater has to have specific qualifications or levels of experience, which may mean that only qualified staff or senior staff can use the test, or may require that all test administrators undertake a training course. Training courses can be a major financial outlay. Training courses for specific tests can vary in both length and cost and may involve a one-day training session, a part-time course, or a week-long residential course. In addition, some tests require administrators to undertake follow-up training to stay up to date or to be re-calibrated as a rater. AHPs should also estimate the ongoing costs for any supplies that need to be replaced for each assessment, for example, food for a kitchen assessment, paper, or scoring forms. Some tests have copyrighted scoring forms, and you should estimate the cost of replacement test forms if copyright does not allow these to be photocopied.

Time

The most obvious time factor to consider is the time required to administer the test. Some standardised assessments comprise lengthy test batteries. These testing procedures can be tiring for patients. For example:

- Poor stamina can affect test performance and impact the reliability of test results. A test manual should indicate the range of time taken by subjects undertaking the test and/or recommend the length of time you should make available for testing.
- You need to allow for the time required to prepare for test administration each time, such as the time needed for setting up the test environment and materials, or for purchasing supplies (e.g. food for a meal preparation assessment).
- Time required to score the test, interpret results, and write up any reports also needs to be estimated.
- Another time factor, which can be overlooked when considering clinical utility, is the initial time required to learn to administer the test. This might be through attendance on a training course or be undertaken individually by reading the test manual and practising test administration, for example, through role play with colleagues.

Some tests incorporate timings into the scoring of test items, but this does not always add to the clinical usefulness of the measure. For example, McAvoy (1991) that 'activities that are timed, as in the Northwick Park Index, are of little value when safety or control or quality of movement are the key issues, but these qualities are not included in [m]any of the standardised forms' (p. 385).

Energy and Effort

The ease with which the AHP can learn to administer the test and the ease of each test administration will influence how much a test is used in a service. Some tests seem complex initially and administration is hard to 'get to grips with', but most tests become easier to administer with practice, so that an 'expert' administrator can undertake the test without undue effort. Some physical assessments, where a service user may require a lot of assistance with mobility and transfers, can place a high physical demand on the AHPs administering the test.

Portability

AHPs need to decide in advance the settings in which a test is to be used as some tests are heavy and/or bulky. If testing is always to occur in a department, then a test with lots of heavy equipment may be appropriate. However, if AHPs will need to use the test in several different environments (for example, on the ward, in a day hospital, or in the person's home, school, or work setting) then portability becomes critical.

You need to consider how easy it will be to move the test between potential testing environments. If the test has many components and does not come with its own case, you may need to purchase some kind of bag or case for carrying. The health and safety of staff must be ensured, so if the test is very heavy it may be worth purchasing a trolley for pulling/pushing it between test environments. For example, the Chessington Occupational Therapy Neurological Assessment Battery (COTNAB; Tyerman et al. 1986) comes in a large wooden box on castors and when packed with all the required test equipment is very heavy. AHPs tend to administer the COTNAB in their therapy department or outpatient clinic environment, as it is very difficult to transport it between hospital wards or in the community between clients' homes.

Acceptability

The concept of acceptability overlaps with face validity. AHPs should consider whether the assessment fits with the philosophy, theoretical frameworks, and practice used within the therapy service or by a particular clinician. Whether the test looks professional is another aspect of acceptability. You also need to identify whether the test will be acceptable to the service user. Will the person see the relevance of the test and is the test likely to cause stress and test anxiety? When judging the acceptability, you should also consider how acceptable the test will be for managers, service purchasers, and lay observers, such as the person's family.

Laver (1994) demonstrated that the Structured Observational Test of Function (SOTOF; Laver and Powell 1995) had good clinical utility. AHPs were sent a covering letter, a copy of the SOTOF manual and test forms, a questionnaire for the AHP to completed related to clinical utility and content validity, a structured interview for the AHP to give to clients to look at face validity, and a stamped addressed return envelope. Sixty-six AHPs responded to the request letter, and a further 38 were recruited through meetings and lectures where the test developer was presenting work on the development of the SOTOF. Forty-four out of the 104 AHP sample completed the study, giving a response rate of 42.3%, which is in line with expected response rates for surveys of 30–40% (Baruch and Holtom 2008).

AHPs used the SOTOF with at least two clients and then completed a postal questionnaire that covered a wide range of clinical utility issues including ease of use, materials, time required, and appropriateness for their clients. The AHP samples included staff of all grades, ranging from a basic grade thorough to a senior AHP, and they were working across a number of different clinical areas, including neurology, gerontology, medical, outpatients, rehabilitation unit, surgery and orthopaedics, and medicine and surgery. Most of the clinical utility questionnaire items used a 5-point rating scale, for example, for the 'Ease of use' section AHPs were asked to rate four questions:

1. Were the SOTOF instructions easy to understand?
2. Were the SOTOF instructions easy to follow?
3. Were the SOTOF protocols easy to follow?
4. Were the SOTOF forms easy to fill in?

Using the same 5-point scale: (1) Impossible, (2) Difficult, (3) Fair, (4) Easy, and (5) Very Easy,
Laver (1994) reported that:

- 54.5% of AHPs rated the SOTOF as fair and 34.1% as easy to understand.
- 52.3% rated the SOTOF instructions as fair and 38.6% as easy to follow.
- 52.3% rated the SOTOF protocols as fair and 34.1% as easy to follow.
- 34.1% rated the SOTOF forms as fair, 50% as easy, and 2.3% as very easy to fill in.

A dichotomous Yes/No scoring system was used to examine the clinical utility of materials required for the SOTOF (Laver 1994), with questions related to the suitability of the materials:

1.	Easy to obtain:	Yes 72.7%	No 22.7%
2.	Appropriate for the client:	Yes 86.4%	No 6.8%
3.	Easy to carry:	Yes 86.4%	No 4.5%
4.	Easy to clean:	Yes 90.9%	No 2.3%
5.	Easy to store:	Yes 88.6%	No 2.3%

AHPs were asked to record the length of time taken to administer the SOTOF. Laver (1994) reported that the majority of AHPs took an hour or less to administer the SOTOF, with AHP times ranging from 30 minutes to 2 hours 15 minutes, and with only four AHPs taking over an hour to complete the test.

See Table 8.1 for ten criteria for good content validity (Terwee et al. 2018b, p. 7). The standards for evaluating the quality of studies on the content validity of a PROM (Terwee et al. 2018a, p. 13):

- Asking patients about the relevance of the PROM items
- Asking patients about the comprehensiveness of the PROM
- Asking patients about the comprehensibility of the PROM
- Asking professionals about the relevance of the PROM items
- Asking professionals about the comprehensiveness of the PROM

EXAMINING VALIDITY AND CLINICAL UTILITY ISSUES: TEST EXAMPLES

In this section, a few assessments are evaluated in terms of their validity and/or clinical utility as examples of the factors that AHPs should consider when reviewing potential tests for their clinical practice.

The Mayers' Lifestyle Questionnaire (2) (Mayers 2003)

Mayers has undertaken studies to examine aspects of the clinical utility, face validity, and content validity of the original Mayers' Lifestyle Questionnaire and contact letter

TABLE 8.1   Ten criteria for good content validity (Terwee et al. 2018b, p. 7).

Area	Question
Relevance	1. Are the included items relevant for the construct of interest?
	2. Are the included items relevant for the target population of interest?
	3. Are the included items relevant for the context of use of interest?
	4. Are the response options appropriate?
	5. Is the recall period appropriate?
Comprehensiveness	6. Are no key concepts missing?
Comprehensibility	7. Comprehensibility
	8. Are the PROM instructions understood by the population of interest as intended?
	9. Are the PROM items and response options understood by the population of interest as intended?
	10. Are the PROM items appropriately worded?
	11. Do the response options match the question?

Source: Terwee et al. (2018b). © 2018, COSMIN.

(1998) and an adapted version for use in mental health services (2003). In the first study, a questionnaire format was used to gather feedback. A sample of 92 occupational therapists asked three clients each, giving a potential sample of 288 clients. Data was returned by 45 AHPs (48.9%) and for 132 (45.8%) clients. Mayers (1998) summarises key issues in three tables divided into comments from AHPs on the usefulness of the contact letter; comments from AHPs on the usefulness of the Lifestyle Questionnaire; and response from clients. In terms of face validity, she reported that 68 of the 132 (51.5%) clients made comments indicating that the tool had been 'easy to complete/understand'. In terms of clinical utility, she reported that:

> *'Twenty-five (55.6%) occupational therapists stated that the Lifestyle Questionnaire was useful and relevant as he or she discussed occupational therapy with clients; 10 (22.2%) said it was not useful. There was no response from the remaining 10 (22.2%)'*

(p. 394).In the second study, an adapted Delphi technique involved a Disability Action Group, comprising six members. For the first phase, each group member was sent questions to consider (see Box 8.1) and a copy of the contact letter and Lifestyle Questionnaire to read and complete. For the second stage, group members met, and each person presented his or her ideas in turn. In the final stage, the group discussed the issues raised, and priorities were identified and ranked. Both individual written reflections from the first stage and group discussions were analysed.

In the discussion, Mayer's (1998) reflects on the results of the two studies and notes changes that were made to the tool as a result of feedback from AHPs, clients, and the Disability Action Group. She concluded that the 'Lifestyle Questionnaire gives the client the opportunity to state his or her individual need(s) and to prioritise these' (p. 397).

- What was your initial reaction when you read the contact letter and Lifestyle Questionnaire?

- Do you think that a client would have a clearer idea of the role of the community occupational therapist after reading the contact letter?

- Do you think you would have any problems with the wording and with completing the Lifestyle Questionnaire (it may help you to answer this question by completing it yourself)?

- Do you think that having the opportunity to prioritise your needs beforehand would prepare you better for the community occupational therapist's first visit?

Source: Mayers (1998). © 1998, SAGE Publications.

Mayers reported that original version of the Mayers Lifestyle Questionnaire (1998) was found to be suitable for people with problems caused by physical disability. Following requests from community occupational therapists working with clients with enduring mental health problems, the tool was modified, and the application of the adapted version, Mayers' Lifestyle Questionnaire (2), was examined (Mayers 2003). As part of this study, Mayers examined aspects of clinical utility, content validity, and face validity. Out of a volunteer sample of 83 AHPs who received copies of the tool, 33 returned clinical utility and content validity data; in addition, these AHPs submitted face validity feedback from a total sample of 75 clients who had completed the Lifestyle Questionnaire. Data was collected via AHP and client questionnaires. Questions for AHPs are provided in Box 8.2, and questions for clients are provided in Box 8.3.

Mayers (2003) reported that 28 (84.8%) AHPs reported that the Lifestyle Questionnaire had been useful, and 23 (69.7%) had indicated that the tool would be helpful for the majority of their clients. In her paper, she provides summary tables of comments related to these questions. In terms of reasons why the tool might not be useful, only one factor was identified by more than one AHP; this related to the length of the questionnaire being quite long for people with poor concentration. Mayers also summarised the important areas or topics AHPs identified as omitted in the content validity question. Of these, only two areas were identified by more than one AHP, eight (24.2%) suggested the inclusion of a 'comment box after the final column', and two suggested an item on 'coping with physical/mental health problems'.

In terms of face validity, Mayers (2003) reported that 67 (89.3%) of the clients who completed the questionnaire said that it included all areas that were important to them and that affected their quality of life. In addition, clients had been asked to use asterisks (*) to mark those items on the questionnaire that indicated their top priorities, and 51 (68%) of the sample did this. Mayers listed the 14 top priorities provided by clients in a table and notes that these are similar to areas identified by a number of authors in her literature review. Following the analysis, Mayers made some changes to the wording of a number of items. At least one client prioritised each item; therefore, all the original items were included in the final version. Overall, the study supported the clinical utility, content validity, and face validity of the measure. Mayers notes that a larger sample would have been desirable and has continued to send out evaluation forms when copies of the test are requested.

Clinical Utility

The purpose of the Lifestyle Questionnaire is for clients to identify, record, and prioritise their needs before you commence intervention.

(i)   Has this been useful to you?

(ii) If 'yes', please state 'how' and 'why'

(iii) If 'no', please give reasons.

Clinical Utility

Do you think the Lifestyle Questionnaire will be helpful for the majority of your clients?

(i) Yes/No

(ii) If no, please give reasons.

Content Validity

Having used the Lifestyle Questionnaire, please state any important area(s) or topics(s) that you think have been omitted.

Source: Mayers (2003). © 2003, SAGE Publications.

Each therapist was asked to record feedback on the following three questions from three clients who had completed the Lifestyle Questionnaire:

Did the wording of the Lifestyle Questionnaire include all areas that affect your quality of life and are important to you? Yes/No.

If 'no', please indicate any area that has been omitted.

Please state any problems that you had in completing the Lifestyle Questionnaire.

Source: Mayers (2003). © 2003, SAGE Publications.

Rivermead Perceptual Assessment Battery (RPAB)

RPAB (Bhavnani et al. 1983) was designed to assess deficits in visual perception following stroke or head injury. Normative data enables the AHP to evaluate whether a person has difficulty with visual perceptual tasks greater than that expected prior to brain damage. The aspects of visual perception addressed by the battery can be summarised under eight headings: form constancy, colour constancy, sequencing, object completion, figure-ground discrimination, body image, inattention, and spatial awareness. The test comprises 16 short subtests. Fifteen of these tests are timed activities administered at a table on a layout guide and comprise activities such as picture cards, block designs, jigsaws, and drawing. The RPAB has been found to lack ecological validity (Laver 1994). The test environment is very structured and formal, and the activities used lack everyday meaning as they are not drawn from clients' normal repertoire of tasks. Age appropriateness was also considered a weakness. Some of the tasks, such as the object matching subtest which includes toy cars, were perceived as childish by some clients (Laver 1990). Another issue involves the timing of the written and drawn subtests. Many patients with stroke experience hemiparesis to an upper limb; in some cases, this affects a previously dominant hand. In these circumstances, the patient has to perform the subtests using a non-dominant hand to hold the pen. As assessment usually occurs as soon as possible after diagnosis, and precedes intervention, the patient rarely has had an opportunity to practice writing with the non-dominant hand prior to testing. Therefore, many patients were found to fail these tests because of the length of time taken rather than actual ability (Cramond et al. 1989). Further limitations include the difficulty of administering the test to clients with severe cognitive impairment (short-term memory, attention, and concentration are required) or aphasia. The formality of the test administration procedures increases test anxiety and can have detrimental effects on performance. Many older clients have visual and auditory acuity loss because of primary ageing. The RPAB protocol does not permit the repetition of instructions or the use of additional verbal and visual cues; some clients fail subtests, as they do not comprehend the instructions. The colour-matching task has been criticised (Laver 1990). There is poor differentiation between the colours of some items on the tasks. RPAB involves the differentiation of several pieces in blue and green shades as colour vision alters with ageing owing to yellowing of the lens, which affects the perception of the blue-green end of the spectrum; many older clients failed this subtest but could name and point to colours on command. The task requires more complex functioning than the simple identification of colour.

The Middlesex Elderly Assessment of Mental State (MEAMS)

MEAMS (Golding 1989) was developed as a screening test to identify gross impairment of cognitive skills (Golding 1989). MEAMS includes 12 subtests that assess orientation, comprehension, verbal language skills, short-term memory, arithmetic, visual perception, and motor perseveration. This is a useful screening test, which is quick and easy to administer and relatively well accepted by clients (Laver 1994). However, the line drawings used for the remembering pictures subtest are problematic as they are very small and do not account for decreased visual acuity, which is a common deficit occurring as a result of primary ageing. Some subtests, such as the name learning, are age appropriate; photographs of older people are used for this test, and the ability to remember names is a relevant skill. Other subtests, such as the tapping task used to assess motor perseveration, are contrived and lack relevance to everyday activity.

Clifton Assessment Procedures for the Elderly (CAPE)

Pattie and Gilleard developed the CAPE in 1979 [1989] (Pattie 1981). The CAPE is designed to evaluate cognitive and behavioural functioning. The test consists of two parts: the Cognitive Assessment Scale (CAS) and the Behavioural Rating Scale (BRS). These two scales can be used separately or together. The CAS comprises three sections: (a) an information/orientation subtest, an interview covering 12 questions pertaining to orientation of time, place, and person, and three questions on current information; (b) a mental ability test involving counting, reading, writing, and reciting the alphabet; and (c) a psychomotor task requiring the completion of the 'Gibson Spiral Maze' to assess fine motor performance and hand–eye coordination. The BRS is administered as a survey to the primary carer (for example, nurse or relative) of the patient. Questions on this scale relate to four main areas: Physical Disability, Apathy, Communication Difficulties, and Social Disturbance.

The limiting aspect of the CAPE is the Psychomotor subtest. Pattie (1988) has acknowledged that 'at a practical level some users have questioned the usefulness of the Gibson Spiral Maze' (p. 72), and Bender (1990) refers to the maze as 'the least successful element of the CAS' and reports that 'many clinicians manage without it' (p. 108). The maze is not drawn from the usual repertoire of activities carried out in everyday life by older people and lacks ecological validity. The score from the maze indicates level of impairment and does not identify causes for dysfunction. Fine motor performance and hand–eye coordination are complex skills based on the interaction of motor, sensory, cognitive, and perceptual functions. A complex range of deficits, including comprehension, apraxia, loss of visual acuity, and restricted range of movement, could affect performance on this test. Clinicians, therefore, need to observe the performance of the test informally to identify cues pertaining to performance component dysfunction. Further assessment is required to evaluate the specific type of neuropsychological dysfunction.

The CAPE writing task has greater ecological validity than the maze, as clients need to be able to sign their name for financial independence. However, the task indicates the ability/inability to perform the task. The dysfunction could arise from a range of deficits and requires further investigation. The information/orientation questions do not indicate the effects of cognitive impairment on occupational performance, and some people find it demeaning to be asked such questions. The BRS is based on report rather than AHP observation, and thus the reliability of the results is dependent on the observational skills and memory of the respondent selected. Pattie (1988) admits that administrators of the CAPE have disputed the factor structure of the BRS and also queried the CAPE grading system.

APPLYING CONCEPTS OF VALIDITY TO YOUR OWN PRACTICE

Now turn to Worksheet 8.1 found on pp. 265–267.

For this reflection, you will need to select a published assessment, which could be an assessment/test that you are already using in your practice. Often, AHPs inherit assessments when they start work in a different clinical setting or department; this exercise will be especially useful if you are using a test that was already available in your department and which you have not critiqued. You might select a test that you are considering purchasing/using in the future. If you are a student, select a test you have seen used on clinical placement or one available at your university or college. Look to see what information (test manual, journal articles, handouts from training courses, etc.) is available on your chosen test. If there is very little, which can be the case when you have inherited an assessment, you might need to conduct a literature search in order to complete the worksheet.

The worksheet takes you through a series of questions about different types of validity and prompts you to record key evidence and to form opinions about whether the published evidence indicates adequate levels of validity for your clinical needs.

WORKSHEET 8.1　Reflecting on Validity

	YES	NO
Name of the test:		
Full reference		
Is there evidence of **content validity**?		
Describe study, brief summary of method (e.g. content analysis of literature, expert panel review), any sample details, and findings:		
Do you feel confident that this test measures what it says it does?		
Have the domains to be measured been weighted to reflect their relative importance to the overall content area?		
Is this test attempting to measure a theoretical construct?		
If Yes, is there evidence of construct validity?		
Describe study and findings: method (e.g. exploring the relationship between hypothesised variables, factor analysis), sample used, statistics calculated, results:		
Is the level of construct validity acceptable for your clinical practice?		
Does this test attempt to distinguish between individuals/groups, diagnostic categories, etc.?		
If Yes, is there evidence of *Discriminative validity*?		
Describe study and findings: method, sample size, clinical sample used, statistics calculated, results:		
Is the level of discriminative validity adequate for your clinical practice?		

(Continued)

WORKSHEET 8.1 (Continued)

	YES	NO
Name of the test:		
Full reference		
Was this test originally developed as a research tool or for use in a different clinical setting?		
If Yes, is there evidence of *External validity?*		
Describe study and findings: method, sample size, clinical sample used, statistics calculated, results:		
Are you confident that this test will be valid for your clinical setting?		
Is there evidence of *criterion-related validity?*		
Is the test used to make predictions about future ability, functioning in a different environment, etc.?		
If Yes, is there evidence of *predictive validity?*		
Describe study and findings: method, sample size, clinical sample used, statistics calculated, results:		
What would be the likely consequences and problems associated with your predictions not being valid?		
Is the predictive validity adequate for your clinical setting?		
Does this test measure the same or similar traits/behaviours as other existing and recognised test(s)?		
If Yes, is there evidence of *concurrent validity?*		
Describe study and findings: method, concurrent measure(s), sample size, clinical sample used, statistics calculated, results:		
Is the level of concurrent validity adequate for your clinical setting?		

Name of the test:

Full reference	YES	NO
Is there evidence of *face validity?* Describe study and findings: method, sample size, clinical sample used, statistics calculated, results:		
Does you think this test will be acceptable to your clients, their families, and colleagues who will view the results?		
If Yes, is there evidence of *Clinical utility?* Describe study and findings: method, sample size, clinical sample used, statistics calculated, results:		
Are you confident that this test will be useful in your clinical setting?		

REVIEW QUESTIONS

8.1   Describe one method to examine the content validity of a test.

8.2   Define construct validity.

8.3   List one type of criterion-related validity, and describe a method for evaluating this type of criterion-related validity.

8.4   What is predictive validity and why is it important to AHPs?

8.5   What is face validity and why should AHPs consider it?

8.6   What factors would you examine if you wanted to evaluate a test's clinical utility?

You will find brief answers to these questions at the back of this book on p. 445.

REFERENCES

Anastasi, A. (1988). *Psychological Testing*, 5e. New York. NY: Macmillan.

Asher, I.E. (1996). *Occupational Therapy Assessment Tools: An Annotated Index.* Amer Occupational Therapy Assn.

Bartram, D. (1990). Reliability and validity. Chapter 3. In: *Testing People: A Practical Guide to Psychometrics* (eds. J.R. Beech and L. Harding). Windsor, Berks: NFER-Nelson.

Baruch, Y. and Holtom, B.C. (2008). Survey response rate levels and trends in organizational research. *Human Relations* 61 (8): 1139–1160. https://doi.org/10.1177/0018726708094863.

Baum, C. and Edwards, D.F. (1993). Cognitive performance in senile dementia of the Alzheimer's type: the kitchen task assessment. *American Journal of Occupational Therapy* 47 (5): 431–436. https://doi.org/10.5014/ajot.47.5.431.

Bayley, N. (1993). *Bayley Scales of Infant Development.* San Antonio. TX: Psychological Corporation.

Bender, M.P. (1990). Test review – Clifton assessment procedures for the elderly. In: *Assessment of the Elderly* (eds. J.R. Beech and L. Harding). NFER-Nelson Publishing Company.

Bhavnani, G., Cockburn, J., Whiting, S., and Lincoln, N. (1983). The reliability of the Rivermead perceptual assessment and implications for some commonly used assessments of perception. *British Journal of Occupational Therapy* 46 (1): 17–19. https://doi.org/10.1177/030802268304600109.

Clemson, L., Fitzgerald, M.H., and Heard, R. (1999). Content validity of an assessment tool to identify home fall hazards: the Westmead home safety assessment. *British Journal of Occupational Therapy* 62 (4): 171–179.

Cramond, H.J., Clark, M.S., and Smith, D.S. (1989). The effect of using the dominant or nondominant hand on performance of the Rivermead perceptual assessment battery. *Clinical Rehabilitation* 3 (3): 215–221. https://doi.org/10.1177/026921558900300306.

Crocker, L. and Algina, J. (1986). *Introduction to Classical and Modern Test Theory.* Orlando, FL: Holt, Rinehart and Winston.

Cronbach, L.J. and Meehl, P.E. (1955). Construct validity in psychological tests. *Psychological Bulletin* 52 (4): 281.

Davis, D.S., Quinn, R.O., Whiteman, C.T. et al. (2008). Concurrent validity of four clinical tests used to measure hamstring flexibility. *The Journal of Strength & Conditioning Research* 22 (2): 583–588. https://doi.org/10.1519/JSC.0b013e31816359f2.

DeGangi, G.A. (1995). *Infant/Toddler Symptom Checklist: A Screening Tool for Parents.* Psychological Corp.

DeGangi, G.A. and Greenspan, S.I. (1989). *Test of Sensory Functions in Infants (TSFI)*. Los Angeles: Western Psychological Services.

DeGangi, G.A., Poisson, S., Sickel, R.Z., and Santman Wiener, A. (1995). *Infant/Toddler Symptom Checklist: A Screening Tool for Parents*. San Antonio (TX): Therapy Skill Builders, Psychological Corporation.

Donnelly, S. (2002). The Rivermead perceptual assessment battery: can it predict functional performance? *Australian Occupational Therapy Journal* 49 (2): 71–81. https://doi.org/10.1046/j.1440-1630.2002.00308.x.

Duncan, P.W., Studenski, S., Chandler, J., and Prescott, B. (1992). Functional reach: predictive validity in a sample of elderly male veterans. *Journal of Gerontology* 47 (3): M93–M98. https://doi.org/10.1093/geronj/47.3.M93.

Dunn, W. and Daniels, D.B. (2002). Initial development of the infant/toddler sensory profile. *Journal of Early Intervention* 25 (1): 27–41. https://doi.org/10.1177/105381510202500104.

Fitzpatrick, R. (2004). Measures of health status, health-related quality of life and patient satisfaction. In: *Outcome Measures in Orthopaedics and Orthopaedic Trauma*, 2e (eds. P. Pynsent, J. Fairbank and A. Carr), 54–63. CRC Press.

Golding, E. (1989). *The Middlesex Elderly Assessment of Mental State: MEAMS*. Thames Valley Test Company.

Haynes, S.N., Richard, D., and Kubany, E.S. (1995). Content validity in psychological assessment: a functional approach to concepts and methods. *Psychological Assessment* 7 (3): 238.

Jeffrey, L.I. (1993). Aspects of selecting outcome measures to demonstrate the effectiveness of comprehensive rehabilitation. *British Journal of Occupational Therapy* 56 (11): 394–400. https://doi.org/10.1177/030802269305601103.

Kirshner, B. and Guyatt, G. (1985). A methodological framework for assessing health indices. *Journal of Chronic Diseases* 38 (1): 27–36.

Laver, A.J. (1990). The Rivermead perceptual assessment battery. In: *Assessment of the Elderly* (eds. J.R. Beech and L. Harding). NFER Nelson: Windsor. ISBN: 9780700512577.

Laver, A. J. (1994). The development of the Structured Observational Test of Function (SOTOF) (Doctoral dissertation, University of Surrey). https://ethos.bl.uk/OrderDetails.do?uin=uk.bl.ethos.259917 available to borrow from Royal College of Occupational Therapists, London

Laver, A.J. and Powell, G.E. (1995). *The Structured Observational Test of Function (SOTOF)*. NFER Nelson https://ray.yorksj.ac.uk/id/eprint/1903.

Law, M. (2004). *Outcome Measures Rating Form*. Ontario, Canada: CanChild Centre for Disability Research https://canchild.ca/system/tenon/assets/attachments/000/000/371/original/measguid.pdf.

Lawton, M.P. and Brody, E.M. (1969). Assessment of older people: self-maintaining and instrumental activities of daily living. *The Gerontologist* 9 (3_Part_1): 179–186. http://www.eurohex.eu/bibliography/pdf/Lawton_Gerontol_1969–1502121986/Lawton_Gerontol_1969.pdf.

Letts, L., Scott, S., Burtney, J. et al. (1998). The reliability and validity of the safety assessment of function and the environment for rehabilitation (SAFER tool). *British Journal of Occupational Therapy* 61 (3): 127–132. https://doi.org/10.1177/030802269806100309.

Lewis, C.B. and Bottomley, J.M. (2008). *Geriatric Rehabilitation: A Clinical Approach*. Pearson Prentice Hall.

Mayers, C.A. (1998). An evaluation of the use of the Mayers' lifestyle questionnaire. *British Journal of Occupational Therapy* 61 (9): 393–398. https://doi.org/10.1177/030802269806100903.

Mayers, C.A. (2003). The development and evaluation of the Mayers' lifestyle questionnaire (2). *British Journal of Occupational Therapy* 66 (9): 388–395. https://doi.org/10.1177/030802260306600902.

McAvoy, E. (1991). The use of ADL indices by occupational therapists. *British Journal of Occupational Therapy* 54 (10): 383–385. https://doi.org/10.1177/030802269105401009.

McDowell, I. (2006). *Measuring Health: A Guide to Rating Scales and Questionnaires*. USA: Oxford University Press.

Melzack, R. (1987). The short-form McGill pain questionnaire. *Pain* 30 (2): 191–197. https://doi.org/10.1016/0304-3959(87)91074-8.

Molloy, D.W., Alemayehu, E., and Roberts, R. (1991). Reliability of a standardized mini-mental state examination compared with the traditional mini-mental state examination. *The American Journal of Psychiatry* 148 (1): 102–105. http://citeseerx.ist.psu.edu/viewdoc/download?doi=10.1.1.467.4169&rep=rep1&type=pdf.

Pattie, A.H. (1981). A survey version of the Clifton assessment procedures for the elderly (CAPE). *British Journal of Clinical Psychology* 20 (3): 173–178. https://doi.org/10.1111/j.2044-8260.1981.tb00515.x.

Pattie, A.H. (1988). Measuring levels of disability: The Clifton assessment procedures for the elderly. In: *Psychological Assessment of the Elderly* (eds. J. Wattis and I. Hindmarch), 61–81. Churchill Livingstone.

Pattie, A.H. and Gilleard, C.J. (1989). *Clifton Assessment Procedures for the Elderly (CAPE)*. Hodder and Stoughton.

Prinsen, C.A., Vohra, S., Rose, M.R. et al. (2016). How to select outcome measurement instruments for outcomes included in a "Core outcome set" – a practical guideline. *Trials* 17 (1): 449. https://doi.org/10.1186/s13063-016-1555-2.

Pynsent, P., Fairbank, J., and Carr, A. (2004). *Outcome Measures in Orthopaedics and Orthopaedic Trauma*. CRC Press.

Scudds, R.A., Fishbain, D.A., and Scudds, R.J. (2003). Concurrent validity of an electronic descriptive pain scale. *Clinical Rehabilitation* 17 (2): 206–208. https://doi.org/10.1191/0269215503cr601oa.

Streiner, D.L., Norman, G.R., and Cairney, J. (2015). *Health Measurement Scales: A Practical Guide to their Development and Use*. USA: Oxford University Press.

Terwee, C.B., Prinsen, C.A., Chiarotto, A. et al. (2018a). COSMIN methodology for evaluating the content validity of patient-reported outcome measures: a Delphi study. *Quality of Life Research* 27 (5): 1159–1170. https://doi.org/10.1007/s11136-018-1829-0.

Terwee CB, Prinsen CAC, Chiarotto A, de Vet HCW, Bouter LM, Alonso J, Westerman MJ, Patrick DL, Mokkink LB (2018b) COSMIN methodology for assessing the content validity of PROMs: User manual version 1.0. Available from: https://cosmin.nl/wp-content/uploads/COSMIN-methodology-for-content-validity-user-manual-v1.pdf

Tyerman, R., Tyerman, A., Howard, P., and Hadfield, C. (1986). The Chessington OT Neurological Assessment Battery Introductory Manual. *Nottingham*: Nottingham Rehab Limited 3 (5): 7–9. www.ukmobilityhealthcare.co.uk/COTNAB-Battery.

Tyson, S.F. and Connell, L.A. (2009). How to measure balance in clinical practice. A systematic review of the psychometrics and clinical utility of measures of balance activity for neurological conditions. *Clinical Rehabilitation* 23 (9): 824–840. https://doi.org/10.1177/0269215509335018.

Welk, G. (2002). *Physical Activity Assessments for Health-Related Research*. Human Kinetics.

Whiting, S., Lincoln, N.B., Bhavnani, G., and Cockburn, J. (1985). *The Rivermead Perceptual. Assessment Battery Manual*. Windsor: NFER-Nelson.

Wolf, H. (1997). Assessments of activities of daily living and instrumental activities of daily living: their use by community-based health service occupational therapists working in physical disability. *British Journal of Occupational Therapy* 60 (8): 359–364. https://doi.org/10.1177/030802269706000809.

Wright, J., Cross, J., and Lamb, S. (1998). Physiotherapy outcome measures for rehabilitation of elderly people: responsiveness to change of the Rivermead Mobility Index and Barthel Index. *Physiotherapy* 84 (5): 216–221. https://doi.org/10.1016/S0031-9406(05)65552-6.

Zamanzadeh, V., Rassouli, M., Abbaszadeh, A. et al. (2014). Details of content validity and objectifying it in instrument development. *Nursing Practice Today* 1 (3): 163–171. http://npt.tums.ac.ir/index.php/npt/article/view/24.

RESOURCES

COnsensus-based Standards for the selection of health Measurement Instruments – COSMIN

COSMIN is an initiative of an international multidisciplinary team of researchers with a background in epidemiology, psychometrics, medicine, qualitative research, and healthcare, who have expertise in the development and evaluation of outcome measurement instruments. https://www.cosmin.nl/about

CHAPTER 9

Reliability

OVERVIEW

This chapter will define the main types of reliability of relevance to allied health professionals (AHPs) – test–retest reliability, inter-rater reliability, intra-rater reliability, internal consistency, and parallel form reliability – and consider how these are evaluated and what levels of reliability are considered acceptable for practice. The chapter will also explore the concepts of rater severity, sensitivity, specificity, and responsiveness. Standard error of measurement and floor and ceiling effects will be described.

QUESTIONS TO CONSIDER

1. How do I ensure that my measurements are reliable?
2. How can I ensure that my outcome measures are responsive to a clinically relevant degree of change?

INTRODUCING THE CONCEPT OF RELIABILITY

It is critical for AHPs to consider the reliability of an assessment. Frequently, AHPs will wish to evaluate the effectiveness of a treatment or intervention programme by retesting a patient on an assessment administered prior to treatment, to establish whether desired changes in function have occurred. It is, therefore, important that changes in a patient's performance on the test are not affected by the time interval or by the rater. The degree of established reliability tells the AHP how accurately the scores obtained from an assessment reflect the true performance of a person on the test (Opacich 1991). When an AHP uses a test with evidence of high levels of reliability obtained through a robust reliability study design, they can be confident that the scores obtained on the test will reflect their client's true performance.

Principles of Assessment and Outcome Measurement for Allied Health Professionals:
Practice, Research and Development, Second Edition. Alison J. Laver-Fawcett and Diane L. Cox.
© 2021 John Wiley & Sons Ltd. Published 2021 by John Wiley & Sons Ltd.

If an assessment was very reliable, an AHP could obtain the same result each time they used that assessment under exactly the same conditions. In reality, the results obtained from the vast majority of assessments will differ across administrations owing to error. Pynsent and colleagues (2004, p. 4) describe measurement as an equation in which:

$$\text{Measurement} = \text{true value} + \text{error}$$

Reliability data is used to provide an index of the amount of measurement error in a test. The aspects of people evaluated by AHPs are open to many variables that may act as 'sources of error' during an assessment. Pynsent (2004, p. 4) lists four main sources of error:

1. error from the rater,
2. from the instrument itself,
3. random error, and
4. error from the patient.

Errors can occur because of the way the AHP administers, scores, and interprets the results of a test. Errors can also occur because of fluctuating or temporary behaviour in the person being tested. For example, the client may guess the answer or may remember the answer from a previous test administration. Errors can occur when the person is distracted during testing. In addition, a person's true ability may not be demonstrated during assessment if his performance is impacted by test anxiety. Potentially confounding variables may include the person's motivation, interests, mood, and the effects of medication. Because such variables may influence the person's performance to some degree, they can never be completely discounted. Therefore, AHPs need to know how likely it is that these potential sources of error will influence the results obtained on a test (de Clive-Lowe 1996).

DEFINING RELIABILITY

In broad terms, the 'reliability of a test refers to how stable its scores remain overtime and across different examiners' (de Clive-Lowe 1996, p. 359), and reliability studies are undertaken to try to separate measurement errors from the person's true value or score on a measure (Pynsent 2004). Often, 'numerical data are associated with quality, reliability, and credibility' (Krohne et al. 2014, p. 8). The main types of reliability of relevance to AHPs are test–retest reliability, inter-rater reliability, intra-rater reliability, internal consistency, and parallel form reliability. Other terms such as agreement, concordance, repeatability, and reproducibility are sometimes used in the test literature to describe aspects of reliability (Pynsent 2004).

Moss (1994, 2004) defines reliability as:

consistency, quantitatively defined, among independent observations or sets of observations that are intended as interchangeable.

(p. 6, 1994)

Or

the degree to which measures are free from error and therefore yield consistent results (i.e. the consistency of a measurement procedure).

(Thanasegaran 2009, p. 35)

Reliability should be examined at the test development stage if a measure is being designed either to be used by more than one AHP and/or to be administered more than once to provide a measure of outcome (Biasutti 2019). Many test developers present reliability data in the test manual and related publications. This knowledge is produced through studies of reliability. The methodology required to evaluate reliability varies depending upon the type of reliability to be examined. The basic method involves a test being administered by different AHPs to large numbers of people at different times, and statistical analyses of the similarities and differences in the scores, obtained from these various test administrations, are calculated. The AHP needs to be able to understand the differences between various types of reliability, ascertain whether these have been adequately studied, and judge whether the quoted reliability is adequate for the context of their clinical practice.

RELIABILITY COEFFICIENTS AND STANDARD ERROR OF MEASUREMENT

A *reliability coefficient* is used to indicate the extent to which a test is a stable instrument that is capable of producing consistent results. Reliability is usually expressed as a correlation coefficient and varies between zero and one. *Correlation* is the term used to describe a 'measure of association that indicates the degree to which two or more sets of observations fit a linear relationship' (McDowell 2006, p. 711). Various statistical formulae can be used for estimating the strength of correlation and produce *correlation coefficients*. Correlation in the broadest sense is a measure of an association between variables (Schober et al. 2018, p. 1763). For all methods, a finding of no correlation is indicated by zero (0) and means that no relationship was evident in the two sets of data being compared. Perfect reliability is represented by a coefficient of 1.0, but in real life this is hardly ever achieved. The most common method of assessing internal consistency reliability estimates is through the use of coefficient alpha (Thanasegaran 2009). There are three different measures of coefficient alpha; one of these is Cronbach's coefficient alpha. Cronbach's alpha is actually an average of all the possible split-half reliability estimates of an instrument (Crocker and Algina 1986).

The AHP, therefore, needs to judge the acceptable amount of error when making clinical decisions from test results. For ordered test variables, as measured on ordinal or interval scales (see Chapter 4), the correlation statistic is cited with a positive or negative sign and can range from minus one to plus one (−1.0 to +1.0). This indicates whether the correlation is negative or positive. Very few test administrations will produce perfect correlation, unless they are two different measures of the same thing. For example, a person's height measured in feet and inches should have perfect correlation as when measured in metres and centimetres (Munro 2005). Negative correlations are obtained when one test variable has the opposite effect to another; for example, 'the correlation between the outside temperature and the size of our heating bill over a year should show a near-perfect negative correlation. A near-zero correlation is likely to be found between our height and the size of our heating bill' (Saslow 1982, p. 193). In testing, a negative correlation indicates 'that the same individual will score high on one test and low on another' (Asher 1996, p. xxxi). So, the closer the reliability coefficient is to 1.00, the more reliable is the test.

LEVEL OF SIGNIFICANCE

Some authors refer to level of significance when reporting their reliability studies. Asher (1996) states that the level of significance is obtained through a statistical procedure that 'identifies the amount of objectivity of data by determining the probability that chance influences the results' (p. xxxi). The lower the level of significance reported, the greater the confidence that you may place in the results. In therapy psychometric literature, the most frequently cited levels of significance are 0.05, which equals a 5% chance; and 0.01, which equals a 1% chance. Figures are often cited with a less than sign (<). Levels of <0.001 and <0.0001 are considered highly significant.

ERROR OF MEASUREMENT

A score that would represent entirely all observations of an individual's behaviour on a test is known as the person's *universe score* or *true score* (Asher 1996). No one test administration can represent the person perfectly, and a person's test scores are expected to vary to some degree from one test administration to another. AHPs rarely have time to administer more than once at baseline and once for each follow-up measurement. Therefore, AHPs need to be able to generalise from the results of a single test administration. The following formula (Royeen 1989, p. 55) is often used: $X = t + e$, where:

X = the observed score

t = the true score

e = the error score.

The goal then 'is to reduce or identify the controllable error to establish confidence that the observed score approximates the true score' (p. 55). Error of measurement is identified by checking the agreement between an original test score and subsequent scores (Asher 1996).

Standard Error of Measurement (SEM)

No measurement is perfectly accurate, but it is accurate within certain error margins. The lower the error margin, the more confidence we can place in the measure; the higher the error margin, the more we need to think about whether we are addressing the right problem, whether we need to delay a decision and search for further confirmation or refutation of our ideas (Raju et al. 2007). Some test manuals provide details of the SEM, and this can be very useful to AHPs in deciding how accurate the test result is likely to be and how much to rely upon this result in decision making.

SEM is the estimate of the 'error' associated with a person's obtained score on a test when compared with his/her hypothetical 'true' or 'universe' score (Harvill 1991). A range of scores can be calculated from this figure, and this is known as a *confidence interval* (Bowling 2014). The confidence interval represents the range of scores within which you can be highly confident that the person's true score lies. The usual confidence interval used is 95%, which means that you can be 95% confident that the true score lies within the interval (range of scores) calculated. To develop a confidence interval, it is assumed that the scores obtained by a population on a test will be distributed along a normal curve. In a normal curve, 95% of scores lie within 1.96 standard deviations (sd) of the mean. To calculate a 95% confidence interval for a client's score, the AHP will need to look up the reported SEM from the test manual.

For example, a manual may state that the AHP can be x (e.g. 95%) per cent certain that a person's true score lies in the range of the obtained score plus or minus y (e.g. 3). The AHP takes the SEM value y and multiplies it by desired confidence

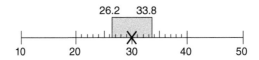

FIGURE 9.1   Example confidence interval: Justin's Confidence Interval for Section B. Auditory Processing (10 month old). *Source*: Dunn (2002). © 2002, Pearson.

interval *x* (i.e. for a 95% interval, multiply *y* by 1.96 sd). Dunn (2002) in the Infant and Toddler Sensory Profile Manual provides a good example as shown below.

Example of Calculating a Confidence Interval for a 10-Month-Old

Justin's section raw score total for Section B. Auditory Processing = 30
SEM for this score = 1.93 (note this is provided in the manual, Dunn (2002), Table 6.2, p. 62)

$$1.96 \times 1.93 = 3.78$$

Subtract 3.78 and add 3.78 to Justin's raw score to get the 95% confidence interval. For Justin these numbers would be:

$$30 - 3.78 = 26.2$$
$$30 + 3.78 = 33.8$$

This calculation gives you 95% confidence that Justin's true score lies somewhere between 26 and 34 (p. 63) (see Figure 9.1)

A number of therapy assessments have been subjected to Rasch analysis, and this statistical procedure can be used to report the reliabilities of each item in terms of standard error. Fisher (2010), in the 7th edition of the Assessment of Motor and Process Skills (AMPS) manual, discusses the advantages of this approach as the many-faceted Rasch analysis computer programme reports the reliabilities of each skill item, task, and rater calibration and person measure in terms of standard errors. When considered from the perspective of person-centred measurement, the reporting of person-by-person standard errors of measurement has two advantages. First, rather than applying a single standard error of measurement to an entire sample, we are able to apply a specific standard error of measurement to each person. Second, knowledge of each person's error of measurement enables us to determine when that person has made significant gains, beyond chance, as a result of participation in intervention (Fisher and Merritt 2012).

TYPES OF RELIABILITY

There are several types of reliability that the AHP should consider. The main forms of reliability of relevance to AHPs described in the psychometric and therapy literature (for example, Berchtold 2016, Crocker and Algina 1986; Hartman-Maeir et al. 2009) include:

- test–retest reliability,
- inter-rater reliability,
- intra-rater reliability,
- parallel form reliability (equivalent/alternate form), and
- internal consistency.

Test–Retest Reliability

Test–retest is a term used to describe the properties of measurement tools evaluated twice on different time occasions (Berchtold 2016, p. 1). Stability is an important concept for AHPs as we need to know whether a behaviour or level of function is stable or has changed over time. In psychometric terms, stability is linked to reliability and relates to whether an assessment can measure the same behaviour or construct repeatedly (Berchtold 2016). One aspect of repeatability, of concern to AHPs, is how consistently an assessment can repeat results over time. In order to pick up real changes in function, an AHP needs to know whether the assessment they plan to use at several time points during intervention to monitor their client's function will provide reliability in terms of stability across time. Therefore, tests used as outcome measures should have adequate test–retest reliability.

Test–retest reliability is the correlation of scores obtained by the same person on two administrations of the same test and is the consistency of the assessment or test score over time (Anastasi 1988). This type of reliability is important because AHPs need to examine whether their interventions have been effective, and to do this they administer tests on two or more occasions to monitor changes following treatment. Test–retest reliability is calculated using the correlation between two administrations of the test to the same people with a defined time interval between the two test administrations. When the same clients and AHP are used for a reliability study and the results obtained are consistent over time, then a test is said to have test–retest reliability (Polit 2014). An acceptable correlation coefficient for test–retest reliability is considered to be 0.70 or above (Paiva et al. 2014).

A big question that faces researchers, and needs to be considered by AHPs interpreting reported test–retest data, is: *how much time should be allowed between test administrations?* There is no perfect answer because the populations assessed on therapy assessments and the purposes of assessments vary considerably. When choosing the most appropriate time interval between test administrations, the purpose of the test should be considered along with the way in which test scores are to be used (Crocker and Algina 1986). The time period selected needs to be long enough so that any effects from practice, or remembering the answers to test items, should have faded. However, it cannot be so long that a genuine change in function or ability occurs, because then any difference in scores obtained from the test and the retest would result from changes to the person's true scores. The time interval also needs to reflect the likely interval between testing selected by AHPs to measure outcomes in clinical practice. For example, a test of infant development will need a short period between test administrations because there is likelihood that maturation will cause frequent changes in an infant's ability and test performance. In addition, it is unlikely that a young infant will remember his previous responses to test items (Crocker and Algina 1986). Adults, however, are likely to remember their responses over quite long periods, and so test developers will need to leave a longer period between test administrations. This may be done when the group of people being tested have a condition that is associated with little or very slow changes in function. However, when a shorter time period is required between test administrations, they will have to develop an alternative form of the test (see the section on parallel form reliability below).

Inter-Rater Reliability

Inter-rater reliability refers to the agreement between or among different AHPs (raters) administering the test. AHPs need to be sure that any change in a person's performance on a test represents a genuine change in the person's performance and is not caused by a different test administrator. A reliable measure needs to ensure objectivity by using a method of assessment (van de Pol et al. 2010) which is not influenced by the emotions, or personal opinion of the rater. This is important because service users often move between therapy services, for example, from an acute ward to a rehabilitation ward, from inpatient service to community services such as a day hospital or outpatient service, from an intermediate care/rapid response service to longer-term support by a community team. Therefore, a person might be given the same assessment on a number of occasions, but each time a different AHP administers the test.

Inter-rater reliability is calculated using the correlation between the scores recorded by two or more AHPs administering the test to the same person at the same time. An acceptable correlation coefficient for inter-rater reliability is considered to be 0.90 or above (Gwet 2014). Many test manuals and journal articles reporting psychometrics deal with inter-rater reliability and AHPs should expect to have easy access to such data when a test is likely to be administered by more than one AHP.

Intra-Rater Reliability

Intra-rater reliability refers to the consistency of the judgements made by the same AHP (test administrator/rater) over time. AHPs often use tests that require some degree of observation and/or clinical judgement (Mumby et al. 2007). So they need to know that differences in results obtained for different clients, or the results for the same client obtained at different times, represent a genuine change in the person's performance, or real differences between clients, and is not the result of a fluctuation in the AHP's own consistency in giving and scoring the test. In studies of intra-rater reliability, the interval between ratings by the same examiner is usually brief, and the assessment requires some observation or judgement on the part of the rater (Mumby et al. 2007). One factor that may impact inter-rater and intra-rater reliability is the AHPs' level of experience. When reviewing reliability studies, look to see whether the AHPs used were of the same grade/level of experience or whether the sample used AHPs of mixed seniority.

Rater Severity

Some test developers have considered the variation in how lenient or stringent AHPs are when judging a person's performance on an observational assessment; this is known as rater severity (Bundy et al. 2001; Zhu et al. 1998). For example, AHPs wishing to use the AMPS (Bernspång 1999) are required to attend a rigorous five-day training course so that they can be calibrated for rater severity. AHPs view a series of videotapes of AMPS tasks being administered. Some AHPs are found to be more lenient in their scoring and give clients higher scores than more severe raters. Knowledge of rater severity scoring the AMPS is accounted for in the determination of the person's ability measure, thus reducing the chance that inter-rater variability will confound the 'true' measure of the person's function (Fisher 2003).

Parallel Form Reliability (Equivalent or Alternate Form)

Parallel or Alternate form reliability examines the correlation between scores obtained for the same person on two (or more) forms of a test. A parallel form is an alternative test that differs in content from the original test but which measures the same thing to the same level of difficulty (Costa et al. 2012). Parallel forms are used for retesting where a practice or learning effect might impact the test results. Parallel forms are particularly useful when the client group will need regular reassessment, has a condition which is associated with rapid improvements/decline in function, or where improvement in scores owing to a practice effect will skew the test results. Several terms are used to describe parallel test forms, and you may also see these referred to as *equivalent forms* or *alternate forms*. Reliability studies and statistics for this type of reliability can, therefore, be referred to as parallel form reliability, equivalent form reliability, or alternate form reliability. Parallel form reliability is calculated using the correlation between two forms of the same test. The correlation coefficient obtained from two sets of scores drawn from parallel (equivalent/alternate) test forms can be called the *coefficient of equivalence* (Crocker and Algina 1986). An acceptable correlation coefficient for parallel form reliability is considered to be 0.80 or above (Salkind 2010, p. 162).

Internal Consistency

Revicki (2014) states that internal consistency reflects the extent to which items within an instrument measure various aspects of the same characteristic or construct. A basic principle of measurement is that 'several related observations will produce a more reliable estimate that one' (Fitzpatrick 2004, p. 55). If this is to be the case, then the related observations will need to measure aspects of a single construct, attribute, or behaviour. When two or more items are included in a test, to measure the same construct or element of behaviour, a comparison can be made between these items to see if they produce consistent results. The more observations of a particular behaviour are made within a test, the more likely it will be that the observed behaviour is not a random incident (Cromack 1989). However, AHPs do not want overly long tests that will tire or bore their clients. So test developers need to select the optimum number and type of test items to adequately evaluate the construct or behaviour of concern. Internal consistency studies enable a test developer to ascertain whether all the items in a test are measuring the same construct or trait. This is known as the *homogeneity* of test items. Items must measure the same construct if they are to be a homogenous item group, and a test is said to have item homogeneity when people perform consistently across the test items. Items may test the same performance domains and constructs, but vary in difficulty. Studies of internal consistency examine both item homogeneity and item difficulty, and study the effect of errors caused by content sampling. Such studies are undertaken to help the test developer ascertain how far each test item or question contributes to the overall construct or behaviour being measured (McDowell 2006).

You may see the term *item-total correlation* used in literature related to internal consistency. This is where the correlation of each test item with the total test score has been used as an indication of the internal consistency/homogeneity of the scales (Streiner 2003). Internal consistency coefficients are reported by some test developers and help AHPs to consider how homogenous the item responses are within a scale or assessment (Dunn 2002). Cronbach's alpha is one of the most frequently used statistical methods for evaluating the internal consistency of a test (Streiner 2003). Values of between 0.70 and 0.90 are considered optimal, although 0.80 or above is acceptable (Vaske et al. 2017). So, when reviewing coefficients for internal consistency, you are looking for values of at least 0.70 and preferably 0.85 and above.

Another method of evaluating internal consistency is the *split-half method* (Streiner 2003). The test is administered once, and items are divided into two halves, which are then correlated with each other. A correction for the shortened length of the tests can be applied. The extent to which the two halves are comparable and the degree to which each represents the whole test is considered to be an estimate of the internal consistency. Some test developers calculate a coefficient alpha; this provides an average of all possible split-halves (Dunn 2002). A variant of the split-half method is the *even-odd system*, which involves the test developer comparing the even-numbered test items with the odd-numbered test items (Daniel et al. 2015).

METHODOLOGICAL ISSUES

There is no gold standard for conducting reliability studies, and methodology and sample sizes vary widely across reported studies. Therefore, in addition to examining the reliability coefficient stated for a test, it is important that an AHP who is deciding whether the test has acceptable levels of reliability review the methodology and sample sizes used. This information is usually published in test manuals or journal articles.

Methodology varies considerably across inter-rater reliability studies. Some test developers only evaluate the reliability of the scoring of the assessment through a method that involves different therapists scoring videotaped administrations of a test, whereas other test developers consider the reliability between AHPs for both test administration and scoring. This is especially important for tests where the AHP uses an element of judgement to guide test administration, such as the provision of prompts or cues or deciding where to start or stop the administration of hierarchical test items.

For example, the inter-rater reliability of the Rivermead Perceptual Assessment Battery (*RPAB*; Whiting et al. 1985) was evaluated using the videotaped assessment of six people scored by three occupational therapists, and Matthey et al. (1993) suggest that the small 'sample sizes used by the RPAB authors to calculate the reliability coefficients ... [make] the reliability data questionable' (p. 366). The methodology used by Russell et al. (1993) to evaluate the inter-rater reliability of the Gross Motor Function Measure (*GMFM*) was more robust as they examined the reliability of testers administering and scoring the test. However, their sample size was still small as they had three pairs of AHPs administer and score the GMFM with a sample of 12 children. Laver (1994) undertook two studies to examine the inter-rater reliability of the Structured Observational Test of Function (*SOTOF*; Laver and Powell 1995). In the first study, 14 pairs of AHPs (n = 28) administered the SOTOF to 14 people with a primary diagnosis of stroke. In the second study, four AHPs formed different pairings to administer the SOTOF to a mixed sample of 23 subjects (7 patients with a primary diagnosis stroke, 15 with dementia and 1 with head injury). This gave combined inter-rater reliability data for 32 AHPs and 37 patients. In both studies, one AHP administered the test while the second AHP observed the administration, and then both AHPs scored the patient independently.

The experience of the AHPs involved in the studies should also be considered in order to identify whether a newly qualified AHP will obtain results consistent with those of an experienced senior AHP. In the RPAB manual (Whiting et al. 1985), the level of experience of the three AHPs used for the study is not stated. However, this data is provided for the GMFM and the SOTOF inter-rater reliability studies. Both studies reported that their samples comprised AHPs with a broad range of experience. In the GMFM study (Russell et al. 1993), the six AHPs had paediatric experience ranging from 2.5 to 18 years. In the sample for the first SOTOF inter-rater reliability study (Laver 1994), AHPs' experience with elderly clients ranged from 1 to

15 years, and the sample comprised 8 basic grade AHPs, 11 senior II AHPs, 3 senior I AHPs, 3 head IV, 1 head III, 1 deputy head, and 1 AHP who did not specify her grade (n = 26). In the second study, the sample (n = 4) comprised one basic grade, one senior II, and one head occupational therapist, and the test developer, who was working as a senior lecturer (and had previously been a Senior I OT).

Test Specificity

AHPs also need to consider the specificity and sensitivity of tests. Trevethan (2017) describes this as '… the ability of a screening test to detect a true negative, being based on the true negative rate, correctly identifying people who do not have a condition, or, if 100%, identifying all patients who do not have the condition of interest by those people testing negative on the test' (p. 2, see Figure 9.2). Test specificity is important because AHPs want only those people who exhibit a specific behaviour or functional deficit to be identified on a test. A *false positive* result occurs when someone who does not have a deficit is identified on a test as having the deficit. A *false negative* result occurs when a person who has a deficit is not shown to have that deficit through his performance on the test. Specificity, therefore, has been defined as 'the proportion of non-cases according to the agreed diagnostic criteria who are negative' on a test (Green et al. 2005, p. 10). AHPs need to be aware of the risk of a false negative result because this can lead to a person not receiving a correct diagnosis or assessment of the problem, which in turn can result in required treatment being withheld and the person's condition deteriorating unnecessarily.

A specific test minimises the number of false positive results that occur when the test is used and will not identify people who do not exhibit the behaviour or deficit being examined (Opacich 1991). Both types of errors can lead to negative consequences for an individual. A false positive test might result in a person being incorrectly diagnosed and given an inappropriate treatment or suffering discrimination because of the label assigned as a result of the false positive test. In some cases, this could have a serious consequence; a person might be given unnecessary medication and suffer from side effects needlessly, or be refused employment or insurance because of his diagnosis.

		Status of the person According to "gold standard"		
		Has the condition	Does not have the condition	
Result from test	Positive	a True positive	b False positive	Row entries for determining **positive predictive value**
	Negative	c False negative	d True negative	Row entries for determining **negative predictive value**
		Column entries for determining **sensitivity**	Column entries for determining **specificity**	

FIGURE 9.2   Diagram showing sensitivity, specificity, and positive and negative predictive values. *Source*: Adapted from Trevethan (2017).

A good test manual will provide details of potential levels of error, enabling AHPs to consider the risk of a false positive or false negative result occurring when they administer the test. For example, the Infant and Toddler Symptom Checklist Manual (DeGangi et al. 1995) provides a table illustrating the 'Classification Accuracy for Cut-off Scores' (p. 41) and provides false positive (labelled as false delayed) and false negative (labelled as false normal) percentages for all five age bands covered by the test. These percentages varied considerably across the age bands; for example, for children aged 19–24 months, the false positive risk was only 3%, and a 0% false negative rate indicated that the test should identify accurately all infants with a problem. However, for children in the 25–30 month age band, a false positive rate of 13% and a false negative rate of 14% are given. AHPs therefore would be wise to use this test in conjunction with other measures in this age group.

Test developers of therapy assessments often decide that a false negative result will have a greater potential risk to the individual than a false positive result and will select test items in order to minimise false negative scores. For example, DeGangi et al. (1995), authors of the Infant and Toddler Symptom Checklist, reported that 'the cut off scores for each subtest were chosen to minimise the false-normal error rate, judged to be the more serious of the two types of error from the perspective of screening and diagnostic decision making' (p. 42).

Abidin (1995) identified three different types of false negative data in parent populations when he analysed his research and clinical experience using the Parenting Stress Index (*PSI*). He describes these as Type I False Negative, Defensive Individuals; Type II False Negative, Dishonest Respondents; and Type III False Negative, Disengaged Parents. In the PSI manual, descriptions of the three False Negative Types are provided to assist AHPs in interpreting extremely low PSI Total Stress Scores (scores falling below the 15th percentile), to decide whether the test results reflect a true picture of a parent under a low level of stress or whether further investigation is required to examine a hypothesis that the parent falls under one of the three False Negative Types. In order to assist test administrators to identify false negative scores related to defensive responding, Abidin developed a PSI defensive responding scoring system using 15 of the PSI items that are highlighted by shading on the scoring part of the answer sheet. A cut-off score is given, and parents with this score or below are considered to be responding in a defensive manner; the test administrator then knows that the results must be interpreted with caution.

Test Sensitivity

Test sensitivity is important because a sensitive test will identify all those people who show the behaviour or deficit in question. Trevethan (2017) describes this as '... the ability of a screening test to detect a true positive, being based on the true positive rate, reflecting a test's ability to correctly identify all people who have a condition, or, if 100%, identifying all people with a condition of interest by those people testing positive on the test' (p. 3). An alternative definition is 'the proportion of cases according to the agreed diagnostic criteria who are positive' on the test (Green et al. 2005, p. 10). A sensitive test will minimise the chance of false negative results occurring and can identify what it was designed to test.

If a test is not sensitive enough to the target of therapy, then changes that have occurred may be missed, and this can be problematic if intervention appears to be ineffective when significant change has actually occurred. This is sometimes referred to as the degree of *responsiveness* of a test. 'Responsiveness to change can also be considered a fundamental characteristic of the evaluation instruments, designed to measure longitudinal change through time' (de Yébenes Prous et al. 2008, p. 240). The responsiveness of a test is critically important to AHPs because they often need to measure changes in aspects of people's functioning, for example, when evaluating the impact of intervention or monitoring the effects of medication. When using evaluative measures, the AHP should ensure that the test used is responsive to picking up both the type and amount of change in behaviour or function that is anticipated, or desired, as the result of the intervention. It is important that measures can identify clinically important change, even if this is quite small (Pynsent et al. 2004).

Although an increasing number of therapy measures are now backed by studies of their reliability and validity, one of the most important psychometric properties for AHPs to consider is sensitivity to clinically relevant change over time to establish the effects of their interventions.

Various methods are used to examine responsiveness to change. The simplest method is the calculation of percentage change. Effect sizes and relative efficiency are also accepted methods for comparing the responsiveness to change of different tests (van der Zee et al. 2011). Effect size can be applied to evaluate continuous data. Pynsent (2004) states that 'the effect size is usually quoted as a measure of sensitivity to change for instruments whose sample means are reasonably normally distributed' (p. 5), and he provides the following equation:

$$\text{Effect size index} = \frac{\text{Mean at time 1} - \text{mean at time 2}}{\textit{Standard Deviation}\left(\textit{SD}\right)\textit{at time 1}}$$

McDowell (2006) describes how the likelihood ratio is used by some test developers in relation to specificity and sensitivity analyses:

> Likelihood ratio 'is an approach to summarizing the results of sensitivity and specificity analyses for various cutting points on diagnostic and screening tests. Each cutting point produces as value for the true positive rate (i.e. sensitivity) and the false positive rate (i.e. specificity). The ratio of true to false positives is the likelihood ratio for each cutting point'
>
> (p. 713).

When reviewing research into the responsiveness of tests, AHPs should be aware that the larger the effect size, the more responsive the test is to clinical change. An effect size of 0.2 or below is considered small, 0.5 is considered a moderate effect size, and 0.8 or more is considered a large effect size (Sullivan and Feinn 2012). Relative efficiency is particularly useful when you have two potential outcome measures for your service and wish to select the one that will provide the greatest responsiveness. There are both parametric (using a t statistic) and non-parametric (using the z statistic derived from the Wilcoxon sign rank test) methods for calculating the relative efficiency between tests. Regardless of the method used, a score of 1 specifies that the responsiveness of the two tests being compared is the same. Scores greater than or less than one indicate that one test is more responsive than the other. To allow comparison of the responsiveness of different tests, raw scores may need to be transformed. For example to provide comparable scores out of 100, we would divide the person's actual score by the total possible score and then multiply this figure by 100 (Wright et al. 1998).

Wright et al. (1998) compared the responsiveness to change of the Rivermead Mobility Index (*RMI*) and the Barthel Index (*BI*) in a sample of 50 people receiving physiotherapy. They reported that both 'the RMI and the BI are responsive to changes in older people having physiotherapy (effect sizes 1 and 0.87 respectively)' (p. 216). They also used both parametric and non-parametric methods to calculate the relative efficiency of the two tests and reported that 'parametric calculation of relative efficiency of the RMI versus the BI was 1.42; non-parametric methods gave a result of 1.25 for the same comparison' (p. 219). 'In both cases, a result greater than 1 would indicate the RMI to be more responsive than the BI' (p. 218). Therefore, they concluded that the 'RMI was more efficient at measuring outcome than the BI' (p. 216).

Floor and Ceiling Effects

Floor and ceiling effects can impact the accuracy of an assessment. Measurement of outcome can be confounded when service users either improve or deteriorate beyond the range of functioning tested by the outcome measure. Therefore, *AHPs* need to consider the range of ability expected from their client population and select a suitable measure so as to ensure that their clients will be unlikely to perform above or below the measurement range of the tests used in their service. A ceiling effect occurs when the person scores the maximum possible score on a test, and the test does not reflect the full extent of his ability. A floor effect occurs when a person obtains the minimum score on a test, and the test does not reflect the full extent of the person's deficits. The size of the ceiling and floor effects is established by examining the percentage of a clinical sample obtaining either maximum or minimum scores. When deciding whether any reported ceiling or floor effects could impact the use of a measure for your clients, it is important to look at both the sample used in the study (diagnosis, age range, etc.) and the setting in which a test is being used (community, inpatient, outpatient, etc.). For example, Wright et al. (1998) examined the floor and ceiling effects of the RMI and the BI at three time periods: pre-admission, on admission, and at discharge. They used a sample of 50 people receiving physiotherapy for a range of orthopaedic, neurological, and cardiorespiratory conditions. They reported that when patients were scored before admission, 44% achieved the maximum possible score on the BI and 31% scored the maximum possible score on the RMI, indicating that both tests had a ceiling effect when used with patients in the community. However, when the samples were measured on admission to a rehabilitation ward, the 'scores on the BI were evenly distributed around the mid-point of the scale [and] there was no evidence of a floor or ceiling effect' (p. 218). But on admission 'the average score of the RMI was below the mid-point of the scale and ... 6% scored the minimum value [and] a floor effect was demonstrated' (p. 218). At discharge the BI was found to have a 'mild ceiling effect' (p. 219) with 4% of their sample scoring the maximum value, and the RMI was found to have a 'minor floor effect' with 6% of subjects obtaining the minimum score. Wright, Cross, and Lamb concluded that 'floor and ceiling effects are evident in both the RMI and BI respectively, and ... that this could limit their usefulness for in-patients'. They also stated that the BI is limited in its usefulness as an outcome measure in a community-based population because of the marked ceiling effect.

Floor and ceiling effects can be particularly relevant for certain client populations (Lim et al. 2015).

RELIABILITY STATISTICS

The following section provides a brief discussion on reliability statistics to help AHPs look at cited correlations critically and make informed judgements about the level of reliability of an assessment, and whether this is adequate for their practice. This section is by no means intended as an exhaustive presentation of reliability statistics, and any AHP conducting a reliability study should only use this as a starting point and refer to statistics textbooks and manuals for more detailed guidance.

Statistics is the application of mathematical formulae to order, interpret, and analyse a set of empirical data. Statistics enable us to describe the characteristics of our data and to draw inferences from it. Statistical analyses allow the test developer, and the AHP who will be the test administrator, to determine whether the results are owing to significant effects or to chance factors (Asher 1996). As an AHP you *need to know* enough about reliability statistics to make an *informed decision* about the value of a test for your clients. Just because a test is published does *not* mean it has adequate reliability! There are several statistical procedures used in reliability studies, and although many produce correlation coefficients, the numbers they produce are not necessarily equivalent and of identical merit. The following section will briefly present some of these statistical procedures and will discuss how the statistics they produce compare.

As stated earlier, reliability is usually expressed as a correlation coefficient ranging from −1.0 to +1.0. When you are examining reliability figures quoted in test manuals and the psychometric literature, the closer the number is to +1.0 the stronger is the reliability of the measure. It is rare to obtain reliability statistics of +1 or very close to +1. Fox (1969, as cited in Asher 1996) categorised correlations into four levels:

- Correlations from 0 to ±0.50 are low.
- Correlations from ±0.50 to 0.70 are moderate.
- Correlations from ±0.70 to 0.80 are high.
- Correlations greater than ±0.86 are very high.

The acceptable level of reliability does vary depending on the type of reliability being examined and must be examined in the context of the variables being correlated (Asher 1996):

- *Test–retest reliability*: An acceptable correlation coefficient for test–retest reliability is considered to be 0.70 or above (Opacich 1991).
- *Internal consistency*: An acceptable correlation coefficient for internal consistency is 0.85 and above (McDowell 2006).
- *Inter-rater reliability*: 0.90 or above is considered an acceptable level (Opacich 1991).
- *Parallel Form reliability*: Coefficients ranging in the 0.80 and 0.90s are acceptable for equivalent (alternate/parallel) form reliability (Crocker and Algina 1986).

So, when reviewing the reliability literature, you are looking for values of at least 0.70 and preferably 0.80 and above.

The Statistic Can Influence the Result

This section explores the different statistical methods used to produce reliability statistics and explains some of the disadvantages and advantages of these methods, which AHPs should take into account when evaluating whether the reliability of a measure is adequate for their clinical practice.

There is debate in the therapy literature concerning the 'correct' statistic to use to estimate reliability. The statistic chosen should relate to the level of measurement of the scale used in the test. For example, different statistics should be applied to dichotomous nominal data compared to continuous interval data. Kappa (Tooth and Ottenbacher 2004), coefficient alpha (Henson 2001), and per cent agreement (Teyhen et al. 2012) are described in the therapy and rehabilitation literature. All these statistics have a ceiling value of 1.00 or 100% and so depending on the type of reliability being evaluated and the statistic used, you should be looking for values of 0.70–1.00 (75–100%).

Percentage agreement (P) is an expression of the probability of a consistent decision. Percentage agreement is the simplest measure of consistency. It is often applied to criterion-referenced tests that use 2-point ordinal scales involving mastery decisions (for example, unable versus able, or independent versus dependent). P can be defined as the proportion of subjects consistently classified as either master–master (able-able) or nonmaster-nonmaster (unable-unable) using two criterion-referenced measurements.

Intra-class correlation coefficients (ICC) is used to produce measures of consistency or agreement of values within cases. It is useful when more than two raters have been involved in collecting data, for example, in an inter-rater reliability study (whereas Pearson's *r* is used to compare the ratings of a number of assessments undertaken on a sample by only two raters). Pynsent (2004) states 'ICC should be used for continuous data to measure agreement between or within methods or raters. There are other measures available but the ICC is appropriate and the most commonly used' (p. 4).

Pearson product–moment correlation coefficient is used to measure the degree of linear relationship between two sets of observations. Values obtained range from −1.00 to +1.00 (Crocker and Algina 1986). Pearson's *r* is used for ratio- or interval-level data (McDowell 2006). As r indicates the strength of the linear relationship, the highest value of +1.0 occurs when all data points fall exactly on the line. Tooth and Ottenbacher (2004) discussed the limitations of this statistic applied to reliability studies. Pynsent (2004) provides a good example of this problem:

> *If a mercury thermometer was compared with a digital thermometer and the mercury device measured exactly the same as the digital equipment but 2° lower, then Pearson's coefficient would be 1, suggesting 100 per cent agreement. It is always worth plotting the results to find systematic biases when comparing data.*
>
> (p. 4)

Cohen's Kappa (K) provides a statistical method for producing a 'coefficient of agreement between two raters, kappa expresses the level of agreement that is observed beyond the level that would be expected by chance alone' (McDowell 2006, p. 713). The Kappa value is easy to interpret; it uses the proportion of agreement and gives the advantage of accounting for chance agreement. Kappa provides a transformation of P to a new scale in which the points 0 and 1 are interpretable. A value of 1 indicates that decisions are as consistent as those based on perfectly statistically dependent scores (Crocker and Algina 1986). A value of 0 does not mean that decisions are so inconsistent as to render the item worthless, but that the decisions are no more consistent than decisions based on statistically independent scores. 'The coefficient K can assume negative values ... which corresponds to the situation in which there is an inverse relationship between the scores on the two forms' (Crocker and Algina 1986, p. 201). Pynsent (2004) recommends the use of Kappa when binary results are to be compared (i.e. paired/dichotomous data usually labelled as 1 and 0), and when analysing ordinal data a weighted kappa can be applied where the amount of disagreement is weighted.

Tooth and Ottenbacher (2004) have stated that kappa (κ statistic) is 'now more widely used in reliability and agreement studies reported in the medical and rehabilitation literature' (p. 1371); Kappa was preferred to per cent agreement as it corrects for chance agreement. Discrepancies were found between the average kappa values and the average percentage agreement indexes evaluated in their study; all the reliability coefficients in their study had a ceiling value of 1.00 or 100%, kappa had an approximate average value of 0.5 compared to per cent agreement, which had an approximate average of 0.75 (75%).

Examining Reliability Data: Test Examples

When making a decision whether to use a test or not based on reliability data, it is important to obtain as much of the evidence as possible. Most test developers will report initial reliability studies in the test manual or journal articles. For some tests, additional reliability data is available, either from later studies undertaken by the test developers or by independent researchers. Studies may not be directly comparable if they evaluate reliability with different diagnostic groups or age groups. But a range of studies will help to build up a picture of the reliability of a measure. The AHP should look for consistency across studies and take particular note of significant differences in reported levels of reliability.

CONCLUSION

In conclusion, a good measure must have demonstrated validity and reliability. A target analogy can be used to see how a measure may have none, both, or only one of these psychometric properties.

In a target analogy for reliability and validity (Figure 9.3), the 'Bull's eye' represents the true outcome to be measured, and each arrow represents a single application of the outcome instrument.

In this figure, the 'Bull's eye' (which is the shaded circle in the middle of each target) represents the true outcome to be measured, and each arrow represents a single application of the outcome instrument. In Figure 9.3(a), none of the arrows

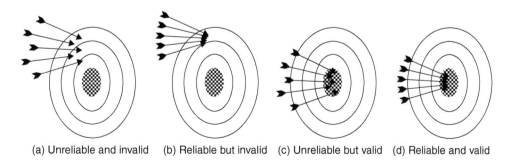

(a) Unreliable and invalid   (b) Reliable but invalid   (c) Unreliable but valid   (d) Reliable and valid

FIGURE 9.3 A target analogy for reliability and validity. Pynsent (2004). *Source*: Pynsent et al. (2004). CRC Press © 2004, Taylor & Francis.

have fallen within the bull's eye and the arrows are spread quite widely; this figure represents a measure that is neither valid nor reliable. In Figure 9.3(b), the arrows are clustered very closely together, indicating a reliable measurement, but they are not hitting the bull's eye, so although reliable the measure is not measuring what it sets out to measure and is not valid. In Figure 9.3(c), all the arrows fall within the bull's eye, indicating good validity, but the spread of the arrows is still quite wide, so reliability could be improved. Finally, Figure 9.3(d) represents a valid and reliable measure; all the arrows have fallen within the shaded bull's eye, and they are clustered close together.

Please now turn to Worksheet 9.1 found on p. 289.

For this reflection you will need to select a published assessment. This could be a test that you are already using in your clinical practice. Often AHPs inherit assessments when they start work in a different clinical setting or department; this will be exercise particularly useful if you are using a test that was already available in your department and which you have not critiqued. You might select a test that you are considering purchasing/using in the future. If you are a student, select a test you have seen used on clinical placement or one available at your university or college. Look to see what information (test manual, journal articles, handouts from training courses, etc.) is available on your chosen test. If there is very little, which can be the case when you have inherited an assessment, you might need to conduct a literature search in order to complete the worksheet.

The worksheet takes you through a series of questions about different types of reliability and prompts you to record key evidence and to form opinions about whether the published evidence indicates adequate levels of reliability, specificity, sensitivity, and responsiveness for your clinical needs.

REVIEW QUESTIONS

9.1   What is reliability?

9.2   What is the difference between inter-rater reliability and intra-rater reliability?

9.3   Define test–retest reliability.

9.4   What would be an acceptable correlation coefficient for test–retest reliability?

9.5   What is responsiveness, and why is it important if you want to measure outcomes?

You will find brief answers to these questions at the back of this book on p. 445.

Name of the test:
Full reference

	Yes	No
Is there evidence of test–retest reliability?	Yes	No
Describe study and findings – method, sample size, clinical sample used, statistics calculated, results:		
Is the level of reliability adequate (0.70 or above) or good (0.80 or above)?		
Do you feel confident that you can apply this test reliably over time?		
Is there evidence of inter-rater reliability?	Yes	No
Describe study and findings: method, rater/AHP sample size and description, clinical sample used, statistics calculated, results:		
Is the level of reliability adequate (0.80 or above) or good (0.90 or above)?		
Do you feel confident that you can apply this test reliably across different AHP raters?		
Is there evidence of internal consistency?	Yes	No
Describe study and findings – method, sample size, clinical sample used, statistics calculated, results:		
Is the level of internal consistency adequate (0.85 or above)?		
Do you feel confident that this test has homogeneity?		
If the test has a parallel (equivalent) form, is there evidence of parallel form reliability?	Yes	No
Describe study and findings – method, sample size, clinical sample used, statistics calculated, results:		
Is the level of reliability adequate (0.70 or above) or good (0.80 or above)?		

Name of the test:
Full reference

Do you feel confident that the parallel form can be used reliably?	
Test specificity: Is there evidence of test specificity?	Yes / No
Describe study and findings – method, sample size, clinical sample used, statistics calculated, results:	
What is the false positive rate?	
What would be the likely consequences and problems associated with a person being wrongly identified as having a problem on this measure?	
Is the test specificity adequate for your clinical setting?	
Responsiveness to change: Is there evidence of responsiveness to change?	Yes / No
Describe study and findings – method, sample size, clinical sample used, statistics calculated, results:	
Do you feel confident that this test can detect the type and amount of anticipated and/or desired change in your client group?	
Floor and ceiling effects: Is there evidence that the test has floor and/or ceiling effects?	Yes — Floor Effects / Yes — Ceiling Effects / No
Describe study and findings – method, sample size, clinical sample used, statistics calculated, results:	
Do you think that these effects will result in any of your clients failing or passing all test items?	
Standard error of measurement (SEM): Does the test manual/related literature report on the SEM?	Yes / No
Does it provide details on how you would use the SEM to calculate a confidence interval for a client's score?	
Do you feel confident about calculating confidence intervals using this test?	

REFERENCES

Abidin, R.R. (1995). *PSI: Parenting Stress Index*. Psychological Assessment Resources.

Anastasi, A. (1988). *Psychological Testing*, 5e. New York. NY: Macmillan.

Asher, I.E. (1996). *Occupational Therapy Assessment Tools: An Annotated Index*. Amer Occupational Therapy Assn.

Berchtold, A. (2016). Test–retest: agreement or reliability? *Methodological Innovations* 9 https://doi.org/10.1177/2059799116672875.

Bernspång, B. (1999). Rater calibration stability for the assessment of motor and process skills. *Scandinavian Journal of Occupational Therapy* 6 (3): 101–109. https://doi.org/10.1080/110381299443681.

Biasutti, M. (2019). Self-assessing music therapy: the validity and reliability of the music therapy practice scale (MTPS). *The Arts in Psychotherapy* 63: 40–45. https://doi.org/10.1016/j.aip.2019.03.006.

Bowling, A. (2014). *Research Methods in Health: Investigating Health and Health Services*. UK: McGraw-Hill Education.

Bundy, A.C., Nelson, L., Metzger, M., and Bingaman, K. (2001). Validity and reliability of a test of playfulness. *The Occupational Therapy Journal of Research* 21 (4): 276–292. https://doi.org/10.1177/153944920102100405.

de Clive-Lowe, S. (1996). Outcome measurement, cost-effectiveness and clinical audit: the importance of standardised assessment to occupational therapists in meeting these new demands. *British Journal of Occupational Therapy* 59 (8): 357–362. https://doi.org/10.1177/030802269605900803.

Costa, A.S., Fimm, B., Friesen, P. et al. (2012). Alternate-form reliability of the Montreal cognitive assessment screening test in a clinical setting. *Dementia and Geriatric Cognitive Disorders* 33 (6): 379–384. https://doi.org/10.1159/000340006.

Crocker, L. and Algina, J. (1986). *Introduction to Classical and Modern Test Theory* (eds. Holt, Rinehart and Winston). New York, USA: Part of Macmillan group as Holt McDougal.

Cromack, T.R. (1989). Measurement considerations in clinical research. In: *Clinical Research Handbook: An Analysis for the Service Professions* (ed. C.B. Royeen), 47. Slack Incorporated.

Daniel, F., da Silva, A.G., and Ferreira, P.L. (2015). Contributions to the discussion on the assessment of the reliability of a measurement instrument. *Referência-Revista de Enfermagem* 4 (7): 129–137. https://www.redalyc.org/pdf/3882/388243209007_2.pdf.

DeGangi, G.A., Poisson, S., Sickel, R.Z., and Santman, W.A. (1995). *Infant/Toddler Symptom Checklist: A Screening Tool for Parents*. San Antonio (TX): Therapy Skill Builders, Psychological Corporation.

Dunn, W. (2002). *Infant/Toddler Sensory Profile: user's Manual*. Pearson.

Fisher, A. G. (2003). *Assessment of motor and process skills. Administration and Scoring Manual*. AMPS Overview | Center for Innovative OT Solutions

Fisher, A.G. (2010). *Assessment of Motor and Process Skills Volume 2: User Manual*, 7e. USA: Fort Collins. Three Star Press.

Fisher, A.G. and Merritt, B.K. (2012). Conceptualizing and developing the AMPS within a framework of modern objective measurement. In: *Assessment of Motor and Process Skills*, vol. 1, 14–11. https://www.innovativeotsolutions.com/wp-content/uploads/2018/07/ampsChapters14–15.pdf.

Fitzpatrick, R. (2004). Measures of health status, health-related quality of life and patient satisfaction. In: *Outcome Measures in Orthopaedics and Orthopaedic Trauma*, 2e (eds. P. Pynsent, J. Fairbank and A. Carr), 54–63. CRC press.

Green, D., Bishop, T., Wilson, B.N. et al. (2005). Is questionnaire-based screening part of the solution to waiting lists for children with developmental coordination disorder? *British Journal of Occupational Therapy* 68 (1): 2–10. https://doi.org/10.1177/030802260506800102.

Gwet, K.L. (2014). *Handbook of Inter-Rater Reliability: The Definitive Guide to Measuring the Extent of Agreement among Raters.* Advanced Analytics, LLC https://books.google.co.uk/books?hl=en&lr=&id=fac9BQAAQBAJ&oi=fnd&pg=PP1&dq=inter-rater+reliability+coefficient&ots=UVgsdCzp7a&sig=cPf1-1kf2Zqjt5vqbRe-GdYP_oY#v=onepage&q=inter-rater%20reliability%20coefficient&f=false.

Hartman-Maeir, A., Harel, H., and Katz, N. (2009). Kettle test – a brief measure of cognitive functional performance: reliability and validity in stroke rehabilitation. *American Journal of Occupational Therapy* 63 (5): 592–599. https://doi.org/10.5014/ajot.63.5.592.

Harvill, L.M. (1991). Standard error of measurement. *Educational Measurement: Issues and Practice* 10 (2): 33–41. https://www.csus.edu/indiv/b/brocks/Courses/EDS%20245/Handouts/Standard%20Error%20of%20Measurement.ITEM.pdf.

Henson, R.K. (2001). Understanding internal consistency reliability estimates: a conceptual primer on coefficient alpha. *Measurement and Evaluation in Counseling and Development* 34 (3): 177–189. https://doi.org/10.1080/07481756.2002.12069034.

Krohne, K., Torres, S., Slettebø, Å., and Bergland, A. (2014). Everyday uses of standardized test information in a geriatric setting: a qualitative study exploring occupational therapist and physiotherapist test administrators' justifications. *BMC Health Services Research* 14 (1): 72. https://doi.org/10.1186/1472-6963-14-72.

Laver, A. J. (1994). *The development of the Structured Observational Test of Function (SOTOF)* (Doctoral dissertation, University of Surrey). https://ethos.bl.uk/OrderDetails.do?uin=uk.bl.ethos.259917

Laver, A.J. and Powell, G.E. (1995). *The Structured Observational Test of Function (SOTOF).* NFER Nelson.

Lim, C.R., Harris, K., Dawson, J. et al. (2015). Floor and ceiling effects in the OHS: an analysis of the NHS PROMs data set. *BMJ Open* 5 (7): e007765. https://doi.org/10.1136/bmjopen-2015-007765.

Matthey, S., Donnelly, S.M., and Hextell, D.L. (1993). The clinical usefulness of the Rivermead perceptual assessment battery: statistical considerations. *British Journal of Occupational Therapy* 56 (10): 365–370. https://doi.org/10.1177/030802269305601003.

McDowell, I. (2006). *Measuring Health: A Guide to Rating Scales and Questionnaires.* USA: Oxford University Press.

Moss, P.A. (1994). Can there be validity without reliability? *Educational Researcher* 23 (2): 5–12. https://doi.org/10.3102/0013189X023002005.

Moss, P.A. (2004). The meaning and consequences of "reliability". *Journal of Educational and Behavioral Statistics* 29 (2): 245–249. https://journals.sagepub.com/doi/pdf/10.3102/10769986029002245?casa_token=kTPr4fR9LOMAAAAA:bS-dOlSkDsjXLfzeunLBQn7vowmiAFj-6cVLIIxikIuTro8keEY48mVBlr0JUFRrtycln1WqgwU.

Mumby, K., Bowen, A., and Hesketh, A. (2007). Apraxia of speech: how reliable are speech and language therapists' diagnoses? *Clinical Rehabilitation* 21 (8): 760–767. https://doi.org/10.1177/0269215507077285.

Munro, B.H. (2005). *Statistical Methods for Health Care Research*, 5e, vol. 1. Lippincott Williams & Wilkins.

Opacich, K.J. (1991). Assessment and informed decision-making. In: *Occupational Therapy: Overcoming Human Performance Deficits* (eds. C. Christiansen and C.M. Baum), 354–372. McGraw-Hill Professional.

Paiva, C.E., Barroso, E.M., Carneseca, E.C. et al. (2014). A critical analysis of test-retest reliability in instrument validation studies of cancer patients under palliative care: a systematic review. *BMC Medical Research Methodology* 14 (1): 8. https://doi.org/10.1186/1471-2288-14-8.

van de Pol, R.J., van Trijffel, E., and Lucas, C. (2010). Inter-rater reliability for measurement of passive physiological range of motion of upper extremity joints is better if instruments are used: a systematic review. *Journal of Physiotherapy* 56 (1): 7–17. https://doi.org/10.1016/S1836-9553(10)70049-7.

Polit, D.F. (2014). Getting serious about test–retest reliability: a critique of retest research and some recommendations. *Quality of Life Research* 23: 1713–1720. https://doi.org/10.1007/s11136-014-0632-9.

Pynsent, P., Fairbank, J., and Carr, A. (2004). *Outcome Measures in Orthopaedics and Orthopaedic Trauma*. CRC Press.

Pynsent, P. (2004). Choosing an outcome measure. In: *Outcome Measures in Orthopaedics and Orthopaedic trauma*, 2e (eds. P. Pynsent, J. Fairbank and A. Carr), 1–7. London: Arnold.

Raju, N.S., Price, L.R., Oshima, T.C., and Nering, M.L. (2007). Standardized conditional SEM: a case for conditional reliability. *Applied Psychological Measurement* 31 (3): 169–180. https://doi.org/10.1177/0146621606291569.

Revicki, D. (2014). Internal consistency reliability. In: *Encyclopedia of Quality of Life and Well-Being Research* (ed. A.C. Michalos). Dordrecht https://doi.org/10.1007/978-94-007-0753-5_1494: Springer https://link.springer.com/referenceworkentry/10.1007%2F978-94-007-0753-5_1494.

Royeen, C.B. (ed.) (1989). *Clinical Research Handbook: An Analysis for the Service Professions*. Slack Incorporated.

Russell, D., Rosenbaum, P., Gowland, C. et al. (1993). *Gross Motor Function Measure Manual*, 1–23. Hamilton, ON: Neurodevelopmental Clinical Research Unit, McMaster University.

Salkind, N.J. (ed.) (2010). *Encyclopedia of Research Design*, vol. 1. Sage.

Saslow, C.A. (1982). *Basic Research Methods*. Addison Wesley Publishing Company.

Schober, P., Boer, C., and Schwarte, L.A. (2018). Correlation coefficients: appropriate use and interpretation. *Anesthesia & Analgesia* 126 (5): 1763–1768. https://doi.org/10.1213/ANE.0000000000002864.

Streiner, D.L. (2003). Starting at the beginning: an introduction to coefficient alpha and internal consistency. *Journal of Personality Assessment* 80 (1): 99–103. https://doi.org/10.1207/S15327752JPA8001_18.

Sullivan, G.M. and Feinn, R. (2012). Using effect size – or why the P value is not enough. *Journal of Graduate Medical Education* 4 (3): 279–282. https://doi.org/10.4300/JGME-D-12-00156.1.

Teyhen, D.S., Shaffer, S.W., Lorenson, C.L. et al. (2012). The functional movement screen: a reliability study. *Journal of Orthopaedic & Sports Physical Therapy* 42 (6): 530–540. https://doi.org/10.2519/jospt.2012.3838.

Thanasegaran, G. (2009). Reliability and validity issues in research. *Integration & Dissemination* 4: 35–40. https://pdfs.semanticscholar.org/9d59/0efc7d31e979ceeac73ad7472f3e4e4d3884.pdf.

Tooth, L.R. and Ottenbacher, K.J. (2004). The κ statistic in rehabilitation research: an examination. *Archives of Physical Medicine and Rehabilitation* 85 (8): 1371–1376. https://doi.org/10.1016/j.apmr.2003.12.002.

Trevethan, R. (2017). Sensitivity, specificity, and predictive values: foundations, pliabilities, and pitfalls in research and practice. *Frontiers in Public Health* 5: 307. https://doi.org/10.3389/fpubh.2017.00307.

Vaske, J.J., Beaman, J., and Sponarski, C.C. (2017). Rethinking internal consistency in Cronbach's alpha. *Leisure Sciences* 39 (2): 163–173. https://doi.org/10.1080/01490400.2015.1127189.

Whiting, S., Lincoln, N.B., Bhavnani, G., and Cockburn, J.E. (1985). *Rivermead Perceptual Assessment Battery*, 61. Windsor: NFER-NELSON.

Wright, J., Cross, J., and Lamb, S. (1998). Physiotherapy outcome measures for rehabilitation of elderly people: responsiveness to change of the Rivermead mobility index and Barthel index. *Physiotherapy* 84 (5): 216–221. https://doi.org/10.1016/S0031-9406(05)65552-6.

de Yébenes Prous, M.J.G., Salvanés, F.R., and Ortells, L.C. (2008). Responsiveness of outcome measures. *Reumatología Clínica* (English Edition) 4 (6): 240–247. https://doi.org/10.1016/S2173-5743(08)70197-7.

van der Zee, C.H., Kap, A., Mishre, R.R. et al. (2011). Responsiveness of four participation measures to changes during and after outpatient rehabilitation. *Journal of Rehabilitation Medicine* 43 (11): 1003–1009. https://doi.org/10.2340/16501977-0879.

Zhu, W., Ennis, C.D., and Chen, A. (1998). Many-faceted Rasch modeling expert judgment in test development. *Measurement in Physical Education and Exercise Science* 2 (1): 21–39. https://doi.org/10.1207/s15327841mpee0201_2.

CHAPTER 10

Selecting and Appraising Assessments and Outcome Measures

OVERVIEW

This chapter discusses ways of identifying, appraising, and selecting appropriate assessment and outcome measures for practice, service evaluation, or research. It describes the process for undertaking critical appraisal of underpinning evidence, psychometric studies, and measurement properties through test critique. A detailed critique of the Parenting Stress Index (PSI; Abidin 1995) is given as an example. Worksheets to guide you through undertaking test critique are provided at the end of the chapter.

QUESTIONS TO CONSIDER

1. How do I define what type of assessment or outcome measure is needed?
2. Where do I find information about assessments and outcome measures?
3. What do I need to consider when critically appraising an assessment or outcome measure?
4. How do I decide if an assessment or outcome measure is appropriate for my practice and/or research?

This chapter will help you to think about the questions to consider when identifying and appraising the evidence base underpinning assessments and outcome measures. The decision to use a particular assessment or outcome measure should be conscious and the result of informed evidence-based reasoning. There is a wide choice of standardised tests from which an allied health professional (AHP) can choose. AHPs often require a 'toolkit' of several assessments and measures to meet the needs of their clients and service, and we should not make high-stakes decisions on the basis of a single measure of the person's performance. It is critical that AHPs should select the most appropriate measures for their clients, and financial considerations often place limits upon the number that can be purchased for a service. Therefore, careful consideration needs to be given before purchasing. You should repeat your review of the evidence periodically (for example, every one to two years) as additional evidence related to the assessments and outcome measures used in your practice might be available, and more appropriate ones may have been published. Objective criteria should be used to make an informed choice. This can be a daunting task, so where do you start when trying to find the 'right' measure to evaluate the effectiveness of your interventions? This four step process helps to ensure rigorous decision making: preparing, finding, appraising, and selecting (see Figure 10.1).

The first step, 'Preparing to review assessments and measures and conceptual considerations' addresses the question 'How do I define what type of assessment or outcome measure is needed'. In this step, decisions regarding the purpose and use of the desired assessment or outcome measure are made, and these decisions then focus the search strategy in the next step, 'Finding potential assessments and outcome measures'. This second step addresses the question 'Where do I find information about assessments and outcome measures?'

Once you have identified pertinent sources of information (e.g. from colleagues, test manuals, journal articles), the next challenge can be the varying quality of test development and psychometric studies. Just because an assessment or outcome measure is published or in the public domain does not mean it is evidence based and without flaws. For example, in a systematic review of patient-reported outcome measures (PROMs) for people with voice disorders, Francis et al. (2017) reported several common deficiencies among 32 identified measures including: '(a) a lack of patient involvement in the item development process, (b) lack of robust construct validity, and (c) lack of clear interpretability and scaling' (p. 62).

Some challenges to a rigorous evidence base can be the following: information on an assessment's measurement properties is scarce; psychometric studies were conducted with small samples; and/or different studies report conflicting results. So, AHPs need to develop critical appraisal skills and become informed consumers of the

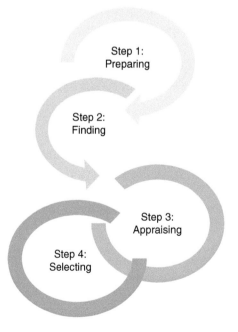

FIGURE 10.1   Process for choosing the most appropriate assessment or outcome measure.

psychometric research literature. The third step in the process involves drawing all available evidence together, appraising the evidence, and summarising this in a test critique. This step addresses the question 'What do I need to consider when critically appraising an assessment or outcome measure?' The fourth, and final, step addresses the question 'How do I decide if an assessment or outcome measure is appropriate for my practice and/or research?' The factors that need to be taken into consideration include those related to the client or research sample group, the AHPs or researchers who will be administering the assessment or measure, the quality of the underpinning evidence base, and the clinical or research setting.

STEP 1: PREPARING TO REVIEW ASSESSMENTS AND MEASURES AND CONCEPTUAL CONSIDERATIONS

How Do I Define What Type of Assessment or Outcome Measure Is Needed?

Two important aspects to consider at this stage are the construct to be measured (i.e. outcome or domain) and the client or research population (also called the target population; Prinsen et al. 2016). When thinking about the population, factors to identify can include the age group; diagnosis, disease characteristics, and symptoms; and ethnicity and culture. For some assessments, level of education is also a consideration.

Often the review and selection of new assessments and outcome measures is undertaken as a team. When working with others, it is important to 'agree on a standard set of data that should be collected and recorded routinely' (Royal College of Physicians 2012, section 3.11.1, p. 30).

It can be useful consider and discuss the following questions with colleagues to focus your search (Royal College of Occupational Therapists 2019):

1. What are the conditions and needs of your service users, and what aspects of their circumstances, functioning, and participation do you need to assess in detail?
2. What assessments are currently used in your local team or service?
   - Are they appropriate to the conditions and needs of your service user/s?
   - Are the assessments respected and their findings valued in care planning meetings and case conferences?
   - Is sufficient time allowed for administering them?
   - What aspects of functioning, participation, or symptoms do they measure?
   - Are they standardised?
   - Do staff receive training to keep up to date in using those assessments?
3. What resources are available to fund any licences and related materials (e.g. test sheets) for using the required assessment tools, and for staff training to use the tools correctly?
4. Will the assessment be recorded on paper and/or in a digital care record? Health and social are services are increasingly using digital care records and reducing their use of paper records. However, you may need to record the assessment data on paper and then again in the digital care record.

(p. 1)

STEP 2: FINDING POTENTIAL ASSESSMENTS AND OUTCOME MEASURES

Where Do I Find Information About Assessments and Outcome Measures?

There are a number of avenues you can explore to identify potential assessments and outcome measures for your service; these include:

- Accessing the expertise of colleagues.
- Using your local hospital, university, or professional association's library to search in journals and books.
- Searching the Internet as there are many useful websites on specific published measures and on assessment of different conditions. You can access online data bases to search for information about measures (some examples are listed at the end of this chapter in the resources section).
- Attending conferences, study days, workshops, and lectures related to assessment and measurement. If you cannot get the funding to attend, try to access the conference abstracts, many of which are published online; some conference/workshop providers sell the proceedings.
- Looking in catalogues produced by test publishers or visiting their stands if there is an exhibition at a conference or study day.
- Undertaking a literature search (e.g. journal articles, test critiques, reviews, textbooks, test manuals) on one or more of the health databases. Some professional organisations provide access to e-books and journals for members. Useful databases include the following:
  - EBSCO is a provider of research databases, e-journals, magazine subscriptions, e-books, and discovery service to many academic institutions, hospitals, schools, and public libraries. Further information can be found on their website at https://www.ebsco.com.
  - The Cumulative Index to Nursing and Allied Health Literature (*CINAHL*) databases provide a comprehensive database for nursing and allied health literature, and further details can be found on the website at https://www.ebscohost.com/nursing/products/cinahl-databases/cinahl-complete. CINAHL Complete 'provides broad content coverage including 50 nursing specialties, speech and language, pathology, nutrition, general health and medicine'. You may be able to access CINAHL databases through a hospital or university.
  - PubMed is a database that contains biomedical literature from MEDLINE, life science journals, and online books https://www.ncbi.nlm.nih.gov/pubmed.
  - Medline Plus at http://medlineplus.gov is a useful health information site aimed at service users.

The cheapest and easiest way to begin your search is by talking to other AHPs who are working with a similar client group; already using the assessment or outcome measure you are interested in; or leading conference presentations and workshops on aspects of assessment and measurement. You could contact colleagues through specialist interest groups, professional association newsletters, Internet discussion groups, and social media. Professional organisations often operate Specialist Sections, Special Interest Groups (*SIGs*), and AHP email discussion groups to discuss like-minded subjects or clinical areas.

Exploring the Literature for Examples of Tests and Test Critiques

If you are new to conducting a literature search, seek advice from a librarian (e.g. at your hospital or university or professional association's library) or from a colleague who is familiar with searching the literature. Grewal et al. (2016) provide a succinct article on literature search. For readers unfamiliar with appraising articles, this short two-page handout 'Reading Tips for the Clinician: How to Tell Whether an Article Is Worth Reading' (Walker 2002) provides a useful starting point.

Finding journal articles describing outcome measures and their application can be a challenge, because some relevant articles do not mention the specific outcome measure in the article's title, abstract, or key words; which then results in the article not being identified by a key word in the database literature search. So, when searching you may need to use a variety of key words and we recommend searching abstracts as well as titles and, if information is still not being identified, try searching full text.

Some critiques already exist in the form of published reviews in books and journal articles. For example, Asher (2014) provides an annotated index of many standardised and published occupational therapy assessments. Finch et al. (2002) provide detailed test critiques for over 70 measures.

Example Reviews and Critiques in Journal Articles

There are many good systematic reviews and overview articles exploring research on different tests and test critiques in the therapy literature. You can focus your search for assessments by specific profession (e.g. podiatrist assessments); client group (e.g. paediatric measures for children aged 0–10 years); condition (e.g. stroke); symptom (e.g. pain); part of the body (e.g. shoulder); or for use in a particular setting (e.g. patient's home, inpatient). Systematic reviews are useful for selecting measures for research or clinical practice and for identifying gaps in knowledge on the quality of outcome measurement instruments. The Consensus-based Standards for the selection of health Measurement Instruments (*COSMIN*) website (available at: https://www.cosmin.nl) has a collection of systematic reviews of outcome measurement instruments, and reviews are available in a searchable database which contains over 900 reviews. There is also a downloadable manual (Mokkink et al. 2018) for the *COSMIN database of systematic reviews of outcome measurement instruments*, which explains:

1. The scope and content of the COSMIN database
2. How to search the COSMIN database
3. How to save your records of interest and your search strategies

You can limit your searches by level of health, characteristics of the population, and type outcome measurement instrument. The following studies give a range of examples of the type of literature that can prove useful. Van der Leeden et al. (2008) undertook a systematic review of instruments measuring foot function, foot pain, and foot-related disability in patients with rheumatoid arthritis.

O'Connor et al. (2016) identified 88 potential assessments used by AHPs for children with cerebral palsy (CP). In their article, they provide several useful tables, including a summary table that lists 23 assessments under the following categories: domains assessed, standardised procedures available, type of tool, primary purpose of tool, age range for tool administration, acceptable validity for use in the CP population, and International Classification of Functioning, Disability and Health (ICF) domain focus. They found that the most frequently used, well-evidenced assessments focused on gross motor function and they concluded that 'use of evidence-based assessment tools for children with cerebral palsy does not appear aligned with best practice in many settings' (p. 333).

Denman et al. (2017), in a systematic review titled 'Psychometric Properties of Language Assessments for Children Aged 4–12 Years', included the appraisal of 15 comprehensive language tests and presented information related to their underpinning evidence base. Four of the 15 assessments were found to have the strongest evidence of psychometric properties and were recommended for use. Desai et al. (2010) undertook a literature search, review, and critical appraisal of five subjective PROMs used in the assessment of shoulder disability. They considered the evidence for the test development, construct validity, internal consistency, reliability, responsiveness, and the clinical application of each measure, rating the evidence as Good, Fair, or Poor. Hasenstein et al. (2017) considered podiatry clinical outcome measures reported in the research literature over a five-year period in two journals. Their review identified 37 clinical outcome scales, and they reported that the most frequently used measures were 'the American Orthopaedic Foot and Ankle Society scales (54.3%; n = 82), Visual Analogue Scale (35.8%; n = 54), Medical Outcomes Study Short Form Health Survey (any version) (10.6%; n = 16), Foot Function Index (5.3%; n = 8), Maryland Foot Score (4.0%; n = 6), and Olerud and Molander Scoring System (4.0%; n = 6)'.

Another good place to search for possible measures is test publisher's catalogues. The disadvantage of this avenue is that there will almost certainly be some sort of charge for the measures listed. However, if you have some budget available to purchase standardised tests for your service, there are some worthwhile measures available. Test publishers often provide a global statement of the focus of their assessments. Jeffrey (1993) grouped these in to three main categories:

1. Disorder-specific clinical or functional outcomes measures
2. Functional outcome measures suitable for people with a variety of disorders/diagnoses
3. Comprehensive functional measures.

Some publishers specifically deal with tests suitable for AHPs. Helpful catalogues also group tests according to age range (paediatric, adult, older adult), conditions (e.g. mental health, Autistic Spectrum Disorders), and/or domains (e.g. motor, cognitive, sensory, perceptual, behaviour, work placement). You will usually find a brief overview of the test and some summary information. This helps you identify whether you and/or your staff will be qualified to administer the test, whether it may be designed for your client group, how long it should take to administer, whether it comes with standardised equipment, and how much it will cost. The information about qualifications is particularly important as you do not want to waste time purchasing a test that you or your staff are not competent to use and you need to budget in advance for any additional training costs (and/or ongoing purchases for additional packs of record forms). Most catalogues will contain a statement about the general and/or specific qualifications required for test administration; for example, see the 'Qualifications Policy' for the test publisher Pearson (which have a range of clinical assessments, particularly for use by AHPs and psychologists): https://www.pearson-assessments.com/professional-assessments/ordering/how-to-order/qualifications/qualifications-policy.html.

Some publishers list the professions qualified to use the test in their summaries; for example, Thames Valley Test Co has been dissolved so we've adapted sentence 'medical doctor, occupational therapist, physiotherapist' for practitioners wanting to use the Rivermead Assessment of Somatosensory Performance (*RASP*; Winward et al. 2002). Some test publishers require purchasers to register with them before they can buy test materials and allocate a qualification code for different professional groups (see https://www.pearsonclinical.co.uk/AlliedHealth/Allied Health.aspx?utm_source=pearsoncomah&utm_medium=referral&utm_campaign= GBCASP0919COMCO&utm_content=ahassess). When looking for potential tests in catalogues, check for the qualification code first. If a test sounds relevant but has a different code, then contact the publisher and ask for the qualification requirements and opportunities for specific training that would facilitate use of the test. A few publishers/test developers insist that AHPs should attend an approved training course before they can use a specific test.

Catalogue summaries can be a useful starting point, but as tests are often expensive, it is usually worth looking at the test materials before you commit to purchasing them. You can either borrow a test from another service you know is using it, request a review copy from the publisher, or ask if you can order the test on a sale or return basis. Some publishers will provide talks and demonstrations by representatives coming out to your service, as well as providing sample test materials on loan for a trial basis. Other publishers run training events on a specific test or groups of tests.

STEP 3: CRITICAL APPRAISAL OF ASSESSMENT AND OUTCOME MEASURES (TEST CRITIQUE)

When reviewing potential assessments for practice or research, AHPs should examine the original work on the development of the measure and additional psychometric studies, and consider the following aspects: purpose, standardisation, validity, reliability, level of measurement, face validity, and clinical utility. If it is to be used as an outcome measure, then sensitivity to the desired outcome also is important to consider (Jeffrey 1993). Some assessments have been used and evaluated by other authors, and additional useful information may be found in journal articles that describe further exploration of the psychometric properties of a measure or its use with other client populations or cultures. Be aware that a translation of an original test version will not guarantee similar measurement properties (Schellingerhout et al. 2011), so you must critically appraise the quality of the translation process, cross-cultural validation, and the measurement properties of the translated test version you are reviewing. AHPs are likely to experience some challenges in finding a perfect battery of standardised measures for their client group. The robustness of the psychometric properties of a test (such as its validity, reliability, and responsiveness to change) need to be carefully weighed against the pragmatics of your clinical environment and reviewed in terms of face validity and clinical utility factors. This balancing of the scientific versus the practical factors is best undertaken through a formal process known as *test critique*. A number of structured checklists are provided by therapy authors for undertaking test critiques. For example, the 'Outcome Measures Rating Form Guidelines' (Law 2001) followed the headings Focus, Clinical Utility, Scale Construction, Standardisation, Reliability, Validity, Overall Utility, and Materials Used. Detailed descriptions are provided for rating each of these areas.

If specific information is not available for the measure you are reviewing (e.g. for use with a specific population or setting), then you might search for, and consider, indirect evidence. For example, Terwee et al. (2018) provide the example of reviewing an assessment for use with patients with osteoarthritis to assess the hand and only finding psychometric studies conducted with people with other types of upper extremity problems. They comment that this indirect evidence could be considered, but 'will be weighted less than direct evidence obtained in the population of interest' (p. 9).

Why Are Written Test Critiques Useful?

Test Critique

A critical review and discussion about a test. Usually describes the purpose, format, content, psychometric properties and strengths, and limitations of the test.

When reviewing a potential test, we strongly advise you make a written summary of your review in the form of a test critique (for example, using the Worksheet Templates 10.1 or 10.2 at the end of this chapter). Undertaking a written test critique may seem time consuming, but it can be useful for a number of reasons:

1. It helps you to review the test in a systematic manner and look for all the salient information that you need to make an informed decision as to whether this test will be useful in your practice/service.
2. It will help you to reflect on the evidence upon which the test is based and articulate your rationale for selecting or rejecting the test.
3. If you work in a multidisciplinary team, you may need to 'sell' the use of this measure to your colleagues, and providing a written summary of the test can strengthen your case for implementation.
4. A copy of the test critique can be placed in your Continuing Professional Development (*CPD*) portfolio as evidence of new learning, both learning about a new assessment and also as evidence for developing the skill of critiquing tests.
5. As tests are expensive, you may need to make a case to the budget holder for funding to purchase. If you need more than one copy of a test or there is expensive training involved, you may need to make a detailed business case.
6. If you leave the service, a copy of your critique can be archived in your service's records so that any future AHPs can see the evidence for the measures they are inheriting.

When appraising the evidence base, you should search for and review the evidence for the test's measurement properties; a 'measurement property is a quality aspect of an instrument, i.e. reliability, validity and responsiveness. Each measurement property requires its own type of study to assess it' (COSMIN; https://www.cosmin.nl/tools/cosmin-taxonomy-measurement-properties). The psychometric studies which should have been undertaken will depend upon the test's purpose and the proposed use of the scores obtained. Figure 10.2 provides a reminder of the key areas to

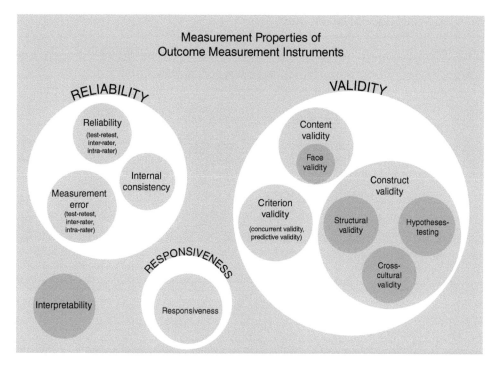

FIGURE 10.2   Measurement properties of outcome measurement Instruments. *Source*: https://www.cosmin.nl/tools/cosmin-taxonomy-measurement-properties/

consider when appraising an assessment's measurement properties; refer back to Chapters 8 and 9 for more specific details.

If you cannot find a useful critique of the test you are interested in already undertaken by another AHP and/or published in the literature, then the series of questions in Table 10.1 will guide you in this process. A comprehensive test critique should involve the examination of many factors, and Table 10.1 provides details of key elements of a test critique and things to think about when undertaking an appraisal.

As a reminder, Table 10.2 provides the COSMIN (Mokkink et al. 2010) definitions of domains, measurement properties, and aspects of measurement properties. For further details related to psychometrics, refer to Chapters 8 and 9.

Table 10.3 details the quality rating and criteria when you are considering the quality of the evidence for an outcome measure, based on the Grades of Recommendation, Assessment, Development, and Evaluation (GRADE 2004) Working Group level of evidence approach, which specifies four categories: high, moderate, low, and very low (Balshem et al. 2011); and the COSMIN checklists (Denman et al. 2017, p. 9; Mokkink et al. 2010; Prinsen et al. 2016, p. 8; Schellingerhout et al. 2011).

Table 10.4 provides an example of a detailed critique of one index, the PSI (Abidin 1995). The catalogue provided the following information on the PSI:

- Overview: Recognise stressful areas in parent–child interactions
- Age range: adult
- Qualification code: CL2
- Administration: individual, 20–30 minutes; short form 10 minutes.

TABLE 10.1   Aspects of test critique.

Appraisal area	Questions and aspects to consider in your appraisal
Purpose	• What is the stated purpose of the test? • Is there information about why and how the measure was developed? • Has it been designed as a descriptive, evaluative, discriminative, and/or predictive measure? *Consider:* Think about the purpose of the test and ways in which it can be used. What do the authors say it was developed for? McDowell (2006) noted that a measure's purpose is not always clearly stated, and it can also be restated slightly differently in different publications. See Chapter 3.
Population	• For what population has the test been designed? Is there a clear description provided of the target population for which the test was developed? • Was the test development study undertaken with a sample representing the target population for which the test was developed? *Consider:* Is it designed for a specific group of people (e.g. with a specified diagnosis; or of a particular age group) or is it a generic assessment/measure? How does the population the test was developed for compare with your clinical population or research sample?
Data collection method	• How is data/information collected? *Consider:* Is the information collected through one method (e.g. self-administered, observation, interview, online survey, pen and paper survey, card sort, app, selecting items on a touch screen) or via multiple methods. Is the method(s) suitable for your client group? For example, if it is self-administered, is the readability appropriate for the age and ability of your clients? See Chapter 2.
Perspective gained	• Whose perspective is the data/information based on? *Consider:* Does the assessment or measure obtain the person's perspective through self-report or the perspective of others through proxy report (e.g. from a carer, parent, teacher, or staff member involved in the person's treatment or care) and/or involve the clinician's judgement (e.g. following observations)? See Chapter 2.
Intended application	• How is the assessment/measure designed to be applied? *Consider:* was it developed for use in clinical practice and/or research; and/or as comprehensive, detailed assessment or a screening tool?
Environment	• Where was the assessment/measure designed to be used? • Is there a clear description provided for the context where the test is to be used? *Consider:* In what environments and settings can the test be administered?
Materials and equipment required	• What equipment, materials, and consumables will be required? *Consider:* Are these easy to obtain? How much do these cost to purchase?

TABLE 10.1 (Continued)

Appraisal area	Questions and aspects to consider in your appraisal
Content	• What domains are covered? What types of items are there? *Consider:* Do the domains cover all theoretical constructs of interest for your clinical or research population? Do the domains cover all the observable behaviours you wish to measure in your clinical or research population? Are there any gaps between what domains are covered by the assessment and the domains you need or want to assess?
Levels of function	• What levels of function are assessed/measured? (for example: body function and structure, activities, participation, environmental factors) *Consider:* Are there any gaps between what levels of function and functional test items are covered by the assessment and the person's function you need to assess? See Chapter 11.
Level of measurement and scoring method	• What scoring system is used and what level of measurement is provided by this scoring system? *Consider:* Does the measure provide data at a nominal, ordinal, interval, or ratio level? Are different test items measured using a variety of formats resulting in more than one level of measurement being used? Are the scores easy to score, analyse, and interpret? See Chapter 4.
Adequacy of standardisation	• Is the test standardised? • Is it a norm-referenced or a criterion-referenced test? • What criteria are used if it is a criterion-referenced measure? • Is there an adequate description of norms if it is a normative test? *Consider:* Does the test have a manual with clear instructions for administering and scoring? If it is a norm-reference test, is the normative sample representative of the clients with whom you will use the test? See Chapter 7.
Validity	• Is there a clear description provided of the construct or content to be measured? • Is the origin of the construct clear: was a theory, conceptual framework, or disease model used or a clear rationale provided to define the construct to be measured? • Is it clear that all the assessment's content (e.g. items, tasks, observations, parameters) is relevant, comprehensive, and comprehensible with respect to the construct of interest and the target population' (COSMIN 2019)? • Has validity been established? What evidence is there about its validity with your client population? *Consider:* Depending on the purpose and content of the assessment, different types of validity may be relevant to consider, which can include: content, concurrent, convergent, construct, predictive, and criterion. See Chapter 8.

(Continued)

TABLE 10.1   (Continued)

Appraisal area	Questions and aspects to consider in your appraisal
Face validity	• Does the test look like it tests what it says it tests from the perspective of the person undertaking the test, their family, or informal carers, and other people involved in the person's rehabilitation and management? • How acceptable is it for your clients or research participants? *Consider:* Have the opinions of people similar to your clinical or research participant group be sought regarding their experiences of undertaking the assessment and what they believe is its purpose? See Chapter 8.
Reliability	• Does the test have acceptable levels of reliability? What evidence is there about its reliability with your client population? *Consider:* How accurately do scores reflect a true performance of the individual? Is the test stable across time and raters? See Chapter 9.
Responsiveness, specificity, and sensitivity	• Is there information about how responsive the measure is to meaningful clinical change? *Consider:* Is the test responsive to the amount of change likely to be achieved through the clinical or research interventions to be delivered? See Chapter 9.
Clinical utility and feasibility	• Does the test have good clinical utility? • How feasible is it for use in clinical practice? *Consider:* Time required for administration and scoring; and ease of administration and scoring. See Chapter 8.
Qualifications needed for administration and training issues	• What qualifications are needed by the test administrator and is additional training required to administer the test? *Consider:* Some tests take time to learn to administer and score; some may only be administered by an AHP with particular credentials.
Cost and accessibility	• How do you obtain a copy? • What does it cost? • What are the copyright requirements for use and distribution? *Consider:* Cost to purchase the test, test materials, or consumables (e.g. food for a kitchen assessment), and/or cost for training to learn to administer the test need to be considered. Does the test require specific equipment and materials that are costly, technical, or difficult to transport?
References for test and related evidence base	You might put the full reference for a test manual or a journal article describing the test here or a link to a summary article, critique by other authors, or a website that lists related publications. For example, a link to Aus-TOMs related publications for the underpinning evidence base available from: https://austoms.files.wordpress.com/2018/03/austoms-ot-publications.pdf

TABLE 10.1   (Continued)

Appraisal area	Questions and aspects to consider in your appraisal
Website and further resources	Some assessments/measures have useful websites, for example https://austoms.com/about
Strengths and limitations	Summarise your findings into a list of strengths and weaknesses in order to facilitate a comparison of possible options and help you decide upon your final choice of what test to use for your service or specific client.

TABLE 10.2   Definitions of domains, measurement properties, and aspects of measurement properties.

Term

Domain	Measurement property	Aspect of a measurement property	Definition
Reliability			The degree to which the measurement is free from measurement error
Reliability (extended definition)			The extent to which scores for patients who have not changed are the same for repeated measurement under several conditions: e.g. using different sets of items from the same Health Related-Patient Reported Outcomes (HR-PRO) (internal consistency); over time (test–retest); by different persons on the same occasion (inter-rater); or by the same persons (i.e. raters or responders) on different occasions (intra-rater)
	Internal consistency		The degree of interrelatedness among the items
	Reliability		The proportion of the total variance in the measurements which is due to 'true'^{a} differences between patients
	Measurement error		The systematic and random error of a patient's score that is not attributed to true changes in the construct to be measured
Validity			The degree to which an HR-PRO instrument measures the construct(s) it purports to measure

(Continued)

TABLE 10.2   (Continued)

Term			
Domain	Measurement property	Aspect of a measurement property	Definition
		Content validity	The degree to which the content of an HR-PRO instrument is an adequate reflection of the construct to be measured
		Face validity	The degree to which (the items of) an HR-PRO instrument indeed looks as though they are an adequate reflection of the construct to be measured
	Construct validity		The degree to which the scores of an HR-PRO instrument are consistent with hypotheses (for instance, with regard to internal relationships, relationships to scores of other instruments, or differences between relevant groups) based on the assumption that the HR-PRO instrument validly measures the construct to be measured
		Structural validity	The degree to which the scores of an HR-PRO instrument are an adequate reflection of the dimensionality of the construct to be measured
		Hypotheses testing	Idem construct validity
		Cross-cultural validity	The degree to which the performance of the items on a translated or culturally adapted HR-PRO instrument are an adequate reflection of the performance of the items of the original version of the HR-PRO instrument
	Criterion validity		The degree to which the scores of an HR-PRO instrument are an adequate reflection of a 'gold standard'
Responsiveness			The ability of an HR-PRO instrument to detect change over time in the construct to be measured
	Responsiveness		Idem responsiveness

TABLE 10.2   (Continued)

Term			
Domain	Measurement property	Aspect of a measurement property	Definition
Interpretability[b]			Interpretability is the degree to which once can assign qualitative meaning – that is, clinical or commonly understood connotations – to an instrument's quantitative scores or change in scores

[a] The word 'true' must be seen in the context of classical test theory (CTT), which states that any observation is composed of two components: a true score and an error associated with the observation. 'True' is the average score that would be obtained if the scale were applied an infinite number of times. It refers only to the consistency of the score, and not to its accuracy.

[b] Interpretability is not considered a measurement property, but an important characteristic of a measurement instrument.

Source: Mokkink et al. (2010). © 2010, Elsevier

TABLE 10.3   Rating the quality of evidence.

Quality rating	Rating code	Criteria
High	++++ (four plus)	Consistent findings in multiple studies of at least good quality OR one study of excellent quality AND a total sample size of ≥70 people
Moderate	+++ (three plus)	Conflicting findings in multiple studies of at least good quality OR consistent findings in multiple studies of at least fair quality OR one study of good quality AND a total sample size of ≥50 people
Low	++ (two plus)	Conflicting findings in multiple studies of at least fair quality OR one study of fair quality AND a total sample size of ≥30 people
Very low	+ (one plus)	Only studies of poor quality OR a total sample size of <30 people
Conflicting evidence	± (one plus over one negative)	Conflicting findings across different studies (i.e. different studies with positive and negative findings)
Unknown	?	No studies found
Not evaluated	NE	Evidence not sought and appraised

Sources: Balshem et al. (2011); Denman et al. (2017); Mokkink et al. (2010).

TABLE 10.4   Test critique example: critique of the Parenting Stress Index (PSI) undertaken by Alison Laver-Fawcett (ALF).

Critique Area	Comments
Name of test, **authors**, and **date of publication**	Parenting Stress Index (PSI). Reference: Abidin (1995).
Publisher: Where to obtain test. Cost (if any)	UK distributor Harcourt Assessment. Complete kit (includes manual, 10 reusable item booklets, 25 hand-scored answer/profile forms) (Note: ALF reviewed the full test version). Updated cost details (March 2021) The Parenting Stress Index, Fourth Edition Short Form (PSI-4-SF) PSI-4 Short Form Kit (includes PSI-4 Professional Manual and 25 Short Form Record/Profile Forms $192.00. Source: Psychological Assessment Resources Inc. Available from: Parenting Stress Index, Fourth Edition Short Form | PSI-4-SF (parinc.com)
Population: For what population has the test been designed	Adults: Parents of children aged 1 month to 12 years. References are provided for research using the PSI with a wide range of child populations including those with birth defects (e.g. spina bifida, congenital heart disease), communication disorders (e.g. hearing impairment, speech deficits), attention deficit hyperactivity disorder (ADHD), autism, developmental disability, learning disability, premature infants, at-risk/abused children, and other health problems (such as asthma, diabetes, and otitis media). Originally developed in the United States with norms mainly based on a white American population, the PSI has since been used in a number of cross-cultural studies and has been translated into Spanish, Chinese, Portuguese, Finnish, Japanese, Italian, Hebrew, Dutch, and French.
Purpose(s) of test: Stated purpose and uses	The manual states that the 'PSI was designed to be an instrument in which the primary value would be to identify parent–child systems that were under stress and at risk for the development of dysfunctional parenting behaviour or behaviour problems in the child involved' (Abidin 1995, p. 6). Uses: The author describes the PSI as a screening and diagnostic tool, so the primary purpose is to provide descriptive information. Predictive validity studies (see below) allow for some predictive assessment uses. Several studies are summarised in the manual which have found the PSI to discriminate between different groups of children and of parents. Some of the test–retest reliability data shows acceptable levels, thus allowing for the full PSI to be used as an outcome measure for evaluative purposes, but coefficients varied considerably across four studies, and careful attention should be paid to the length of the period between baseline testing and the follow-up evaluative test. However, the short form (PSI/SF) can be used as an evaluative measure with more confidence.
Data collection method(s) used	Self-report tool. The parent is given a seven-page reusable item booklet containing a front sheet with scoring instructions and 120 questions. The parent is given a separate answer sheet/profile form. The parent circles his/her answer for each of the 101 PSI items and on the 19 item Life Stresses scale if required. The AHP then tears off the perforated edge and opens up the form. Inside answers are transformed to numerical scores which are summed and then plotted on the profile.

TABLE 10.4   (Continued)

Critique Area	Comments
Level(s) of function addressed by test	Reflecting on the National Center for Medical Rehabilitation Research (NCMRR) model of levels of function/dysfunction, we think that most of the sub-scales address the societal limitation level because they address interactions between humans in their environment through exploration of the child–parent system, the parent–spouse system, and the parent–social environment context. The test looks at domains such as Role Restriction and Isolation, which clearly fall within the level of societal limitation. The PSI has two sub-scales that provide data at the impairment level: the Child Domain of 'Mood' and the Parent Domain of 'Depression'. The Parent sub-scale of 'Health' covers the concept of health in a very broad way and might capture health problems at several levels, including the pathophysiology level.
Testing environments where test can be used:	PSI can be used as a clinical and/or research tool. References provided for research where the PSI has been applied in a range of settings including: well-child clinics/well-care paediatrics clinic; private paediatric group; parenting clinic for consultation on child behaviour; early parenting groups for mothers abusing drugs and/or alcohol; preschool training project; and parenting skills programme
Scoring method and levels of measurement:	For most items, an ordinal scale is used. The majority of items are scored on a 5-point Likert type scale: strongly agree; agree; not sure; disagree; and strongly disagree. Some items use a 4-point or 5-point scale with specific choices for that question, for example, 'I feel that I am: 1. a very good parent; 2. a better than average parent; 3. an average parent; 4. a person who has some trouble being a parent; 5. not very good at being a parent'. The Life Stresses scale uses a dichotomous nominal 2-point 'yes' or 'no' scale to rate whether any of the 19 listed events have occurred in the person's immediate family in the last 12 months (e.g. marriage, pregnancy, legal problems, began new job, death of immediate family member).
Qualifications needed to administer the test and additional training requirements/ costs:	Catalogue lists as 'CL2'. Manual states that non-graduates can administer the PSI, but examiners of scores and interpretation of PSI scores should be undertaken by people with 'graduate training in clinical counselling or educational psychology or in social work or related fields' (Abidin 1995, p. 3).
Standardisation: Is it standardised? Test development details	Yes, the test has been standardised and comprises a standardised item booklet and answer sheet. I (ALF) reviewed the 3rd edition. Earlier editions were published in 1983 and 1990. Test development began in 1976. Content was based on a literature review of research in psychology and psychiatry into stressors linked to dysfunctional parenting. Out of the original 150 test items, 95 were related to at least one research study. Initial test development took place at the University of Virginia over three years during which the PSI was piloted on a group of 208 mothers of children under three years in a parenting clinic linked to a group of paediatricians in Virginia. Test went through several revisions. Factor analyses were conducted on PSI items, and the final version of 101 items finalised.

(Continued)

TABLE 10.4   (Continued)

Critique Area	Comments
Is it a **normative-or criterion-referenced** test? Details of criteria or norms:	The PSI is a normative assessment. Original norms based on 2633 mothers (age 16–61 years, mean age 30.9) of children aged 1 month to 12 years (mean 4.9 years; SD 3.1) and comprising 76% white, 11% African American, 10% Hispanic, and 2% Asian women. The sample was drawn from several US states (Virginia, Massachusetts, New York City, North Carolina, and Wisconsin) and from a range of settings: well-child-care paediatric clinics, public school day centres, health maintenance programme, private and public paediatric clinics, and public schools. Opportunistic sample (not random or stratified). Normative data was also presented for 200 fathers aged 18–65 years (mean age 32.1 years) comprising 95% white and 5% African American men. The manual reports that 'the data from this sample would suggest that fathers earn lower stress scores on many PSI scales when compared to mothers' (Abidin 1995, p. 25). In the manual, norms are also presented for a sample of 223 Hispanic parents. References are given for cross-cultural studies for populations of Bermudan, Chinese, French Canadian, Hispanic, Irish, Israeli, Italian, Japanese, and Portuguese parents. Percentile scores can be calculated for all PSI sub-scales, the Child Domain and the Parent Domain, and the Total Stress Score.
Reliability data:	The PSI Manual provides details of studies to evaluate the internal consistency and test–retest reliability of the PSI. Data is variable and details of studies brief, making it difficult to draw firm conclusions about the reliability of the PSI and its use as an outcome measure. *Test–retest reliability:* The PSI Manual provides brief summaries of four test–retest reliability studies. It is difficult to draw firm conclusions from the data, and there was considerable variation across studies, both in terms of the period between the initial and post-test administrations and in the retest reliability data obtained from each study. Accepted values for test–retest reliability are coefficients of 0.70 or above (Benson and Clark 1982; Laver-Fawcett 2002; Opacich 1991). *Parent Domain* scores are consistent across three of the four studies and fall just at an acceptable level: 0.69 (Zakreski 1983, n = 54 parents, retest period over 3 months), 0.70 (Hamilton 1980, n = 37 mothers, retest period 1 year), 0.71 (Burke 1978, n = 15 mothers, retest period 3 weeks), with a much higher value of 0.91 reported by Abidin (1995, n = 30 mothers retest periods 1–3 months). Across the four studies, concerning variability was found for the test–retest reliability of the *Child Domain* which ranged from 0.55 Hamilton (1980) and 0.63 (Abidin 1995), which would be perceived as unacceptably low levels of reliability, to 0.77 (Zakreski 1983) and 0.82 (Burke 1978), which are acceptable. Test–retest reliability data for the *Total Stress Scoring* was provided from three studies and ranged from 0.65 (Hamilton 1980), which is slightly lower than acceptable levels, to 0.88 (Zakreski 1983) to 0.96 (Abidin 1995), which is a highly acceptable reliability level. Given the nature of the construct being studied, one would expect some changes to occur, especially over longer periods, so I would suggest that an AHP should consider the time intervals for reassessment required to measure outcomes and look at the data for the study that used the most comparable retest period. Test–retest reliability data for the PSI short form from two studies produced acceptable levels of reliability. *Internal consistency:*

TABLE 10.4   (Continued)

Critique Area	Comments
	A table is given showing coefficient alpha calculations for the Child Domain, Parent Domain, Total Stress Score, and all sub-scales calculated from the normative sample data (n = 2633 and from a study by Hauenstein et al. (1987) using a sample of 435. Accepted values for internal consistency are 0.80 or above (Benson and Clark 1982; Laver-Fawcett 2002; Opacich 1991). Coefficients from the normative sample ranged from 0.70 to 0.83 for the Child sub-scales and 0.90 for the *Child Domain* (47 items) and 0.70 to 0.84 for the Parent sub-scales, 0.93 for the *Parent Domain* (54 items), and 0.95 for the *Total Stress Score* (101 items). Abidin (1995) reports that Hauenstein and colleagues obtained similar values, and their data ranges from 0.57 for the Health sub-scale to 0.95 for the Total Stress Score.
Validity data:	Yes, various validity studies have been undertaken by the test developer and other researchers, and summaries and references are given in the manual.
	Content validity: Content was initially based on a literature review. A panel of six professionals rated each item for relevance of content and adequacy of construction. A reference (Burke 1978) is cited for more details of the initial content validation process. Factor analytic studies are reported, and Abidin (1995) reports that data 'supports the notion that each subscale is measuring a moderately distinct source of stress' (p. 32).
	Concurrent validity: Extensive research has been undertaken by different researchers. In Appendix C, the manual lists references for research providing PSI correlations with 92 different measures including the Bayley Scales of Infant Development (3 studies, e.g. Hanson and Hanline 1990); Beck Depression Inventory (9 studies, e.g. Donenberg and Baker 1993); Child Behaviour Checklist (18 studies, e.g. Kazdin 1990); and the Peabody Picture Vocabulary Test – revised (2 studies, e.g. Wilfong et al. 1991).
	Predictive validity: The manual provides details of a predictive validity study that 'examined the relationship of PSI scores to children's subsequent behavioural adjustment in a sample of 100 White, middle-class mothers with children between 6 and 12 months at the time of the initial testing with the families. They were followed up 4 ½ years later' (Abidin 1995, p. 37). The manual reports that the PSI 'Life stress, Child Domain, and the Parent Domain PSI scores were significant predictors of subsequent child functioning in relation to conduct disorders, social aggression, attention problems, and anxiety withdrawal' Abidin 1995, p. 38).
	Discriminative validity: References are given for studies using the PSI with a variety of clinical populations. For example, Moran et al. (1992) found that the PSI discriminated between children with developmental delay and normally developing children, and Cameron and Orr (1989) found that the PSI discriminated between children with delayed mental development and the normative sample. LaFiosca (1981) reported 'that the PSI was able to identify correctly 100% of the parents of normal children and 60% of the parents of the children who were seen at a child development clinic, when the 90th percentile of the PSI Total Stress Score was used as a cut-off. Further, significant mean differences were found for the Total Stress Score, the Child and parent Domain scores, and for the majority of subscales' (Abidin 1995, p. 38).

(Continued)

TABLE 10.4   (Continued)

Critique Area	Comments
Clinical utility (ease of use and scoring, portability, cost, training issues, settings, etc.)	The test can be used with a wide range of child–parent populations and can be administered during a clinic appointment or given to the parent to take home and complete independently. It could be used for inpatient, outpatient, and community-based practice settings. The PSI Manual is laid out in a logical way, and it was easy to find the information I wanted when I needed it. The main text is well referenced and fairly easy to read. There are additional numbered references in the Appendix and useful lists of 'PSI correlations with other measures' and for uses of 'PSI in research with special populations' which are cross-referenced to the numbered references. The manual reports that the PSI takes approximately 20 minutes to complete. It took my husband, the mother who tried the PSI for my critique, and I less time, at about 15 minutes each. The three of us found it straightforward to complete and easy to understand. The test accounts for Defensive responding, and the AHP can easily calculate a defensive responding score for the Parent Domain and interpret the data accordingly. The test allows for a small amount of missing data, and a formula is given for calculating sub-scale and domain scores if data is omitted. The AHP conversion of raw scores to sub-scale, domain, total stress, and percentile scores coring was quite easy to do, and it took me about 15 minutes to sum the scores in each sub-scale and domain, calculate the total score, and plot scores on the profile to transform raw scores into percentiles. It took only another minute to look up the age-based norms in the Appendix. The amount of time required for interpretation will depend on the complexity of the results and the therapist's familiarity with the PSI and manual. Chapter 3 'Interpretation and Interventions' of the PSI manual provides helpful summarises related to each sub-scale and domain with guidance as to what percentile levels would indicate a need for further intervention/referral and with ideas for intervention approaches. As the scoring of responses is done on a separate form to the PSI item question booklet, the person completing it needs to carefully track the correspondence between the item numbers on the answer form and on the item booklet; as most items are scored using the same scale (SA, A, NS, D, SD), it is quite easy to miss one out and continue going down the score sheet, and it is only when the parent reaches a question with a different scoring format that he/she will realise that the item they are scoring on the answer sheet does not correspond with the item question in the booklet. The introductory kit (www.hogrefe.co.uk) is £240. AHPs in a team/department could share one manual, and there are 10 reusable item booklets enabling 10 parents to be assessed simultaneously. No additional training is required, and we would suggest that an AHP should allow at least 1 hour to familiarise themselves with the manual and another hour to complete the PSI themself (or have a colleague, family member, friend complete an answer form) and score and interpret a practice set of data prior to using the test with clients.

TABLE 10.4   (Continued)

Critique Area	Comments
Face validity (for AHPs, service user, others receiving results)	I felt the PSI had good face validity, both as an AHP administering, scoring, and interpreting the test and as a mother of two young children completing the PSI. I felt the questions were relevant to me as a mother. As an AHP, there was a clear theoretical base for the sub-scales and domains, and I felt I was assessing parents' perceptions of their children's behaviours and of their own situations and coping. I provided the mother who tried the PSI for my critique a short face validity survey to complete on the PSI (see blank copy below). She rated the PSI as 'Easy' (as opposed to difficult), 'Interesting' (as opposed to boring), and 'Relevant' (as opposed to irrelevant) and 'Undemanding' (as opposed to stressful). She commented that the PSI was 'very interesting as it was about me for a change rather than just my child'. The mother did not find any questions unclear or ambiguous, and she answered all questions and indicated that there were no questions that she did not feel comfortable answering. When asked if she found it useful to reflect on the PSI questions, she answered: 'Yes, it made me think about a few of the answers I gave, perhaps highlighting a few areas'.
Summary of **strengths**:	Strong underlying research and theory base to the development of the PSI. Extensive research into the validity of the PSI and uses in different cultures and with a wide range of conditions. Fairly easy to complete for most parents and not too time intensive (about 15–20 minutes). Straightforward to score and plot the profile (took about 15 minutes). Easy to covert raw score to percentiles on either profile or against age-based norms. Case examples and diagnostic group mean profiles allow for comparison. Manual contains useful information for interpreting scores and planning related intervention. Allows comparison of mother versus father perspectives of child and experience of stress related to parenting. A short form of the PSI, which the manual states takes about 10 minutes to complete, is available as a screening tool if the 15–20 minute administration time is perceived as too long for a particular parent group (e.g. parents having difficulty with concentration) or service requirement (e.g. a service wanted to use the PSI as a screen with all parents). The short form has acceptable levels of test–retest reliability and could be used as an evaluative measure.
Summary of **limitations**:	There is no British normative data, but a wide range of cross-cultural studies indicates that the PSI norms are robust across different populations. Summaries of the psychometric studies are very brief with only a few sentences about the samples and the results, and quite a few of the references cited for important psychometric studies are from unpublished work, making it very difficult for an AHP to access details of these studies. For example, Burke's (1978) unpublished doctoral dissertation is cited as providing 'a detailed description of the initial content validation of the PSI', and the reference for the internal consistency study by Hauenstein et al. (1987) is referenced as an unpublished manuscript. I have concerns about the variability of the reliability data; results from four test–retest reliability studies ranged from 0.55, 0.63, and from 0.77 to 0.82 (see the reliability section above) with half the data being at acceptable levels (over 0.70) and half the data raising causes for concern if the

(Continued)

TABLE 10.4   (Continued)

Critique Area	Comments
	PSI is to be implemented for evaluative purposes (under 0.70). The reasons for the variability in these results are not discussed in the test manual, and it is difficult to hypothesise about the causes of this variability as little detail is given about the methodology used in each study. To compound the problem, three of the four test–retest reliability studies referenced are from unpublished doctoral dissertations. The manual reports parents that with at least fifth grade education were found to understand the instructions; parents with less formal education, learning disability, or cognitive impairment might need support to ensure understanding.
Overall conclusion: Should the test be adopted, piloted, or rejected as an option for your service?	I would recommend this measure to AHPs working in a wide range of paediatric settings. It is a good descriptive measure that provides a useful overview of the parent's perceptions of child behaviours and the parent's overall level and causes of parenting stress. I would suggest AHPs obtain a review/borrowed copy of the PSI first to critique for their particular service and pilot with a few parents prior to purchase. The PSI has some predictive and discriminative uses, but I recommend that AHPs obtain and review the relevant research referenced in the manual before applying in this way. If the PSI is to be used as an evaluative measure, I would recommend AHPs conduct their own test–retest reliability study for the time period that is likely to occur in their clinical practice between baseline assessment and outcome measurement to ensure that the PSI has adequate reliability for this purpose.
References	Abidin (1995). Benson and Clark (1982). Burke (1978). Cited in Abidin (1995). Hamilton (1980). Cited in Abidin (1995). Hauenstein et al. (1987). Cited in Abidin (1995). Kazdin (1990). Zakreski (1983). Cited in Abidin (1995).

Sources: Abidin (1995); Benson and Clark (1982); Burke (1978). Cited in Abidin (1995).

The publisher's brief description of the PSI was as follows:

Identify stressful areas in parent–child interactions with this updated screening and diagnostic instrument. The PSI *was developed on the basis that the total stress a parent experiences is a function of certain salient child characteristics, parent characteristics and situations directly related to the role of being a parent. The* PSI Short Form *is a direct derivative of the 101 item full-length test and consists of a 36-item self-scoring questionnaire/profile. It yields a Total Stress Score from three scales.*
(The Psychological Corporation/Harcourt Assessment Company, Occupational Therapy and Physiotherapy catalogue 2004, p. 61. www.harcourt-uk.com)

Personal reflection of process by Alison Laver-Fawcett (ALF):

I started by reading through the manual, item booklet, and answer sheet and making notes on the test critique form (see Worksheet 10.2). I like to try out tests on myself if at all possible, by completing them myself or role-playing test administration with a colleague, student, or friend. As I was a parent with two small children when the critique was undertaken, this test was relevant to me, so I did it myself and answered the items in relation to my youngest child (then aged 14 months). The manual had some normative data for fathers and stated that 'the data from this sample would suggest that fathers earn lower stress scores on many PSI scales when compared to mothers' (Abidin 1995, p. 25). In my clinical practice and research, I have found it beneficial to use assessments that can be scored by different people involved with my client: the older person and their spouse, the child and their parent, the parent and the child's teacher, or in this case both parents. So asked my husband to complete the PSI too. This gave me two sets of data to try to score and interpret (mother's and father's scores for a child), some clinical utility and face validity information from doing it myself, and a face validity perspective from a father. Based on the information in the manual and trying the test out informally at home, I decided it seemed a useful test. So I approached a mother with a two-year-old child with gross and fine motor skill developmental delay, hemi-hypertrophy, and hearing problems. I explained that I was reviewing this test as an example for this book and asked her if she would be prepared to do the PSI and complete a face validity survey for me. This gave me a third set of data to score and some face validity feedback from a parent whose child was currently receiving occupational therapy and physiotherapy.

Few standardised measures available to AHPs are completely ideal, and you are likely to identify limitations as well as strengths when conducting your own test critiques. Even if you do not find a 'perfect' test, Stokes and O'Neill (1999) advised that 'it may be appropriate to employ an incompletely assessed tool as an alternative to a non-standardised assessment. This may lead to uniformity in the utilisation of scales within departments which in turn will aid in the full evaluation of scales through multi-centre research activities and stem the multitude of "in-house" scales' (p. 562). So, if you find a standardised assessment that covers the assessment domains of interest and has some reasonable psychometric data, albeit with small sample sizes, for example, then it is worth trying this measure. Even better would be to contribute to its ongoing development, perhaps by writing a letter to your professional journal or specialist group newsletter outlining your experience using the test or approaching the test developer or publisher to give your ideas on what further studies would be helpful in your field.

STEP 4: SELECTING ASSESSMENTS AND OUTCOME MEASURES FOR PRACTICE OR RESEARCH

How Do I Decide If an Assessment or Outcome Measure Is Appropriate for My Practice?

The decision to select a new assessment or measure to use in practice or research is based on more than just the best research evidence underpinning those tools you have reviewed. Other factors that need to be taken into consideration include those related to the client group, the AHPs who will be administering the assessment or measure, and the setting (see Figure 10.3).

Questions to consider related to these four areas of client, clinician, evidence, and setting are provided in Table 10.5 below for you to reflect on.

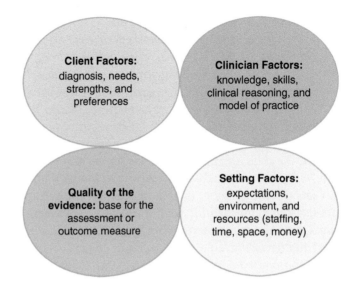

FIGURE 10.3   Factors that influence the choice of assessments and outcome measures in practice.

TABLE 10.5   Questions to consider when deciding to select an assessment or measure for practice.

Factor	Item	What to consider
Client	Relevance	• Will this test be of relevance to my patient population and the areas/locale in which I work? Will the test provide information that addresses the purpose of the assessment/measure required for your practice or research? The information collected must have value, be meaningful to the client, and provide data that informs the intervention and/or will evaluate outcomes. • Who will have access to the test results and benefit from this data, and how will they benefit? • Does the test have good face validity for your client group, service, and/or research participants? • Does the assessment have information about how to introduce it to your client, for example, about the purpose of the assessment and what the person is going to be asked to do? • Are the instructions easily comprehended by the client group? • Will the assessment be suitable for a client with the person's physical ability levels (e.g. do they need to pick up and manipulate objects or be able to write)? • Will the assessment be suitable for a client with the person's mental ability levels (e.g. attention, concentration)?
	Age	• Developmental and chronological age should be taken into account. • If it is a norm-referenced test, the sample used to provide normative data should include people of the same age, gender, and ethnicity.
	Diagnosis specific or generic	• You may choose a test that has been developed for people with a specific diagnosis or to aid the assessment of symptoms. • You may see people with a range of diagnoses and prefer a generic measure.

TABLE 10.5   (Continued)

Factor	Item	What to consider
	Time of day	• Does the client's functioning vary depending on medication, fatigue, or time of day? • If the person experiences variable levels of function, do you need to assess the person's maximum or minimum level of functioning?
Evidence Base	Standardisation	• Could you find evidence of standardisation?
	Reliability	• Could you find evidence of acceptable levels of reliability?
	Validity	• Could you find evidence of acceptable levels of validity? Does the assessment measure what it says it measures? • If it can be used for predictive assessment, does it predict what it was developed to predict? • If it can be used as a discriminative test, does it discriminate between the identified groups or criteria?
Clinician	Role	• What is your role in this setting? • Are there other professionals involved with the person who have undertaken assessments and what information has been obtained already? • What is the AHP's role in this setting? • What role does the assessor take when administering the assessment, e.g. observation, interview, or send out instructions in an email with an embedded link to an online assessment?
	Training and learning to administer	• Do you have the qualifications and competency to undertake this test? • Type of administration and ease of administration. • Clinician's comprehensibility. • Ease of score calculation and interpretation of scores. • Will further training be required? If so, how much does training cost, and how much time will it take? • Would the required funding and time be available?
	Model of Practice	• Do you/the service use a particular model of practice? Are there assessments and outcome measures that have been developed to relate to the chosen model? • Is the assessment/measure you are considering compatible with the model of practice used?
Setting	Feasibility and Utility	• Can the test be administered within your available resources (time, staff, budget, space)? • How long does it take to administer and score? • Can it be administered in the time you have available for this type of assessment? • Is it free? What are the copyright restrictions? What does it cost? Will it be too expensive for my service to purchase? Is the cost worth the benefit for the clients and service?
	Environment	• Where will the assessment be undertaken, e.g. in the person's home or place of residence, an inpatient unit, therapy department, day service, or community venue?

Source: Adapted from Laver-Fawcett (2014).

Lack of budget for purchasing assessments and outcome measures can be a barrier for AHPs in some settings. Although there may be an initial outlay to buy a standardised test, because they are evidence based, valid, and reliable, they improve the effectiveness of assessment, and enable information to be collected in the most efficient way. Copyright restrictions can vary; you will find some assessments and outcome measures are freely available on the Internet. However, pay careful attention, as some require you to submit a registration or request form or provide your contact details, and others ask that the work is cited/acknowledged in a particular way. Some assessments and measures are published in journal articles and are free and easily accessed, and others can be obtained from the directly from the authors (test developer) and used with their permission for free. However, a significant number of measures can only be obtained by purchasing the manual, forms, and any standardised test equipment, and there might also be a requirement to undertake and pay for training before the measure can be purchased. Undertaking a review of the evidence base to provide a detailed critical appraisal can be very useful when making a case to a manager for funding to purchase a new assessment or outcome measure for your service. It is also required in many research grant applications when justifying the selection of measures and the related budget in the grant. Depending on the healthcare system you are working in, another consideration might be whether undertaking this assessment would be reimbursable if a client has insurance.

In particular, the time required to administer, score, and report the findings of an assessment is a key consideration when AHPs are selecting assessments and outcome measures. In a systematic review of the barriers and facilitators, Duncan and Murray (2012) noted that if an outcome measure did not require too much time to document, this increased the chances of it being used in practice. They identified lack of time as a key barrier and related to the 'amount of time required for both patients and AHPs to complete an outcome measure' (p. 5), the size of the AHP's caseload, and institutional restrictions which can restrict the amount of time available for AHPs to spend with patients.

REFLECTION POINT

You can use Worksheet 10.3 to review a test and consider its feasibility for your own practice setting.

How Do I Decide if an Assessment or Outcome Measure Is Appropriate for My Research?

Choosing the right standardised assessment or outcome measure is essential for mixed methods or quantitative research studies, including clinical trials. When deciding the best measure for your research study, there are additional factors, beyond the psychometric properties critically appraised when selecting measures for practice, which need to be considered. Coster (2013, p. 162) cautions that 'the best design and most rigorously executed procedures cannot make up for a poorly chosen measure. Important knowledge about the impact of the intervention may be lost because the selected measure was unable to capture it or, even worse, distorted true results.' So, selecting the correct measure can be critical for ensuring the rigour of your study. There are other considerations which may affect a measure's validity and utility for the study purpose (Coster 2013) or impact staff willingness and capacity to undertake assessment for research. Research outcomes need to be reported 'completely, transparently and competently' (Heneghan et al. 2017, p. 1), and so it is useful to document in detail your decisions regarding the selection of measures and your critical appraisal of their related evidence base during the study design phase.

We recommend the Core Outcome Measures in Effectiveness Trials (*COMET*) initiative (2019) and their website – http://www.comet-initiative.org. This initiative supports the development and application of agreed standardised sets of outcomes, which they refer to as 'Core Outcome Sets' (*COS*). A COS is an agreed minimum set of outcomes that should be measured and reported in all clinical trials of a specific disease or trial population. It is a recommendation of *what* should be measured and reported in all clinical trials (Clarke 2007; COMET Initiative 2019). The COMET website states that

> *these sets represent the minimum that should be measured and reported in all clinical trials of a specific condition, and are also suitable for use in clinical audit or research other than randomised trials. The existence or use of a core outcome set does not imply that outcomes in a particular trial should be restricted to those in the relevant core outcome set. Rather, there is an expectation that the core outcomes will be collected and reported, making it easier for the results of trials to be compared, contrasted and combined as appropriate; while researchers continue to explore other outcomes as well.*
>
> (COMET Initiative 2019)

For randomised controlled trials and outcome studies, an early decision to be taken is how the researcher will operationalise what a 'successful outcome' should be. This can be easier said than done! Wade (2003) highlighted some of the challenges: 'in rehabilitation, outcome is more difficult to measure because (1) usually several outcomes are relevant, (2) relevant outcomes are affected by multiple factors in addition to treatment, and (3) even good measures rarely reflect the specific interest of any individual patient or member of the rehabilitation team, leading to some dissent' (p. 26) (see the sections titled 'The Complexity of Assessment' and 'The Nature of Human Performance' in Chapter 1). The advice provided earlier in this chapter in the section titled 'How Do I Define What Type of Assessment or Outcome Measure Is Needed?' is relevant to this decision. In addition, a challenge for researcher occurs when measuring some constructs such as quality of life, because a number of definitions and measure are available, and a full consensus as to what the measurement of quality of life should entail has yet to be reached (e.g. see Post 2014). Wade (2003) suggested that 'outcome is best measured at the level of behaviour (activities), with other measures being used to aid interpretation'; and currently for rehabilitation and reablement research, this remains useful advice.

Fitzpatrick et al. (1998) recommended eight criteria which researchers 'should apply to evaluate ... patient-based outcome measures for any specific clinical trial: appropriateness, reliability, validity, responsiveness, precision, interpretability, acceptability, feasibility' (p. iii). Although their publication is now over 20 years old, these eight criteria remain relevant today. In addition, another critical consideration is whether a potential measure will be sensitive to the amount of anticipated change if the intervention is successful, so the researcher will need to consider evidence of sensitivity in addition to responsiveness to change. Hypothesising the likely range of obtained scores across the sample is also helpful when looking for evidence of any measurement ceiling or floor effects (for information on sensitivity, responsiveness to change, floor, and ceiling effects, see Chapter 8).

Appropriateness of a Research Measure

Researchers should 'ensure that trial outcomes are relevant, appropriate and of importance to patients in real-world clinical settings' (Heneghan et al. 2017, p. 1). Therefore, the face validity of potential outcome measures should be considered (see Chapter 8). It is essential that research measures should be acceptable to proposed participants. In AHP research, participants are also often patients or people living with a long-term condition, so it is important to avoid, or at least minimise, potential anxiety or distress which might be triggered through undertaking an assessment. For patient-self reported measures, acceptability is also important for obtaining the required high response rate (Fitzpatrick et al. 1998). This reduces the risk of non-response bias occurring. There is less consensus as to what constitutes acceptability, compared to properties such and reliability and validity, and appropriateness and/or face validity is much less reported in the measurement literature. Nonetheless, its importance should not be ignored or underplayed, because otherwise there is a risk that clinical trial outcomes will fail to translate into benefits for patients (Heneghan et al. 2017); see Figure 10.4.

Feasibility of a Measure

In addition to the factors considered regarding the clinical utility of a measure for clinical practice, for research 'it is important to evaluate the impact of different [potential] outcome measures upon staff and researchers in collecting and processing information' (Fitzpatrick et al. 1998, p. 43). You need to consider whether you will have research assistants collecting outcome measure data or whether data will be

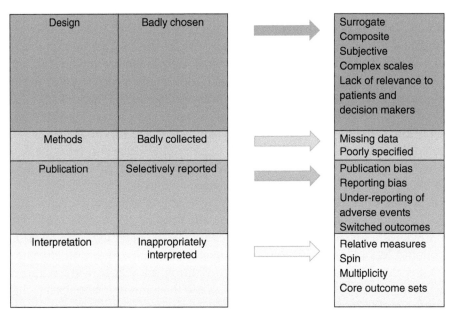

FIGURE 10.4   Why clinical trial outcomes fail to translate into benefits for patients. *Source*: Heneghan et al. (2017).

collected from patients 'in the context of regular clinical patient care'. If the latter, then an excessive additional burden on staff time placed by the expectation of undertaking extra outcome measurement at specified time periods may jeopardise your research and could disrupt routine clinical care. Therefore, if appropriate outcome measurements with a robust evidence base are already routinely used in clinical care and are familiar to staff in that care setting, it can be worth considering using these rather than introducing an unfamiliar measure.

The number and properties of your selected outcome measures will influence the minimum number of people (sample size) required for your study and will need to be taken into consideration when undertaking a power calculation to identify how many participants you will need to recruit to your study. A big enough sample is needed to provide sufficient chance, known as 'power', of detecting the predefined outcome at the hypothesised amount of difference between the baseline and follow-up measures; this is known as the 'effect size' (Walters 2004). However, owing to factors such as ethical, cost, and time considerations, researchers do not want to recruit more participants than needed. So, the 'main aim of a sample size calculation is to determine the number of participants needed to detect a clinically relevant treatment effect' (Noordzij et al. 2010, p. 1388). There are five questions (Walters 2004, pp. 1–2) that need to be answered before a power calculation can be undertaken; these are:

1. What is the main purpose of the trial?
2. What is the principal measure of patient outcome?
3. How will the data be analysed to detect a treatment difference?
4. What type of results does one anticipate with standard treatment?
5. How small a treatment difference is it important to detect and with what degree of certainty?

AHP researchers conducting trials are often supported by a statistician and so will not always have to under the power calculation themselves. However, the statistician will need information about the study to determine which method to use and to conduct the power calculation, so think through these five questions before you meet. For those without access to a statistician, Walters (2004) provides a helpful explanation of four methods which can be used to establish required sample size and power estimation for studies, and illustrates his article using a common health-related quality of life outcome measure, the SF-36 and data from a randomised controlled trial. The four methods described are: '1. assuming a normal distribution and comparing two means; 2. using a non-parametric method; 3. Whitehead's method based on the proportional odds model; 4. the bootstrap' non-parametric method (p. 1).

Coster (2013) provides a detailed explanation of what to consider when selecting outcome measures for research and why. She summarises the factors and questions to ask in a useful appendix to her article. These are provided in Table 10.6.

REFLECTION POINT

You can use Worksheet 10.4 when considering what outcome measure(s) to choose for your research study.

TABLE 10.6   Guiding questions for selecting outcome measures.

Question	Focus	Factors to consider when selecting measures for research
What	Specification of the construct	• Is there a well-specified explanatory model showing how the intervention links to the outcome of interest? • Have the most relevant dimensions or aspects of the outcome been specified clearly?
How	Rationale for selecting the measure	• Does the measurement construct of the instrument match the study's target outcome (as specified by the model)? • Does the instrument address the relevant domains of greatest importance? • Do the items sample the domain at the desired or appropriate level of specificity? • Are the items well suited to the characteristics of the population (i.e. are they free from bias)? • Does the measurement dimension reflect the type of change expected from the intervention? • Do points on the scale match the degrees of variation expected in the sample? • Are item and scale wording appropriate (i.e. meaningful, understandable) for this population? • Does evidence exist that the measure is sensitive to degrees of change expected in this population? • Does evidence exist supporting the ability of the measure to identify meaningful change?
Who	Determination of the most appropriate source of outcome information	• Do the potential providers of outcome information (e.g. professional, caregiver) match the qualifications criteria of the instrument being considered? • If someone other than a professional will be the respondent, is it probable that the respondent will be able to complete the assessment (i.e. has the necessary sensory, literacy, cognitive, physical, and communication abilities)? • Can the measure be adapted if needed to accommodate the functional limitations of the respondent? • Will the identified respondents be available throughout the study period (i.e. for all measurement points)?
When	Determination of when outcomes should be measured	• Does the length of time between assessments match the time period over which this instrument is likely to show effects? • Can the measure be administered as often as required by the study design?

Source: Coster (2013). © 2013, American Occupational Theory Association.

Obtaining Permission to Use a Test for Your Clinical Practice or for Research

Whether, and from whom, you need to obtain permission depends on whether the test is in the public domain and whether there is a cost or training requirement for using the test. If a test has been purchased for use from the author or a publisher, then the permission to use is implicit. However, you might inherit a test when you move to a new service or obtain a copy of a test at a workshop or from a colleague. In these cases, you need to track down who the author is, who has copyright, and whether the test is published. If a test developer has sold the copyright to a publisher, then permission is sought from the publisher, and usually you will be charged to use the test and all related materials. If the assessment has been printed in full in an article where the journal publishers require the author to sign over copyright of the article, then permission may need to be sought from the publisher of the journal. Sometimes the author may have maintained copyright of the instrument prior to publication of the article, and permission then has to be obtained from both the author and the journal publisher. If the instrument has not been published in full (for example, you access a copy being used for research during test development), then the author must be contacted.

Worksheets

At the end of the chapter, you will find templates for a series of worksheets designed to assist you in applying principles of assessment and outcome measurement to your own practice. Now turn to Worksheet 10.1. The worksheet takes you through a series of questions to help you establish whether a test has been standardised. Identify at least one standardised criterion-referenced test and one norm-referenced test suitable for use with your caseload. If you are a student AHP, identify an example of each type of test for a client group you are working with on placement. Use a separate copy of the worksheet to examine each of your selected tests. Examine all the test materials available to you, and try to answer as many of the questions as possible. If you wish to undertaken a detailed evaluation of the strengths and limitations of the tests you have selected, use Worksheet 10.2. For assistance completing the worksheet, there is an example of a completed critique in Table 10.4. Worksheet 10.3 can be used to review a test and consider its feasibility for your own practice setting. Worksheet 10.4 enables you to reflect on the questions posed in Table 10.6 when considering what outcome measure(s) to choose for a research study.

SUGGESTED TASKS

10.1 Give an example of:
   a. a standardised self-report assessment that would be appropriate for your client group and practice setting.
   b. a standardised proxy assessment that would be appropriate for your client group and practice setting.
   c. a standardised observational assessment that would be appropriate for your client group and practice setting.

10.2 Choose a standardised outcome measure of interest to your practice/research/ studies and undertake a literature review and comprehensive test critique using Worksheet 10.2 as a template. Share your critique with your educator, clinical supervisor, mentor, and/or colleagues.

Name of the test:
Full reference

Is there a test manual? YES NO
Comment:

Does the test manual describe the test development process? YES NO
Comment:

Does the test manual describe the purpose of the test and the client group for whom the test has been developed? YES NO
Comment:

Does the test manual provide details of psychometric studies undertaken to establish reliability and validity? YES NO
Comment:

Does the test manual describe the materials needed for test administration or are these included as part of the test package? YES NO
Comment:

Does the test manual describe the environment that should be used for testing? YES NO
Comment:

Is there a protocol for test administration that provides all the instructions required to administer the test? YES NO
Comment:

Name of the test:
Full reference

Is there a test manual? YES NOIs there guidance on how to score each test item? YES NO
Comment:

Is there a scoring form for recording scores? YES NO
Comment:

Is there guidance for interpreting scores? YES NO
Comment:

If it is a norm-referenced test, is the normative sample well described? YES NO NOT APPLICABLE
Comment:

Are there norm tables from which you can compare a client's score with the distribution of scores obtained by the normative group? YES NO
Comment:

WORKSHEET 10.2   Test Critique Form.

Critique Area	Comments
Name of test, authors, and date of publication	
Publisher: where to obtain test. **Cost** (if any)	
For what population has the test been designed	
Purpose(s) of test: Stated purpose and uses	
Data collection method(s) used	
Level(s) of function addressed by test	
Testing environments where test can be used:	
Scoring method and levels of measurement:	
Qualifications needed to administer the test and additional training requirements/costs:	
Standardisation: Is it standardised? Development details	
Is it a **normative-** or **criterion-referenced test?** Details of criteria or norms:	
Reliability data:	
Validity data:	
Clinical utility (ease of use and scoring, portability, cost, training issues, settings, etc.)	
Face validity (for AHPs, service user, others receiving results)	
Summary of strengths:	
Summary of limitations:	
Overall conclusion: Should test be adopted, piloted, or rejected as an option for your service?	

Factor	Item	Comments
Client	Relevance	
	Age	
	Diagnosis specific/generic	
	Time of day	
Evidence Base	Reliability	
	Validity	
Clinician	Role	
	Training	
	Model of Practice	
Setting	Feasibility and Utility	
	Environment	

WORKSHEET 10.4   Reflection on Factors for Selecting Outcome Measures for Research.

Question	Focus	Comments
What	Specification of the construct	
How	Rationale for selecting the measure	
Who	Determination of the most appropriate source of outcome information	
When	Determination of when outcomes should be measured	

REFERENCES

Abidin, R.R. (1995). *Parenting Stress Index (3rd Edition) Professional Manual*. Odessa, FL: Psychological Assessment Resources, Inc.

Asher, I.E. (2014). *Asher's Occupational Therapy Assessment Tools: An Annotated Index*, 4e. Bethesda: American Occupational Therapy Association (AOTA).

Balshem, H., Helfand, M., Schünemann, H.J. et al. (2011). GRADE guidelines: 3. Rating the quality of evidence. *Journal of Clinical Epidemiology* 64 (4): 401–406. https://doi.org/10.1016/j.jclinepi.2010.07.015.

Benson, J. and Clark, F. (1982). A guide for instrument development and validation. *American Journal of Occupational Therapy* 36 (12): 789–800.

Burke WT (1978) The development of a technique for assessing the stresses experienced by parents of young children. Unpublished doctoral dissertation, University of Virginia, Charlottesville.

Cameron, S.J. and Orr, R.R. (1989). Stress in families of school-aged children with delayed mental development. *Canadian Journal of Rehabilitation* 2 (3): 137–144.

Clarke, M. (2007). Standardising outcomes for clinical trials and systematic reviews. *Trials* 8 (39): 1–3. https://doi.org/10.1186/1745-6215-8-39.

COMET Initiative (2019) Core Outcome Measures in Effectiveness Trials. COMET website. Available from: http://www.comet-initiative.org. accessed 27.8.19.

COSMIN (2019) COSMIN Taxonomy of Measurement Properties Available from: https://www.cosmin.nl/tools/cosmin-taxonomy-measurement-properties accessed 21.05.19.

Coster, W.J. (2013). Making the best match: selecting outcome measures for clinical trials and outcome studies. *American Journal of Occupational Therapy* 67: 162–170. https://doi.org/10.5014/ajot.2013.006015.

Denman, D., Speyer, R., Munro, N. et al. (2017). Psychometric properties of language assessments for children aged 4–12 years: a systematic review. *Frontiers in Psychology* 8 (1515): 1–28. https://doi.org/10.3389/fpsyg.2017.01515.

Desai, A.S., Dramis, A., and Hearnden, A.J. (2010). Critical appraisal of subjective outcome measures used in the assessment of shoulder disability. *Annals of the Royal College of Surgeons in England* 92 (1): 9–13. https://doi.org/10.1308/003588410X12518836440522.

Donenberg, G. and Baker, B.L. (1993). The impact of young children with externalizing behaviors on their families. *Journal of Abnormal Child Psychology* 21 (2): 179–198.

Duncan, E.A. and Murray, J. (2012). The barriers and facilitators to routine outcome measurement by allied health professionals in practice: a systematic review. *BMC Health Services Research* 12 (1): 96. https://doi.org/10.1186/1472-6963-12-96.

Finch, E., Brooks, D., Stratford, P.W., and Mayo, N.E. (2002). *Physical Rehabilitation Outcome Measures.: A Guide to Enhanced Clinical Decision Making*, 2e. Toronto: Canadian Physiotherapy Association. ISBN: 0781742412, 9780781742412.

Fitzpatrick, R., Davey, C., Buxton, M.J., and Jones, D.R. (1998). *Evaluating Patient-Based Outcome Measures for Use in Clinical Trials*, vol. 2(14). Winchester, England: Health Technology Assessment https://doi.org/10.3310/hta2140.

Francis, D.O., Daniero, J.J., Hovis, K.L. et al. (2017). Voice-related patient-reported outcome measures: a systematic review of instrument development and validation. *Journal of Speech, Language, and Hearing Research* 60 (1): 62–88. https://doi.org/10.1044/2016_JSLHR-S-16-0022.

GRADE Working Group (2004). Grading quality of evidence and strength of recommendations. *BMJ* 328 (7454): 1490. https://doi.org/10.1136/bmj.328.7454.1490.

Grewal, A., Kataria, H., and Dhawan, I. (2016). Literature search for research planning and identification of research problem. *Indian Journal of Anaesthesia* 60 (9): 635–639. https://doi.org/10.4103/0019-5049.190618.

Hamilton EB (1980) The relationship of maternal patterns of stress, coping, and support to quality of early infant–mother attachment. Unpublished doctoral dissertation, University of Virginia, Charlottesville.

Hanson, M.J. and Hanline, M.F. (1990). Parenting a child with a disability: a longitudinal study of parental stress and adaptation. *Journal of Early Intervention* 14 (3): 234–248.

Hasenstein, T., Greene, T., and Meyr, A.J. (2017). A 5-year review of clinical outcome measures published in the journal of the American Podiatric Medical Association and the Journal of Foot and Ankle Surgery. *Journal of the American Podiatric Medical Association* 107 (3): 176–179. https://doi.org/10.1053/j.jfas.2017.01.023.

Hauenstein E, Scarr S, Abidin RR (1987) Detecting children at risk for developmental delay: efficacy of the Parenting Stress Index in a non-American culture. Unpublished manuscript, University of Virginia, Charlottesville.

Heneghan, C., Goldacre, B., and Mahtani, K.R. (2017). Why clinical trial outcomes fail to translate into benefits for patients. *Trials* 18 (122): 1–7. https://doi.org/10.1186/s13063-017-1870-2.

Jeffrey, L.I.H. (1993). Aspects of selecting outcome measures to demonstrate effectiveness of comprehensive rehabilitation. *British Journal of Occupational Therapy* 56 (11): 394–400. https://doi.org/10.1177/030802269305601103.

Kazdin, A.E. (1990). Premature termination from treatment among children referred for antisocial behavior. *Journal of Child Psychology and Psychiatry, and Allied Disciplines* 31 (3): 415–425.

LaFiosca T. (1981) The relationship of parent stress to anxiety, approval, motivation and children's behavior problems. unpublished doctoral thesis 1981, University of Virginia

Laver-Fawcett, A. (2002). Assessment. In: *Occupational Therapy and Physical Dysfunction: Principles, Skills and Practice* (eds. A. Turner, M. Foster and S.E. Johnson), 633. Edinburgh: Churchill Livingstone.

Laver-Fawcett, A. (2014). Routine standardised outcome measurement to evaluate the effectiveness of occupational therapy interventions: essential or optional? *Ergoterapeuten* 4: 28–37.

Law, M. (2001). Outcome measures rating form guidelines. In: *Measuring Occupational Performance: Supporting Best Practice in Occupational Therapy* (eds. M. Law, C. Baum and W. Dunn). Thorofare, NJ: Slack.

McDowell, I. (2006). *Measuring Health: A Guide to Rating Scales and Questionnaires*, 3e. Oxford: Oxford University Press.

Mokkink, L.B., Terwee, C.B., Patrick, D.L. et al. (2010). The COSMIN study reached international consensus on taxonomy, terminology, and definitions of measurement properties for health-related patient-reported outcomes. *Journal of Clinical Epidemiology* 63 (7): 737–745. https://doi.org/10.1016/j.jclinepi.2010.02.006.

Mokkink LB, Prinsen CAC, Patrick DL, Alonso J, Bouter LM, de Vet HCW, Terwee CB (2018) COSMIN methodology for systematic reviews of Patient-Reported Outcome Measures (PROMs) user manual Version 1.0 Available at: https://www.cosmin.nl/wp-content/uploads/COSMIN-syst-review-for-PROMs-manual_version-1_feb--2018-1.pdf accessed 1.4.19

Moran, G., Pederson, D.R., Pettit, P., and Krupka, A. (1992). Maternal sensitivity and infant-mother attachment in a developmentally delayed sample. *Infant Behavior and Development* 15 (4): 427–442.

Noordzij, M., Tripepi, G., Dekker, F.W. et al. (2010). Sample size calculations: basic principles and common pitfalls. *Nephrology, Dialysis, Transplantation* 25 (5): 1388–1393. https://doi.org/10.1093/ndt/gfp732.

O'Connor, B., Kerr, C., Shields, N., and Imms, C. (2016). A systematic review of evidence-based assessment practices by allied health practitioners for children with cerebral palsy. *Developmental Medicine and Child Neurology* 58 (4): 332–347. https://doi.org/10.1111/dmcn.12973.

Opacich, K.J. (1991). Assessment and informed decision-making. In: *Occupational Therapy: Overcoming Human Performance Deficits* (eds. C.M. Baum and C. Christiansen), 354–372. Slack.

Post, M. (2014). Definitions of quality of life: what has happened and how to move on. *Topics in Spinal Cord Injury Rehabilitation* 20 (3): 167–180. https://doi.org/10.1310/sci2003-167.

Prinsen, C.A.C., Vohra, S., Rose, M.R. et al. (2016). How to select outcome measurement instruments for outcomes included in a "Core outcome set" – a practical guideline. *Trials* https://doi.org/10.1186/s13063-016-1555-2.

Prinsen, C.A.C., Mokkink, L.B., Bouter, L.M. et al. (2018). COSMIN guideline for systematic reviews of patient-reported outcome measure. *Quality of Life Research* 27: 1147–1157.

Royal College of Occupational Therapists (RCOT) (2019). *4 Key Questions to Help Focus Your Search for Relevant Assessment and Outcome Measures*. London: RCOT.

Royal College of Physicians, Intercollegiate Stroke Working Party (2012). *National Clinical Guideline for Stroke*, vol. 20083. London: Royal College of Physicians https://www.strokeaudit.org/Guideline/Historical-Guideline/National-Clinical-Guidelines--for-Stroke-fourth-edi.aspx.

Schellingerhout, J.M., Heymans, M.W., Verhagen, A.P. et al. (2011). Measurement properties of translated versions of neck-specific questionnaires: a systematic review. *BMC Medical Research Methodology* 11 (87): 1–14. https://doi.org/10.1186/1471-2288-11-87.

Stokes, E.K. and O'Neill, D. (1999). The use of standardised assessments by physiotherapists. *British Journal of Therapy and Rehabilitation* 6 (11): 560–565. https://doi.org/10.12968/bjtr.1999.6.11.13928.

Terwee CB, Prinsen CAC, Chiarotto A, de Vet HCW, Bouter LM, Alonso J, Westerman MJ, Patrick DL, Mokkink LB (2018) COSMIN methodology for assessing the content validity of PROMs: User manual version 1.0. Amsterdam, Netherlands: VU University Medical Center. Available from: https://cosmin.nl/wp-content/uploads/COSMIN-methodology-for-content-validity-user-manual-v1.pdf accessed 1.4.19

Van Der Leeden, M., Steultjens, M.P., Terwee, C.B. et al. (2008). A systematic review of instruments measuring foot function, foot pain, and foot-related disability in patients with rheumatoid arthritis. *Arthritis Care & Research* 59 (9): 1257–1269. https://doi.org/10.1002/art.24016.

Wade, D.T. (2003). Outcome measures for clinical rehabilitation trials: impairment, function, quality of life, or value? *American Journal of Physical Medicine & Rehabilitation* 82 (10): S26–S31. https://doi.org/10.1097/01.PHM.0000086996.89383.A1.

Walker, J. (2002). *Reading Tips for the Clinician: How to Tell Whether an Article Is Worth Reading. WCPT Keynotes, EBP Critical Appraisal Skills*. London: World Confederation for Physical Therapy.

Walters, S.J. (2004). Sample size and power estimation for studies with health related quality of life outcomes: a comparison of four methods using the SF-36. *Health and Quality of Life Outcomes* 2 (1): 26. https://doi.org/10.1186/1477-7525-2-26.

Winward, C.E., Halligan, P.W., Wade, D.T., and Basiert Auf Leonardo, T. (2000). *Rivermead Assessment of Somatosensory Performance [RASP]*. Thames Valley Test Company Catalogue.

Wilfong, E.W., Saylor, C., and Elksnin, N. (1991). Influences on responsiveness: Interactions between mothers and their premature infants. *Infant Mental Health Journal* 12 (1): 31–40.

Zakreski JR (1983) Prematurity and the single parent: effects of cumulative stress on child development. Unpublished doctoral dissertation, University of Virginia, Charlottesville.

SUGGESTED RESOURCES

Mokkink LB, Prinsen CAC, Patrick DL, Alonso J, Bouter LM, de Vet HCW, Terwee CB (2018) COSMIN methodology for systematic reviews of Patient-Reported Outcome Measures (PROMs) user manual Version 1.0 Available at: https://www.cosmin.nl/wp-content/uploads/COSMIN-syst-review-for-PROMs-manual_version-1_feb--2018-1.pdf accessed 1.4.19

Mokkink LB, Terwee CB, Patrick DL, Alonso J, Stratford PW, Knol DL, Bouter LM, de Vet HCW (2012) COSMIN Checklist Manual. Available at: http://fac.ksu.edu.sa/sites/default/files/cosmin_checklist_manual_v9.pdf accessed 20.5.19.

Terwee, C.B., Mokkink, L.B., Knol, D.L. et al. (2012). Rating the methodological quality in systematic reviews of studies on measurement properties: a scoring system for the COSMIN checklist. *Quality of Life Research* 21 (4): 651–657.

WEBSITES

- Core Outcome Measures in Effectiveness Trials (COMET): http://www.comet--initiative.org
- Consensus-based Standards for the selection of health Measurement Instruments (COSMIN): https://www.cosmin.nl
- Rehabilitation measures database https://www.sralab.org/rehabilitation--measures/database?population=4636
- Patient-Reported Outcome Measures (PROMS): http://phi.uhce.ox.ac.uk/inst_types.php
- Model of Human Occupation (*MOHO*) Find the assessment tool: https://www.moho.uic.edu/resources/findTheAssessment/home.aspx
- Stroke Engine 'Find an assessment': https://www.strokengine.ca/en/. The Canadian Partnership for Stroke Recovery developed the 'Stroke Engine' website, which has a useful section that lists and reviews relevant assessments. This includes tests used by a range of rehabilitation professionals, including physiotherapists, speech and language therapists, and occupational therapists.

ASSESSMENT AND MEASUREMENT FOR SERVICE EVALUATION AND IMPROVEMENT

CHAPTER 11

Applying Models to Assessment and Outcome Measurement

OVERVIEW

In this chapter, we will describe and discuss the application of different models used in practice for categorising dimensions of functioning and disability. We begin with an overview of systems theory, including open systems theory. The World Health Organisation (WHO) International Classification of Functioning, Disability, and Health (ICF) was published in 2002 (https://www.who.int/classifications/icf/en). The ICF will be explored in greater depth, and examples of assessment domains and measures that provide information at the different levels of function identified will be provided. When applying models, an allied health professional (AHP) often needs to decide at what level to begin assessment, so this chapter will offer an exploration of the merits of a top-down versus a bottom-up approach to AHP assessment. We will also briefly describe the WHO Disability Assessment Schedule 2.0 (WHODAS 2.0, https://www.who.int/publications/i/item/measuring-health-and-disability-manual-for-who-disability-assessment-schedule-(-whodas-2.0)). The chapter concludes with a case study example.

QUESTIONS TO CONSIDER

1. How do I categorise the myriad of information and observational data collected about a person into a meaningful and organised assessment?
2. How do I fit my assessment practice into the wider context of a multidisciplinary team (MDT) and/or inter-agency approach?

WHY USE MODELS?

A *model* is a term used to describe a pattern, plan, chart, or simplified description of a system. Models can be used to aid the gathering and organising of information, and can act as a checklist. AHPs frequently collect multiple pieces of data about a person, their occupations, environment, illness, and problems throughout an assessment process. AHPs also obtain assessment data from different sources (the person, carer(s), other health and social care professionals) as well as from administered standardised tests and from informal observational assessment methods. All this information needs to be documented, organised, and reflected upon in a meaningful way to produce a thorough and useful assessment (see in Chapters 1–3).

It is important for AHPs to understand how their assessment practice fits into the wider context of assessment, intervention, and support provided by other health and social care colleagues, and independent and voluntary service providers. AHPs need to define their areas of expertise and be able to articulate these to their service users, carers (e.g. parents, spouse, or other relative), MDT, referral sources, and other agencies involved in the client's treatment and care. Some practitioners divide the different aspects of assessment for a person and assign them to different members of a MDT. Although this might be pragmatic from the standpoint of reducing repetition for the person being assessed and making the best use of resources, some AHPs view this as a reductionist, rather than a holistic, approach to assessment. When an AHP directs their focus of attention on a specific part of the body, or aspect of functioning, they may be blinkered and fail to see the person as a whole. This can lead to working on goals that are not relevant for the person or a failure to understand the relationship between any illness or dysfunction and other aspects of the person's life. Reductionist thinking can lead to fragmented practice, especially when professionals do not communicate clearly with each other and fail to share information derived from their assessments effectively. Models can be applied to help AHPs gain an overview of the whole and understand how discrete parts can or may interrelate. An explicit application of a model of function can help an individual AHP, an AHP service, or an MDT review their assessment practice and facilitate communication about assessment, outcome measurement, and intervention.

Appling a model of function can assist your assessment process in a number of ways:

- At the stage of problem setting, it can be particularly helpful to categorise the client's problems (identified by the referral or initial interview). It also helps in terms of levels of function/dysfunction and for using the boundaries of a defined level to help focus further on data collection, such as the use of standardised observational tests or to help decide if information needs to be collected from proxy sources.
- When critiquing standardised assessments for use within your service or for a particular client, models and hierarchies describing levels of function/ dysfunction can be useful for identifying and comparing the levels, domains, and scope of different or apparently similar tests.
- Many AHPs work as part of an MDT, and models can be useful to help each team member identify their primary level or domain of concern. In addition, it also helps the team identify areas where there is overlap in the assessment data collected and any gaps or omissions where a level of functioning has not been adequately assessed by team members.

THE COMPLEXITY OF HUMAN FUNCTION

In Chapter 1, we began to explore the challenges of undertaking a rigorous assessment and saw how some of these challenges were linked to the complexity of human functioning and the intricacy of the relationship between a person and his environment. At the start of this chapter on the application of models of function, it is worth thinking about what human functioning entails, because a useful model of function will need to encompass both the breadth and intricacy of human function.

People are individuals with complex systems. Every individual has a unique context, consisting of a multitude of elements and their interactions (Aron 2020). People perform daily activities such as eating, drinking, washing, dressing, cooking, cleaning, and travelling. These activities of daily living (ADL) support their ability to perform other personally selected activities related to work, play, and leisure. The balance or configuration of self-care, work, and leisure activities changes as the individual matures from infancy through adulthood and old age (Kielhofner 1980). Many basic activities become over-learned routines and become part of that person's habitual repertoire of behaviour. *Occupation* is the term used in the occupational therapy literature to describe a person's 'engagement in activities, tasks and roles for the purpose of meeting the requirements of living' (Levine and Brayley 1991, p. 622). This process of engagement is called 'occupational performance' (Christiansen and Baum 1991). The ability to perform activities is dependent on the interrelation of several levels of function. Each activity requires a combination of skills developed because of the normal functioning of the motor, sensory, and cognitive-perceptual systems. The functioning of these systems is in turn dependent on the functioning of individual body components, such as nerves, organs, muscles, and joints. Participation in occupation influences a person's psychological and biological health.

'The physical and psychological consequences of engagement and participation in occupations can range from emotional rewards (such as pleasure and satisfaction) to increased knowledge, wisdom, and a sense of life meaning and are important for a balanced lifestyle' (Matuska and Christiansen 2008, p. 13). Research investigating the effects of sensory deprivation has shown that when sensory stimulus, usually provided through interaction with the physical and social environment, is withdrawn, neurological disorganisation occurs (Rogers 1983).

Individuals can find themselves unable to perform activities independently owing to illnesses, chronic disease, or deficits caused by accidents. Habitual occupational performance is usually taken for granted until an illness, accident, or disabling condition makes performance difficult or impossible. The challenge to independent living caused by these deficits is not just experienced by the individual; the effect of disease on an individual also impacts their family, friends, and colleagues. The impact of an illness, disability, or disease on a person's lifestyle and quality of life can be reduced by the level of support they receive from family, friends, and colleagues, and by the type of health, social, and voluntary services available. The nature of his physical environment also impacts the amount of disability experienced, for example, if their home can be adapted to be wheelchair accessible.

The relationship between these multiple variables is usually very complex and needs to be assessed rigorously. Without accurate assessment, it is impossible to plan effective intervention and management. It is important to establish the limitations of performance and the underlying causes of this limited performance. Limited performance can be caused by impaired skills, dysfunctional systems, and specific motor, sensory, and/or cognitive-perceptual deficits. It is, therefore, essential for AHPs to understand the relationship between an individual's brain and body functioning and their behaviour. To help AHPs approach this task in a logical manner, it can be helpful to organise the assessment process in terms of levels of functioning or impact. Several classification systems that define the range of problems and levels of function/ dysfunction addressed by professionals working in the field of rehabilitation have been proposed. Many models are based on some sort of hierarchy, and we shall begin our consideration of models by looking at the broad hierarchy of living systems.

General Systems Theory and the Hierarchy of Living Systems

General systems theory (Skyttner 2005) forms the foundation of many AHP theoretical frameworks and so is a useful place to begin when considering models of function. For example, the Model of Human Occupation, first published in 1985 (MOHO; Kielhofner 2002), is an occupational therapy model that draws on general systems theory and views humans as open systems. Another example is the Person-Environment-Performance Framework (Christiansen and Baum 1991); in this framework, occupational performance is viewed as a transaction between the individual as an open system and the environment.

General Systems Theory emanates from an interdisciplinary base and involves the integration of natural, social, medical, and scientific disciplines. The systems approach is concerned with the description of systems, which are integrated wholes that derive their essential properties from the interrelationships between their parts (Box 11.1). Therefore, the systems approach does not focus on the parts but on their interrelationships and interdependencies (Capra 1982).

From a structural viewpoint, a system, like a person, is a divisible whole. We can divide the person, conceptually, in terms of separate bones, muscles, organs, and subsystems such as the motor, cardiovascular, and respiratory systems. However, from a functional perspective, a system is an indivisible whole. A system is indivisible functionally, in the sense that some of the essential properties of the system are lost when it is taken apart. When a person experiences some sort of pathology or injury to one part of his body, it can impact the overall functioning and roles of that person. As AHPs we need to understand how a deficit or problem in one part of the person's body or life impacts other parts, and how some disability associated with a deficit, can or cannot be remediated through the physical or sociocultural environment. For example, a man in his mid-70s develops chronic obstructive airways disease (COAD), which leads to a symptom of shortness of breath. This makes it very difficult for him to climb stairs. As a result, he and his wife decide to move to a bungalow. He also has to stop his role of babysitting for his young grandchildren, so that his son and daughter-in-law can go out for the evening, as they live in a three-story house and his grandchildren's bedrooms are located up two flights of stairs.

Systems involving creative, evolutionary, and developmental processes can experience growth. With growth, the system changes in the direction of increasing subdivision into subsystems and sub-subsystems, or differentiation of functions. This is the case for humans, as embryonic development involves the germinated egg progressing from a state of wholeness (a single fertilised egg) to a state of regions that develop independently into specialised organs (Hall and Fagen 1968), such as heart, lungs, and kidneys, which can be viewed as systems in themselves. This process continues after birth, and so AHPs working with children are concerned with the assessment of an infant or child's developmental processes. As such, AHPs will need

---

Box 11.1   Definition of a System

A system is defined as an organised whole comprised of interrelated and interdependent parts. It can be defined as a set of objects together with relationships between the objects and their attributes:

- objects are the components of a system;
- attributes are properties of objects;
- relationships tie the system together.

to consider what would be an expected level of development in different systems, such as the respiratory or motor system, and whether the child has progressed to this expected level of development. In order to do this, AHPs apply discriminative tests, which enable the AHP to compare a child's performance with the norm (expected performance) for children of that age and socio-economic background.

Many systems deteriorate or decay over time, and this is seen in the human ageing process. For example, deterioration occurring in the human visual and auditory system is associated with age, related changes to vision and hearing. AHPs working with older people will need to assess changes in function related to visual and auditory acuity and be able to differentiate these expected ageing processes from changes owing to some sort of pathology.

Subsystems can be recognised at various levels of the organisation of a system; these subsystems constitute Gestalt wholes in themselves and are also organised into a larger Gestalt whole according to the laws of the hierarchy. (Note: The *Concise Oxford Dictionary* defines a *Gestalt* as a 'form, shape, pattern: organised whole or unit – the organised whole as something more than the sum of its parts ...' (p. 379).) The organising laws incorporated by each level are used to describe the levels of a system:

- Each level is perceived as comprising at least one more complex law than the level below.
- Higher levels direct or organise the lower levels.
- Higher levels are dependent upon, or constrained by, lower levels.
- At any level, a phenomenon belonging primarily to that level incorporate characteristics or mechanisms of lower, less complex levels.
- The purpose of a level is found by examining the level above.

For example, in a hierarchy of human performance (as described by Kielhofner 2002), which comprises three levels of volition, habituation, and performance capacity, the lower level of motor coordination at the performance level is controlled by the higher habituation and volitional levels. Volition, at the highest level, is the person's 'pattern of thoughts and feelings' (p. 44), and what a person 'holds as important (values), perceives as personal capacity and effectiveness (personal causation), and finds enjoyable (interests)' (p. 44). Habituation is his 'semi-autonomous patterning of behaviour' which manifests as 'routine, automatic behaviour' that 'is organised in concert with [his] familiar temporal, physical, and social' environments (p. 19). A disturbance or change at one level resonates through the whole system; for example, injury to a muscle at the motor performance level will affect the ability to perform controlled movement. Movements embedded previously as habitual patterns of action, such as driving or brushing teeth, now require focused attention because they cannot be performed with prior ease. The decision to exercise at a volitional level, for example, following an AHP's prescribed set of exercises, will lead to changes in muscle tone and strength and will help to remediate the injured muscle.

Systems may be open or closed. Most natural, or organic systems, are described as open. This means that they exchange materials, energies, or information with their environments. According to Von Bertalanffy (1968), the theory of open systems is part of a general systems theory. The basis of the open system model is the dynamic interaction of its components. Survival of all living things is dependent on some form of action. Even without external stimuli, or input, humans are not a passive, but are intrinsically active systems. An external stimulus, such as a change in the temperature of the external environment, does not effect a reaction in an otherwise inert system (a rock will become hotter or colder in direct response to the external temperature); however, an external stimulus, such as changing temperature, stimulates modification in a highly active system. People, for example, sweat or shiver in order to maintain their body temperature.

The human system is involved with continuous, irreversible cycles of import and export, and construction and destruction of materials. For example, in terms of import and export: we take in oxygen from the air and expel carbon dioxide, and we take in food and drink, extract what our body needs, and expel waste as urine and faeces (see Figure 11.1). Central concepts in the theory of open systems are the concepts of dynamic interaction and feedback. Feedback allows the system to modify its internal components in response to the demands of the external environment. To do this, the system includes a receptor, such as a sense organ, which receives 'information' by nerve conduction. This 'information' is then processed in the system's controlling centre, such as the brain. The processing of information involves the evaluation of the incoming 'message' and the transmission of an outgoing 'response message' to an effector, such as a muscle. The functioning of the effector is fed back to the receptor. This makes the system self-regulating; for example, it guarantees stabilisation or direction of action.

Stephenson (2002) considered the central nervous system (*CNS*) as a complex adapting system (*CAS*) and proposed a model of behaviour based on self-organisation. Stephenson proposes the total integration model (*TIM*) as a new paradigm for physiotherapy, as 'neuroplasticity is explored as the means by which agents in the system interact, with population coding and models of processing being the mechanisms through which behaviour is achieved. Complexity theory is used to construct a holistic model of human behaviour; the TIM. Physiotherapy is placed as a "weighted" stressor within a homeodynamic system, with emergent client behaviour reflecting the aggregate influence of all stressors' (p. 417).

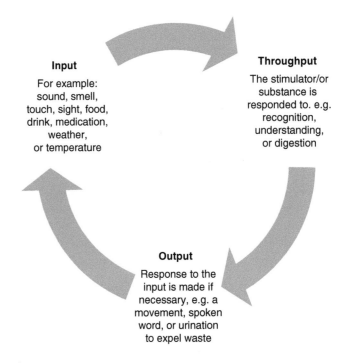

Input

For example: sound, smell, touch, sight, food, drink, medication, weather, or temperature

Throughput

The stimulator/or substance is responded to. e.g. recognition, understanding, or digestion

Output

Response to the input is made if necessary, e.g. a movement, spoken word, or urination to expel waste

FIGURE 11.1   A person as an open system.

The assessment of any complex phenomena requires knowledge of its function as both a part and a whole. AHPs need to encompass a vast field of phenomena from neurons and cells, to organs such as the brain and eyes, to the person as a whole, and to the interaction between people and their social and physical environments. These phenomena can be viewed as an interrelated continuum and can be classified into an ordered hierarchy.

Several taxonomies of phenomena that differentiate levels of complexity have been proposed (Boulding 1956; Von Bertalanffy 1968). Christiansen (1991) described a hierarchy of living systems that could be used by AHPs (see Figure 11.2). Each of the 10 levels in this hierarchy is viewed as a subsystem or component of the next higher level, and there is considered to be increasing complexity as one ascends the hierarchy. The lowest level of the hierarchy of living systems is the level of (i) the atom, followed by (ii) molecules, (iii) cells, and (iv) organs. The level of (v) the person falls in the middle of the hierarchy and is followed by the levels of (vi) the family group, (vii) organisations, and (viii) societies. The highest levels are (ix) *Homo sapiens*, defined as 'biological species which includes existing and extinct humans', and (x) the biosphere, which refers to 'habitable parts of the world for living organisms' (Christiansen 1991, p. 16).

For the majority of AHPs, the prime levels of concern, in this hierarchy of living systems, are the organ level, through the assessment and treatment of functioning of organ systems (such as the musculo-skeletal system), and the person level, through the assessment and treatment of the person's occupational performance. The impact of the person's social supports is explored at the family-group level; this level is of particular concern to those AHPs who educate and support carers, such as the parents of a child with cerebral palsy or the spouse of a person who has experienced a stroke. AHPs work at the organisational level when they signpost or refer service users to other organisations (such as voluntary organisations offering appropriate support or activities) or when liaising with a person's employing organisation to negotiate adaptations to the person's work space or adjustments to their work activities (Madan and Grime 2015). Some AHPs work at an organisational level when providing assessment or training for a group of people, for example, in the areas of lifting and handling or person–job–environment fit. AHPs also contribute at a societal level, for example, by contributing expertise

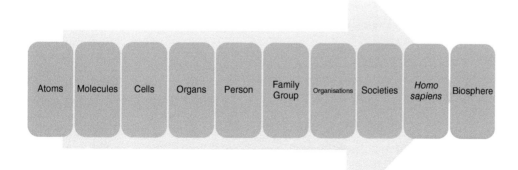

FIGURE 11.2   Hierarchy of living systems. *Source:* Adapted from Christiansen and Baum (1991).

to the development of government policy on topics such as health promotion and social inclusion (Andermann 2016). In terms of the biosphere, AHPs are now challenging us to consider environmental issues such as the development of equipment and the furnishing of AHP departments using recycled materials. Another concern for AHPs is the issue of cleaning and reallocation versus disposal of equipment, and which helps to ensure the minimal amount of waste and the use of non-polluting cleaning chemicals (Gower 2013).

Law and Baum (2005) suggested that AHPs need to understand a number of key concepts to be able to fully appreciate how AHP interventions fit into the larger context of healthcare and rehabilitation. They cite the conceptual frameworks provided by the WHO, the National Center for Medical Rehabilitation Research (*NCMRR*, https://www.nichd.nih.gov/about/org/ncmrr), and the work of Nagi (1991) as examples worthy of consideration. These models will now be described and examples from other health literature used to illustrate how they have been applied by AHPs.

Five-Level Model of Function and Dysfunction

Drawing upon the work of WHO (1980) and Nagi (1991), the NCMRR (1992) broadened the functional and dysfunctional hierarchy to a five-level model. Differentiation was made between pathophysiology, impairment, and functional limitation. Disability remained, and handicap was re-conceptualised as a *societal limitation*. The NCMRR drew upon the expertise of a multidisciplinary group (which included AHPs) to develop their five-level model of function/dysfunction (1992). The NCMRR model's five levels are presented in a hierarchy; see Figure 11.3

The NCMRR model recognised that the progression of dysfunction was not 'always sequential or unidirectional' but should be viewed as a 'complex feedback loop that integrates the whole person as an entity who must adjust to problems in many of these areas simultaneously' (p. 31). The NCMRR has identified the need to apply 'findings from studies of pathophysiology and impairment to the functional limitations they engender' (p. 33). The specification of these five levels of function was an important advance within the field of rehabilitation, as it assisted AHPs and researchers to define their domains of concern and clearly identify which level or levels of function they were addressing in their assessment and intervention. The NCMRR Hierarchy of Dysfunction (1992) was used by Laver (1994) during her doctoral research to develop the Structured Observational Test of Function (*SOTOF*; Laver and Powell 1995). Tables 11.1 and 11.2 show how four of the NCMRR levels were used to assist the categorisation and definition of the test domains and items assessed by the SOTOF.

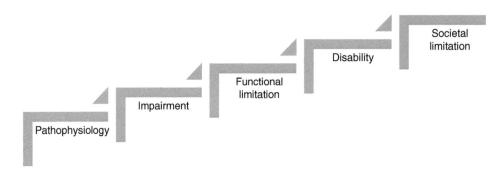

FIGURE 11.3   NCMRR's five-level model of function and dysfunction.

TABLE 11.1 Assessment domains and items covered by the Structured Observational Test of Function (SOTOF).

Level of function/dysfunction	Disability	Functional limitation	Impairment	Pathophysiology
Definition of level	Inability or limitation in performing socially defined activities and roles within a social and physical environment resulting from internal or external factors and their interplay.	Restriction or lack of ability to perform an action or activity in the manner or range considered normal that results from impairment.	Loss and/or abnormality or mental, emotional, physiological, or anatomical structure or function; including secondary losses and pain.	Interruption or interference of normal physiological and developmental processes or structures.
SOTOF assessment question	*HOW?*	*WHAT?*	*WHICH?*	*WHY?*
SOTOF assessment domain	Occupational performance	Specific skill or ability, task sub-components	Performance components	Neurological deficit
SOTOF specific assessment areas	Personal activities of daily living (ADL) – four basic tasks: • Feeding • Washing • Drinking • Dressing	Examples of skill sub-component include: • Reaching • Scanning • Sequencing • Naming	Performance components assessed include: • Perceptual • Cognitive • Motor • Sensory	Example deficits assessed include: • Apraxia • Dysphasia • Agnosia • Spasticity

Source: Adapted from Laver (1994).

TABLE 11.2   SOTOF: Overview of direct and indirect assessment of levels.

Level of dysfunction	Level of living systems	Levels of occupation	Levels of functional assessment
Disability	Person	Occupational performance (activities and tasks)	Task performance
Functional Limitation	Person	Skills	Skill performance
Impairment	Organs	Performance components	Components of task performance
Pathophysiology	(Not addressed)	Neuropsychological functions	(Not addressed)

Source: Laver (1994). © 1994, Alison Jane Laver.

As can be seen in Tables 11.1 and 11.2, the SOTOF (Laver 1994; Laver and Powell 1995) identifies information related to four different levels of functioning:

- **Disability level:** The patient's residual occupational performance in the domain of ADL through structured observation to assess the person's ability to perform simple ADL tasks, such as feeding and dressing.
- **Function Limitation:** The patient's residual and deficit skills and abilities within ADL performance; activity analysis was used to break down each ADL task into its component parts, and these are assessed through structured observation (for example: reaching, scanning, grasping, and sequencing).
- **Impairment:** SOTOF provides a method for identifying the performance components (perceptual, cognitive, motor, and sensory) that have been affected.
- **Pathophysiology:** At this level, a diagnostic reasoning process leads to the identification of the specific neuropsychological deficits that are impacting ADL self-care function (for example: apraxia, agnosia, aphasia, spasticity).

Assessment at each of these four levels is used to address different assessment objectives that are addressed through different assessment questions:

- **Disability level:** *How* does the person perform ADL tasks, independently or dependently?
- **Functional limitation level:** *What* skills and abilities does the person have intact, and what skills and abilities have been reduced or altered by the neurological damage?
- **Impairment level:** *Which* of the perceptual, cognitive, motor, and sensory performance components have been impacted by the neurological damage?
- **Pathophysiology level:** *Why* is function impaired? This involves the identification of *cause* through the naming of the specific neurological deficits and underlying pathology.

For more information on diagnostic reasoning, see Chapter 6.

Laver (1994) also used the NCMRR model as a basis from which to compare and contrast three other observational assessments with the SOTOF (Laver and Powell

1995). The three standardised tests critiqued were the Arnadottir OT-ADL Neurobehavioural Evaluation (*A-ONE*; Árnadóttir 1990), the Assessment of Motor and Process Skills (*AMPS*; Fisher 1993), and the Kitchen Task Assessment (*KTA*; Baum and Edwards 1993). A summary critique of these measures (at the point of their development in 1994) can be found in Table 11.3. Using the NCMRR model as a basis for comparison of the test domains addressed by the four measures:

- The A-ONE was found to address similar domains to the SOTOF across the levels of disability (occupational performance), functional limitation (skills), impairment (performance components), and pathophysiology (neuropsychological deficits); at the level of impairment, both addressed the function of the perceptual, cognitive, motor, and sensory systems.
- The AMPS focused on levels that could be directly observed, and addressed the levels of disability (occupational performance – instrumental ADL) and functional limitation (motor and process skills).
- The KTA provided assessment at the levels of disability, functional limitation, and impairment, but at the level of impairment the KTA focused only on cognitive function.

TABLE 11.3   Critique of A-ONE, AMPS, and KTA.

Test critique criteria	A-ONE	AMPS	KTA
NCMRR (1992) **Levels of function addressed** (*Focus level in italics*)	*Disability* Functional Limitation Impairment Pathophysiology	*Disability* Functional Limitation	*Disability* Functional Limitation
Occupational performance domain	4 Personal ADL tasks: dressing, grooming and hygiene, transfers and mobility, and feeding.	3 Instrumental ADL tasks selected from a list by patient and occupational therapist, for example: making a bed, vacuuming, and fixing a salad.	1 Instrumental ADL task: making cooked pudding. Test focuses on the identification of cognitive components (e.g. initiation, safety, organisation, and sequencing).
Ecological validity related to test environment	Can be performed in patient's own setting at home or in hospital.	Can be performed in patient's own setting at home or in hospital.	Performed in occupational therapist's kitchen or patient's own kitchen.
Ecological validity related to test task and materials	Tasks are basic, universal personal ADL tasks, which are relevant to all ages, both sexes, and patients from different cultural backgrounds.	Patients have some choice in the tasks used, but choice is restricted to a list, and the method for performing task is prescribed.	No choice in task. Method prescribed by instructions. May lack relevance and familiarity for some patients.
Clinical utility related to availability and cost	Test described in a published book, forms have to be purchased, and therapists have to pay to attend a training course. Need to purchase test materials, e.g. food items.	Test outlined in an unpublished manual which is provided by the author on completion of a 1 week training course. Need to purchase test materials.	Test published in *American Journal of Occupational Therapy* (AJOT) and is freely available. No training required. Need to purchase test items.

(Continued)

TABLE 11.3   (Continued)

Test critique criteria	A-ONE	AMPS	KTA
Subject group for whom test designed	Adult and older adult patients with suspected CNS damage.	Adults and older adults.	Adults with suspected dementia.
Normative standards	79 volunteers of both sexes age ranging from 19 to 89. Normative standards for older adults (60+ years) based on a sample of 35.	Studies on various adult populations are still in progress.	No normative data.
Suitability of test for early intervention	Lower-level personal activities of daily living (PADL), but client needs to mobilise to a sink/bathroom.	Higher-level instrumental activities of daily living (IADL), client has to mobilise to gather test items.	Can be used to identify how cognitive deficits impact performance on an IADL task and what cues are required for independent function.

Source: Laver (1994). © 1994, Alison Jane Laver.

McFadyen and Pratt (1997) used Laver's work as a starting point in a review of Measures of Work Performance. Table 11.4 shows how McFadyen and Pratt applied the NCMRR model to provide a conceptual framework for planning assessment and interventions related to work performance.

However, despite its obvious uses, the NCMRR model does not offer an adequate working model for practice and research on its own as it only provides broad descriptions of the levels. A conceptual model of functional performance and performance dysfunction also needs to encompass those personal factors (such as age, gender, and cultural, social, and education backgrounds) that can impact performance. The model needs to account for the social and physical environment available to support (and in some cases hinder) functional performance. Life span, cultural, and environmental issues are considered important within the AHP's domain of concern.

International Classification of Functioning, Disability, and Health (ICF)

One of the most widely recognised and accepted system for defining function was developed by the WHO and was initially called the International Classification of Impairments, Disabilities, and Handicaps, more recently updated to ICF (see resources at chapter end). The purpose was to provide a framework for classifying the consequences of injuries and disease (Hammell 2004). The WHO originally developed in 1980 a three-level hierarchy of dysfunction of Impairments, Disabilities, and Handicap (see https://www.who.int/classifications/international-classification-of-functioning-disability-and-health), updated to a model of disability based on the biopsychosocial model (Engel 1981) with the levels of Body Functions and Structures, Activity, and Participation as can be seen in Figure 11.4.

In ICF, the term *functioning* refers to all body functions, activities, and participation, whereas *disability* is similarly an umbrella term for impairments, activity limitations,

TABLE 11.4 Application of the NCMRR model to measures of, and interventions for, work performance.

Societal limitation	Disability	Functional limitation	Impairment	Pathophysiology
Restriction attributable to social policy or barriers (structural or attitudinal), which limits fulfilment of roles or denies access to services or opportunities	Inability or limitation in performing socially defined activities and tasks within a social and physical environment as a result of internal or external factors and their interplay.	Restriction or lack of ability to perform an action or activity in the manner or range considered normal that results from impairment.	Loss and/or abnormality of mental, emotional, physiological, or anatomical structure or function; including secondary losses and pain.	Interference of normal physiological and developmental processes or structures.
Performance of roles and occupations by the person in societal context	Performance of activity or task by the person in physical and social context.	Performance of sub-components of tasks or activities.	Organs or organ systems.	Cells and tissues.
Example roles: worker, friend, parent, spouse	Performance areas: Productivity, including work-related activities and educational activities; personal and instrumental activities of daily living: leisure activities.	Process components: initiate, organise, sequence, judge, attend, select. Gross motor components: sit, roll, lift, scoop, squat, stand, reach; Fine motor: pinch, grip, grasp, hold, release. Interpersonal components: relate, interact, cope, manage.	Physiological and psychological functioning related to the cognitive and perceptual systems; sensory system; and motor system.	Physiological deficits Neurological deficits Immunological deficits
	Context: physical environment; social environment; cognitive environment.			
Barriers/issues: recreation, attitudes, accommodation, quality of life				
Examples of work performance measures	Examples of work performance measures	Examples of work performance measures	Examples of work performance measures	Examples of work performance measures
Role and interest inventories; Occupational Stress Inventory; Community Profile	Functional Capacity Assessment (FCAs), e.g. ERGOS, EPIC, WEST, Valpar Work Samples.	General Clerical Test (GCT-R); vocational aptitude tests.	McGill Pain Questionnaire, Perceived Stress scale.	Goniometry, Strength capacities.

Source: McFadyen and Pratt (1997). © 1997, SAGE Publications.

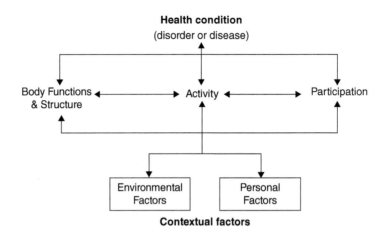

FIGURE 11.4   Representation of the ICF model of disability. Source: WHO (2002). © 2002, World Health Organization.

and participation restrictions. ICF also lists environmental factors that interact with all these components. The formal definitions are provided in the box below.

Body Functions are physiological functions of body systems (including psychological functions).

Body Structures are anatomical parts of the body such as organs, limbs, and their components.

Impairments are problems in body function or structure such as a significant deviation or loss.

Activity is the execution of a task or action by an individual.

Participation is involvement in a life situation.

Activity Limitations are difficulties an individual may have in executing activities.

Participation Restrictions are problems an individual may experience in involvement in life situations.

Environmental Factors make up the physical, social, and attitudinal environment in which people live and conduct their lives.

Source: WHO (2002). © 2002, World Health Organization.

The ICF is a classification system that aims to provide a common language for understanding and researching health and health-related states. The ICF is considered to be a particularly valuable tool for AHPs because it integrates the medical and social models. An example of an AHP outcome measure based on the ICF is the Therapy Outcomes Measure (*TOM*; Enderby et al. 2013). The conceptual foundation from the TOM was based on the WHO model. TOM provides a global measure of health outcomes and can be used with clients across the age range and with a wide variety of diagnoses. Table 11.5 gives an overview of the ICF showing the components, domains, and constructs, and delineating the related contextual factors that require consideration. It also contrasts the positive and negative aspects.

In 2011, Rimmer and colleagues proposed an approach to using the ICF to identify, prevent, and manage *secondary* as well as primary conditions in people with disabilities. They provided potential management strategies for the theoretical consequences of secondary conditions categorised into the three domains of the ICF (see Figure 11.5).

TABLE 11.5   An overview of the ICF (WHO 2001).

	Part 1: Functioning and Disability		Part 2: Contextual Factors	
Components	Body functions and structures	Activities and Participation	Environmental Factors	Personal Factors
Domains	Body functions and structures	Life areas (tasks, actions)	External influences on functioning and disability	Internal influences on functioning and disability
Constructs	Change in body functions (physiological) Change in body structures (anatomical)	Capacity Executing tasks in a standard environment Performance Executing tasks in the current environment	Facilitating or hindering impact of features of the physical, social, and attitudinal world	Impact of attributes of the person
Positive aspect	Functional and structural integrity	Activities Participation	Facilitators	Not applicable
	Functioning			
Negative aspect	Impairment	Activity limitation Participation restriction	Barriers/hindrances	Not applicable
	Disability			

Source: WHO (2001). © 2001, World Health Organization.

Many AHPs welcomed WHO's revised classification; for example, McDonald et al. (2004) stated that 'the ICF is an important and exciting development because of its holistic framework and concentration on function and health, rather than disease-based models of disability, and places the individual ... at the core of the health care process' (p. 299).

The ICF has been adopted by AHPs in many countries (Prodinger et al. 2015). As AHPs are client-centred practitioners, there is a good fit between AHP practice and the ICF model's mandate to place attention in health evaluation and research to insider perspectives of people with disability (McGruder 2004).

The ICF has also met with some criticism. Chard (2004) reports that the ICF definition of disability is based on a concept of function, whereas some people in the disability movement do not accept this definition of disability and consider that the attitudes of individuals and society have a greater link with disability than impairments. Hammell (2004) offers 'a sceptical interrogation of the classificatory practices of the ICF' (p. 408). She reminds AHPs that the ICF offers only a classification system and a scientific coding system and are 'systems for classifying and documenting deviations from assumed norms' and 'are not needs assessments' (p. 410). Hammell reviews literature from disability theorists and warns: 'Although the intent of classifying, measuring and statistically analysing the divergence from assumed norms may, at times, be benign, the consequence for those classified as abnormal can be devastating ... On the basis of classification, disabled people are denied medical interventions ... physically segregated within their communities ... and confined with institutions ...' (p. 409) 'The ICF is not a client-oriented tool, but one to enable professionals to code, to categorise and to compile statistics' (p. 410).

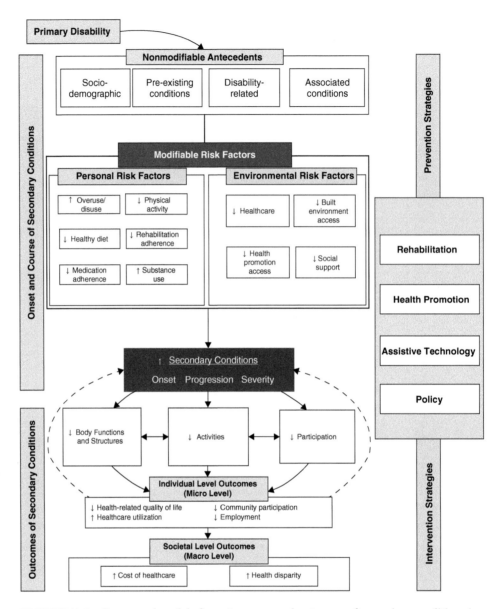

FIGURE 11.5   Conceptual model of onset, course, and outcomes of secondary conditions in people with disabilities. Source: From Rimmer et al. (2011). © 2011, Oxford University Press.

With this in mind, care needs to be taken to maintain an overall holistic focus throughout the assessment process that values the views of the client and carer as paramount throughout and in which the AHP thinks explicitly about their clinical judgements and has a clear rationale for the frameworks they select to help gather data and form these judgements. McDougall et al. (2010) offered a modified ICF model based on a systems perspective which depicts a holistic view that acknowledges the intertwining of health, functioning, life quality, and development, and that these are essential concepts to consider in the lives of all people.

Applying the ICF to AHP Assessment

The WHO (2002) reported that studies showed that diagnosis alone did not predict service needs, length of hospitalisation, level of care, or functional outcomes. In addition, the presence of a disease or disorder is not 'an accurate predictor of receipt of disability benefits, work performance, return to work potential, or likelihood of social integration' (p. 4). A medical classification of diagnoses on its own is not sufficient for making an individual prognosis and treatment plan or for wider service planning and management purposes. What is also required is data about levels of functioning and disability. AHPs with an understanding of the ICF can supplement the information provided by the diagnosis (which may be classified using the International Classification of Disease *ICD*-11 – https://icd.who.int/en) and help to demonstrate how this diagnosis influences the person or diagnostic group in daily life. The model can also provide a framework for exploring how access to physical and social supports has an enabling or disabling effect on an individual or group.

The WHO (2002) provided a section on how the ICF can be applied for service provision at the level of individual clients or at a service or institutional level, and can be applied more widely for a population, community, or at a social policy level. The potential applications of the ICF at the individual, institutional, and social levels are shown in the following box.

ICF Applications: Service Provision

At the individual level

- For the assessment of individuals: *What is the person's level of functioning?*
- For individual treatment planning: *What treatments or interventions can maximise functioning?*
- For the evaluation of treatment and other interventions: *What are the outcomes of the treatment? How useful were the interventions?*
- For communication among physicians, nurses, physiotherapists, occupational therapists, and other health workers, social service workers, and community agencies
- For self-evaluation by consumers: *How would I rate my capacity in mobility or communication?*

At the institutional level

- For educational and training purposes
- For resource planning and development: *What health care and other services will be needed?*
- For quality improvement: *How well do we serve our clients? What basic indicators for quality assurance are valid and reliable?*
- For management and outcome evaluation: *How useful are the services we are providing?*
- For managed care models of healthcare delivery: *How cost-effective are the services we provide? How can the service be improved for better outcomes at a lower cost?*

At the social level

- For eligibility criteria for state entitlements such as social security benefits, disability pensions, workers' compensation and insurance: *Are the criteria for eligibility for disability benefits evidence based, appropriate to social goals and justifiable?*
- For social policy development, including legislative reviews, model legislation, regulations and guidelines, and definitions for anti-discrimination

(continued)

(continued)

> legislation: *Will guaranteeing rights improve functioning at the societal level? Can we measure this improvement and adjust our policy and law accordingly?*
>
> - For needs assessments: *What are the needs of persons with various levels of disability – impairments, activity limitations and participation restrictions?*
> - For environmental assessment for universal design, implementation of mandated accessibility, identification of environmental facilitators and barriers, and changes to social policy: *How can we make the social and built environment more accessible for all persons, those with and those without disabilities? Can we assess and measure improvement?*
>
> *From ICF Beginners Guide, p. 6* https://cdn.who.int/media/docs/default-source/classification/icf/icfbeginnersguide.pdf?sfvrsn=eead63d3_4
>
> *Source:* WHO (2002). © 2002, World Health Organization.

A number of AHP organisations have used the ICF model to assist with the classification of various assessments and measures in terms of the domains and levels of functioning addressed. The [Royal] College of Occupational Therapists (*COT* 2004) provides a table common outcome measures categorised within an ICF framework. This is provided in Table 11.6.

McDonald et al. (2004), offer a detailed case for using the ICF model as a theoretical basis for adaptive seating system assessment and provision. The authors state that the ICF allows them to address the possible conflicts that arise 'between the medical model of reducing or delaying impairment of body functions and structures and the social model of children and families accessing life and environmental situations through mobility and seating equipment' (p. 293). Their paper uses the domains of the ICF to structure their literature review. They conclude that applying the ICF model in clinical practice when providing adaptive seating gives AHPs 'both a

TABLE 11.6 Common AHP outcome measures categorised within an ICF framework.

	Body function/ structure	Activity	Participation	Contextual issues
Barthel Index	✓	✓		
Canadian Occupational Performance Measure (COPM)		✓	✓	
Community Dependency Index			✓	✓
MINI-MENTAL STATE EXAMINATION	✓			
Bayer ADL (B-ADL)		✓	✓	
Structured Observational Test of Function (SOTOF)	✓			
Falls Efficacy Scale		✓	✓	

Source: COT (2004). © 2004, Royal College of Occupational Therapists.

powerful tool for communicating with children and families as well as managers and a basis for evaluating practice' (p. 293).

Fisher (2003) described the relationship of her Assessment of Motor and Process Skills (AMPS) to the ICF (WHO 2002). At the Activities level, AHPs use the AMPS to 'evaluate activity and activity limitations when they implement performance analyses and evaluate the quality of the goal-directed actions performed as part of a complex activity (e.g. daily life task)' (p. 27). At the level of participation, Fisher notes that the 'interpretation of the performance analysis ... yields information at the level of participation' when the AHP addresses the question: 'is the quality and the level of the person's performance at an expected level of achievement given the personal, environmental, and societal factors that may be facilitating or hindering the person's performance?' (p. 27). As an example, she states: 'Once we progress to the idea that a person experiences increased effort and decreased efficiency when buttoning because the size of the buttons on the shirt are hindering his ability to manipulate buttons, we have progressed to analysis at the level of participation' (p. 27).

The Australian Therapy Outcome Measures for Occupational Therapy (Aus-TOMs-OT) closely aligns with the ICF and was developed to measure Impairment, Activity/Activity Limitation, and Distress/Wellbeing, as well as participation/participation restriction outcomes (Abu-Awad et al. 2014). An exploratory study of 60 Dutch physiotherapists by van Dulmen et al. (2017) identified five patient-related outcome measures (PROMs) feasible for use in clinical practice that could be used for identifying an ICF core set which matches the PROMs used.

'Top-down' Versus 'Bottom-up' Assessment Approach

Rogers and Holm (1989) proposed a Functional Assessment Hierarchy comprising four levels (see Figure 11.6). When the AHP is framing the problem, selecting a theoretical framework, and choosing related assessment strategies and tools, an important decision to be made is whether to take a 'top-down' or 'bottom-up'

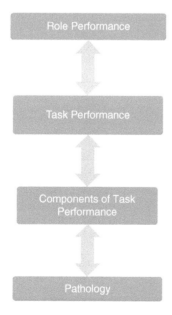

FIGURE 11.6   Hierarchy of functional assessment. *Source:* Rogers and Holm (1989). © 1989, American Occupational Therapy Association, Inc.

approach to the assessment process. Some assessments simultaneously collect data from several levels of function, but usually an assessment tool or strategy just focuses on data at one or two levels of function. For example, the AHP, therefore, has to decide at which level to begin the assessment process. A 'top-down' assessment begins at the *Role Performance* level of the Rogers and Holm (1989) hierarchy and 'determines which particular tasks define each of the roles for that person, whether he or she can now do those tasks, and the probable reason for an inability to do so' (Trombly 1993, p. 253).

- If you were using an NCMRR model (see Figure 11.3) as a framework for assessment, then a top-down approach would start assessment at the levels of societal limitation and disability.
- If you were using the ICF (WHO 2002, see Figure 11.4) model as a framework for assessment, then a top-down approach would start assessment at the levels of participation, contextual, and environment factors.

A 'bottom-up' assessment begins at the levels of *Pathology* and *Components of Task Performance* on the Rogers and Holm Functional Assessment Hierarchy (1989). A bottom-up approach 'focuses on the deficits of components of function, such as strength, range of movement (ROM), balance, and so on, which are believed to be prerequisites to successful occupational performance' (Trombly 1993, p. 253).

- If you were using a NCMRR (1992) model as a framework for assessment, then a bottom-up approach would start assessment at the levels of Pathophysiology and Impairment.
- If you were using the ICF (WHO 2002) model as a framework for assessment, then a bottom-up approach would start assessment at the levels of body structures and functions and impairments.

The 'bottom-up' approach can be associated with a medical model and has been popular in the past (Brown and Chien 2010). Its advantage is that it provides the AHP with important information about underlying performance component functioning of the individual. However, a disadvantage to the 'bottom-up' approach is that the purpose of the assessment, and ensuing treatment plan, may not be obvious to the person and may therefore lack meaning and relevance.

An example of the bottom-up approach is when the occupational therapist detects that a client who is referred to occupational therapy for remediation of occupational dysfunction (e.g. lack of independence in self-care) lacks sitting balance. Because sitting balance is considered to be an ability required to dress independently, the therapist may begin treatment by engaging the client in activities to improve balance. The occupational therapist may not make clear to the client the connection between the component deficit and occupational functioning. The outcome desired by the occupational therapist may or may not be congruent with important goals of the client or even with the client's perceived reason for receiving occupational therapy services. Confusion and dissatisfaction may result.

(Trombly 1993, p. 253)

Rogers (2004) also expresses some reservations about a reliance on a bottom-up approach:

For example, knowing that a client has rheumatoid arthritis, the evaluation may begin with measures of pinch strength. Having ascertained that the client exerts 1.5 pounds of pinch on the right (dominant) and 5 pounds on the left, the practitioner might infer that the client is unable to prepare meals due to inadequate pinch strength. This is a weak diagnostic statement because it is based on prediction or inference about performance supported by impairment testing but not activity testing.

(p. 27)

In contrast, the 'top-down' approach begins at the level of the person as a whole and starts by investigating past and present role competency and by evaluating the person's current ability to perform meaningful tasks from his previous daily activities. Fisher (2003) recommends that AHPs should take a top-down approach:

... we must stress a top-down approach to assessment that begins with the ability of the individual to perform the daily life tasks that he or she wants and needs to perform to be able to fulfil his or her roles competently and with satisfaction. These common daily life tasks are meaningful and purposeful to the person who performs them. In contrast to a bottom-up approach that focuses on impairments and capacity limitations, a top-down approach focus on quality of occupational performance as the person interacts with the physical and social environment in the context of his or her roles.

(p. 2)

A 'top-down' approach helps the AHP to gain an early understanding of the person's values and needs. When the person experiences a discrepancy between previous role and task performance during the assessment process, then he can see the need for treatment and will find greater meaning and relevancy in the resultant treatment plan (Trombly 1993). A 'top-down' approach facilitates the development of a partnership between the AHP and person, in which the person feels valued and understood as a unique individual. Explaining clearly to the person the rationale for both assessment and treatment is essential for joint decision making and the negotiation of goals and is a critical part of client-centred practice (Sumsion 2000).

As an AHP you need to ensure that the person can make a truly informed choice as to whether to engage with the proposed assessment and treatment. If the person understands and accepts the rationale, this helps to build trust and rapport and to enhance his motivation to engage with rehabilitation. The 'top-down' approach, thereby, helps to clarify the purpose of therapy for the person. The approach also helps the AHP form an accurate picture of the person and his problem(s) that is critical for the identification of relevant and meaningful treatment goals. In a review of research and clinical literature pertaining to the Canadian Occupational Performance Measure (*COPM*), Carswell et al. (2004) found that the COPM was 'ideally suited to what ... Trombly ... called the top-down approach to assessment, where occupational performance problems are identified first, and then the underlying causes are further assessed using measures of performance components' (p. 219).

CONCLUSION

The models presented are not assessments in themselves but rather frameworks for assisting healthcare professionals to classify domains and constructs of concern. Models can aid communication between different professionals and can support the identification and documentation of unmet needs. Frameworks such as the NCMRR and ICF enable healthcare professionals to identify when people vary in some aspect of function from culturally specific norms. It is important to remember that some of these models are criticised by people within the disability movement (Chard 2004; Hammell 2004). When using such models for pragmatic reasons to assist in your assessment processes, it is important to maintain a wider systems perspective that keeps considering the whole as well as the parts and stays focused on a client-centred approach.

Case Study – Mary

Mary is an 83-year-old woman living alone who fell in the night when she got up to go to the toilet. She was unable to get herself up and had lain on the floor for four-and-a-half hours. She was found when one of her daughters, Anne, popped in to check on her the next morning. Mary was cold and shaken and complained of severe pain in her left forearm. Anne telephoned her sister Liz for help; she felt her mother needed to go to hospital but also had the responsibility of taking her young children to school. Liz lived in a village a 15 minute drive away. When she arrived she agreed with her sister that their mother needed to see a doctor and discussed the possibility that she could have broken a bone in her arm. They persuaded Mary that she should go to the Community Hospital's Minor Injury Unit (*MIU*) and be checked over. When Liz and Mary arrived at the MIU she was assessed promptly and sent to have her arm X-rayed. The X-ray showed that Mary had sustained a Colles fracture.

So, at the *pathophysiology level* of the NCMRR model of function and at the *body function/structure* level of the ICF, the doctor identified damage to bone; a Colles fracture occurs at the lower end of the radius and occurs with posterior displacement of the distal fragment. Colles fractures are most often sustained when a person is moving forwards with their wrist in supination, for example, reaching out with a hand to help break a fall. Colles fractures are particularly common in older people, and an increased risk of sustaining a Colles fracture is associated with osteoporosis and falls (Padegimas and Osei 2013).

Mary's wrist was put in a plaster cast, which she was told would need to stay on for about six weeks while her fracture healed. Mary wished to return home, but her daughter, Liz, told the doctor in the MIU that her mother would find it very difficult to cope at home alone, particularly as she doubted that her mother would be able to manage her walking frame with a plaster on her arm. Liz was very anxious about her mother being discharged home and keen to see her admitted to hospital, at least for a few days. The daughter reported that she and her sister already needed to visit their mother two or three times a day prior to the fall and that she had been barely coping at home on her own for the last year.

Referral

Staff in the MIU explained to Mary and Liz that there was a Rapid Response Service that might be able to help Mary return home safely. They both agreed, and the unit nurse rang the Rapid Response office, which is on the same site. The social worker was on duty and after taking contact details on the telephone, came to the unit to discuss the situation with Mary and her daughter. The social worker began the EASY-Care method for personalised assessment (https://www.cgakit.com/s-1-easy-care-standard-2010) in the MIU by completing the personal background information section. She also sought some basic details from Mary and her daughter about the home situation prior to the fall and the problems that they both anticipated if Mary did return home with her arm in a plaster cast. She established that Mary definitely did want to return home and had good insight into the constraints that she would be under with the plaster on her arm. The social worker decided that this was an appropriate referral. She explained to Mary that the team could put in visits to help her with aspects of her personal care that she could not manage and that they would try and help her regain her confidence and independence, so that she could continue to live independently in her own home. The social worker also reassured Liz that she would not be expected to do more than she was already doing, and that the team would visit as many times as was necessary to keep her mother safe. When both Liz and her mother agreed to the involvement of the Rapid Response Service, the social worker helped Liz to get her mother to the car and informed them that members of the team would meet them at Mary's house within an hour. The social worker returned to the office to discuss with the occupational therapist (John) and physiotherapist what would be the best approach to maintaining Mary's safety and independence at home.

Initial Visit and First Assessment

When a new referral comes in, the Rapid Response Team allocate the most appropriate workers to undertake the initial assessment. Mary lived in a three-bedroom cottage in a village in the Yorkshire Dales. On presentation, she appeared upset about her fall and her time at the MIU and was extremely anxious about being forced to give up her home and move into a residential or nursing home. She was seated in an armchair by the coal fire. She was still in considerable pain from her arm and she had not yet had any lunch. Her daughter Liz was obviously anxious about the situation.

Interviewing a Proxy to Identify Social Supports and Needs

Kate (Physiotherapist) and John (Occupational Therapist) began the assessment process by introducing themselves to Mary and her daughter and explaining the role of the Rapid Response Service. Liz offered a cup of tea, and the support worker went into the kitchen with her to obtain an informal proxy report of Mary's needs and the current level of care provided by Liz and her sister. At a *societal limitation level* (NCMRR), they needed to assess the support available to Mary to enable her to live safely on her own at home. Liz reported that she and her sister shared the care of their mother and that her need for support had increased significantly over the past year. Mary had not received any regular visits from any health or social services staff prior to her fall. Carer burden needed to be assessed as both Mary's daughters had young children to support and, as their husbands were farmers, they both had responsibilities with farm work. Her daughters would not have the capacity to offer all the support that Mary would require at home while her arm was in plaster.

Collecting Self-Report Data to Obtain History of the Present Condition

Kate began by interviewing Mary in the living room and observed that Mary had an electric armchair that moved her into a semi-standing position to assist transfers. On enquiry, Mary stated that she had purchased the chair three years ago and found it very comfortable and useful. Kate began seeking information at a *pathophysiology level* by asking Mary and her daughter to outline any past medical problems. They reported that Mary had widespread osteoarthritis. She reported that her left hip had been replaced eight years ago and her right knee had been replaced three years ago. Mary had some degree of heart failure, which was monitored by her General Practitioner (*GP*). Kate observed that Mary has signs of oedema, particularly in her feet and calves, and she enquired whether Mary had any problems with swelling. Mary reported that her 'legs felt heavy all the time', and she said that she often had difficulty getting her shoes on because of the swelling. Mary explained that she had been told to keep her legs up, and this was another reason that she had bought the electrically operated chair as it enabled her to get her legs into a raised position. Her daughter informed Kate that Mary had developed cellulitis last year and the District Nurse had visited regularly until it had cleared up. Cellulitis is an acute inflammation of the connective tissue of the skin, caused by infection with staphylococcus, streptococcus, or other bacteria. Cellulitis is most common on the face or, as in Mary's case, the lower legs. Kate undertook an informal observational assessment of Mary's physical function, which included assessment of:

- Strength
- ROM
- Pain
- Posture
- Abnormal tone

When Kate undertook a physical examination of Mary's lower limbs, she found that her left knee was now very stiff with reduced range of movement (ROM), but her replaced knee had good range of movement. Decreased ROM can affect balance when the restricted ROM leads to postural compensations that affect the ability of the person to react quickly to losses of balance.

Initial Informal Observational Assessment

At a *societal limitation level*, John needed to assess the physical home environment, particularly looking for factors which would increase the risk of falls, and factors which would hamper Mary's independence. Mary's house had very steep stairs with a banister on only one side (banister to the left side when going upstairs). John felt that an immediate referral was required to have a banister put up on the wall on the other side so that Mary could have a banister to hold onto with her right hand while both going up and down the stairs. Mary's house had a bathroom and toilet upstairs, and her bedroom was next door to the bathroom. The bathroom had a small shower cubicle in it and a bath. The bedroom contained a single bed and was reasonably spacious.

At a *disability level,* John and Kate needed to assess Mary's ability to perform transfers on and off her chair, bed, and toilet as well as risk-assess the safety of ascending and descending the stairs. They were concerned about how Mary would be able to use the toilet in the night when she would be alone. John explained to Mary that it was important to see how well she could move about her home and to assess her ability to get on and off her chair, bed, and toilet. Mary could use her electric armchair well to get on and off the chair, and she managed to stand safely with the walking frame. However, she had great difficulty walking unaccompanied as she found it hard to lift the frame with her arm in plaster. With the help of one person, she walked to the base of the stairs, but she was not able to safely ascend the stairs as the hand rail was on the side of her fractured wrist. There was no possibility of bringing a bed downstairs as both downstairs rooms were very small. Therefore, Kate asked Mary to try ascending sideways up the stairs, using her good hand on the stair rail. This took a long time but Kate was reassured that at all times Mary was safe. Kate then asked Mary to attempt to get on and off the toilet. This presented her with more difficulties as she was used to pulling herself up using her now fractured arm and the basin. John hypothesised that the purchase of an electrically operated armchair had led to a decrease in quadriceps strength because she no longer had to use muscles actively to go from sitting to standing. Finally, John assessed Mary's transfer on and off the bed. This was not easy as Mary had her wrist in plaster and, because her abdominal muscles were weak, she had difficulty getting from lying to sitting. Mary reported that she usually liked to go to bed quite early (by 9 o'clock). She also reported that she had fallen twice at night.

John had taken a commode in his car in case this was needed. He assessed Mary's ability to transfer on and off the commode independently. However, when he assessed Mary's transfer between her bed and the commode, he felt this was not safe while Mary had her wrist in plaster. Therefore, in order to remain at home while her arm was in plaster, Mary was going to require a night-time visit. Kate asked Mary how often she usually got up in the night to go to the toilet and whether the time varied or was at a similar time each night. Mary reported that she usually got up once, and this tended to be between 3 and 4 a.m. Kate made a note to refer Mary to the neighbourhood night service for a 3 a.m. visit to assist with toileting and decided to leave the commode at the bedside as a transfer from bed to commode would be less demanding for Mary in the night than mobilising across the landing to the toilet. The journey downstairs was safer as the handrail was on the side of the other arm. However, by the time Mary had returned to her seat, she was exhausted and rather tearful.

Mary did have a downstairs toilet, but this was outside in the yard and necessitated a step down at the backdoor and a step up into the toilet. John, therefore, decided to recommend that Mary should have a second commode in her living room for daytime use. Mary would also need assistance to transfer on and off this commode, and regular visits throughout the day would be required to prevent problems with incontinence or risk of falls if Mary attempted the transfer alone.

At the end of the assessment, Kate and John analysed the information collected and considered potential solutions for identified problems. Mary's presenting problems are summarised in Table 11.7.

One model for prioritising areas of need for intervention is Maslow's hierarchy of needs (Maslow 1943). The lowest level of need is the **Physiological level**; at this level, basic needs such as food, drink, warmth, and sleep must be addressed. The next level is the **Safety level**, and the need for security from danger, and providing a roof over your head are considered at this level. Once these basic needs are addressed, the next level is **Social needs**, and this includes experiencing love, belonging, friendship, and being able to engage in social activities. The fourth level

TABLE 11.7 Using the NCMRR model to provide a conceptual framework for describing Mary's presenting problems.

Societal Limitation	Disability	Functional Limitation	Impairment	Pathophysiology
Social Worker: For example, social supports, carer assessment, benefits eligibility	**Occupational Therapist:** For example, tasks, activities, and occupations such as person care, domestic chores, work, and leisure activities	**Physiotherapist:** For example, balance and gait, gross movement patterns such as bridging and rolling – focus on lower limb	**Doctor** Neurological tests for vision, coordination, sensation, and assessment of pain	**Doctor:** For example, diagnosis of the type, location, and possible cause of stroke. Neurological tests for muscle strength and reflexes
Occupational Therapist: For example, roles, physical and social environment to assess person-environment-occupation fit, carer's resources and emotional and physical care-giver burden	**Physiotherapist** For example, mobility and transfers	**Occupational Therapist:** For example, reaching, manipulating, bilateral integration, sequencing task – focusing on upper limb	**Physiotherapist** Motor system (e.g. range of movement) and sensory system (e.g. pain)	**Radiologist:** For example, magnetic resonance imaging (MRI)
	Social Worker For example, level of independence in activities to assess for long-term care needs	**Speech and Language Therapist** Mastication, swallowing, coordination of movements of mouth and tongue	**Speech and Language Therapist** Cognitive and motor functioning	**Physiotherapist** At a tissue level examine specific muscle weakness and tone (spasticity and flaccidity)
	Speech and Language Therapist Eating and drinking	**Psychologist:** For example, recall, attention, recognition	**Psychologist:** For example, cognitive and perceptual functioning	**Speech and Language Therapist** Choking and swallowing reflexes. Diagnosis of neurological deficits: dysphasia and dysarthria
	Nurse: For example, sleep, feeding, washing, and dressing		**Nurse:** For example, blood pressure, temperature, pain	

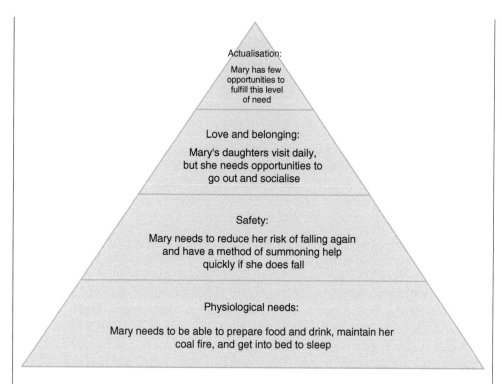

FIGURE 11.7   Mary's needs categorised using Maslow's hierarchy of needs. Source: Based on Maslow (1943).

in the hierarchy is the **Esteem level**; at this level, people need to achieve self-respect, respect from others, and a sense of achievement. Finally, the highest level of needs is **Self-Actualisation**, and this relates to the need for personal growth and development, the opportunity for creativity and for using our talents to their full potential. See Figure 11.7 for the assessment of Mary's hierarchy of needs.

At the most basic physiological level of need, Mary needs to be warm, to eat and drink, to pass urine and move her bowels, to wash and dress, and to sleep. The assessment has identified specific areas of difficulty at this level. At the safety level, the assessment highlighted some significant areas of risk related to difficulties with mobility and transfers. Mary showed that she had insight, cognitive capacity to make an informed choice about areas of risk, and determination to remain in her own home. The problem areas needed both an immediate problem-solving approach and also a more long-term analysis of how the environment might be altered to create a safer living situation. Taking each area of essential need and considering it over a 24-hour period is a useful method of assessing a problem and searching for solutions:

1. **Nutrition**: Breakfast – her daughter will come and organise after taking her children to school. Lunch will be made by a support worker. Evening meal – her other daughter will come at about 6.00 p.m. to prepare Mary's tea.

2. **Elimination:** Mary will need to use the toilet when she wakes, after breakfast, lunchtime, late afternoon, early evening, before going to bed, and during the night. A support worker will assist Mary to get out of bed in morning and use a commode (to be supplied by Rapid Response Service). After breakfast and in the evening her daughters can supervise use of the downstairs commode/toilet. Lunchtime and late afternoon, the support

worker visits can supervise use of the downstairs commode or outside toilet. The evening service will visit between 8 and 9 p.m., supervise going upstairs and use of the toilet, and help Mary out of her clothes and into bed. The night service will visit at 3.00 a.m. and help Mary out of bed and onto the commode (the key will need to be signed for and handed over to night service).

3. **Locomotion/exercise:** Support worker will supervise Mary when she descends the stairs. Mary was told that the support worker will not be standing below her as this would present a risk for the support worker if Mary was to fall on top of her. At the lunchtime and late afternoon visits, the support worker will be instructed to encourage Mary to do some walking around the ground floor of the house and to do some chair-based exercises.

4. **Warmth:** The support worker will light the coal fire in the morning, and Mary's daughters will feed it on their visits as will the support workers.

5. **Cleanliness:** The support worker will supervise washing in the morning, and the evening service will do the same when getting Mary ready for bed.

All these issues were thoroughly discussed with Mary and her daughter. Mary agreed to this proposal as she was still determined that she wanted to stay at home rather than be placed in a recuperation bed in a local residential home.

Identifying Care Needs

At a *societal limitation level*, it was clear that Mary was going to need social care to support her daughters for a considerable length of time, and Kate reflected that this might also be an opportunity to broach the subject of more long-term help to reduce the strain on Mary's daughters. Kate therefore felt that it would be very useful to involve the social worker in this case. There may be possibilities of day care attendance, voluntary sitters, respite care, and ongoing carer support. Kate also felt that the whole living environment could be made safer by a range of adaptations and aids to daily living. He, therefore, wanted the occupational AHP to visit as soon as possible. However, the immediate need was to write a care plan for the support workers and the evening staff and to get the essential items of equipment. While Kate wrote the initial care plan, the support worker returned to the Joint Equipment sub-store at the hospital to get a second commode and get a form for Mary to sign to hand over a key to the house. This key was to be kept in a key safe in the hospital base. Kate informed Mary and her daughter that he would be asking the social worker and the occupational AHP to contact them on the following day.

The Support Worker's Role

When an assessment identifies the need for involvement of the Rapid Response Team's support workers, a care plan is drawn up which is aimed at encouraging independence, and the plan is discussed and agreed with the client. Support workers provide a variety of social care, occupational therapy, physiotherapy, and nursing tasks. They are not asked to perform any tasks without documented training for the specific task and are supervised by the qualified team members. All the support workers can take a monitoring as well as a rehabilitation role as they are trained to re-assess a client's progress prior to continuing their care plan.

If the support worker is concerned that the client has deteriorated since a previous visit, she informs the most relevant person (for example, her supervisor at Rapid Response, the community nursing team, or the client's GP; or will call for emergency services where necessary). Support worker involvement is time-limited to usually no more than six weeks, and Mary and her daughter were made aware of this.

When the support worker returned with the second commode, Kate educated her daughter how to supervise Mary transferring on and off it, and he placed it in the living room. Kate booked a follow-up visit to undertake some more specialist balance tests and to complete a Falls Risk Identification assessment.

When John got back to the team office, he gave the social worker a verbal description of Mary's first assessment and then began inputting the information that he had gathered so far onto the patient electronic record system.

Physiotherapy Assessment of Balance and Risk of Falls

Balance problems can result from a wide range of causes, and it is very important to assess balance to identify the root cause of any balance disorder (Sherrington and Tiedemann 2015). Browne and O'Hare (2001) give three important reasons for assessing balance:

1. 'First, it is an aid to understanding how the postural control system works' (p. 489); this addresses an assessment question at the level of *impairment*.
2. Second, it is an aid to clinical diagnosis and the assessment of treatment efficacy' (p. 489), and so may help with providing a diagnosis at the *pathophysiology* or *impairment* levels, and it provides a baseline for outcome measurement across the level(s) where intervention will be targeted.
3. 'Thirdly, it can be used to identify elderly people with a history of falls and areas where they are at risk of falling' (p. 489). This risk assessment provides predictive data that can inform the intervention and help identify those people who might most benefit from a falls programme to reduce their future risk of falls.

Physiotherapy Assessment

A guidance document written on behalf of the Chartered Society of Physiotherapy (*CSP*) by Goodwin and Briggs in 2012 suggested the following outcome measures for assessing balance:

- Berg Balance Scale
- Timed Up and Go Test
- Performance-Oriented Mobility Assessment (often called the Tinetti Scale)
- 180° turn
- Four-square step test

On this occasion, Kate used the Timed the Timed up and go test, the Performance-Oriented Mobility Assessment (known as the Tinetti Scale), and a Four Test Balance Scale (Finnegan et al. 2018; Goodwin and Briggs 2012; NICE 2013).

In addition, Kate used the Modified Falls Efficacy Scale (*m-FES*, Hill et al. 1996). Kate used these tests to establish a baseline of appropriate outcome measures, to enable an evaluation of the impact of any intervention.

Occupational Therapy Assessment

John visited Mary the following morning with the support worker to undertake a more thorough assessment of Mary's abilities in all personal and domestic ADL; this was an observational assessment undertaken at a *disability level* (NCMRR 1992). The occupational AHP planned to assess Mary's ability to:

- get dressed/undressed;
- wash;
- transfer on/off the bed, upstairs toilet, chair in living room, chair in kitchen, outside toilet;
- get up and down stairs;
- get in and out the front and back doors;
- prepare a drink and snack; and
- access help in the event of another fall.

During this assessment, John had two considerations:

1. A short-term analysis as to what Mary would be able to manage during the six weeks her arm was to be in plaster and an assessment of what aids, equipment, and support would be required to maintain Mary safely at home during the period

   In the short-term, John identified a need for a toilet frame for both the upstairs and downstairs toilets. These frames would both raise the seat by three inches, which would decrease the power needed by the quadriceps to get Mary up into standing, and also provide arms that Mary could use to push up on rather than pulling herself using the basin. John also tried a bed rail inserted under the mattress and on the side of Mary's non-fractured arm. This enabled Mary to pull herself up into sitting over the side of the bed with less difficulty and also gave her something to hold onto as she transferred to the commode. John amended the care plan to ask the night staff to supervise this transfer and if it was done safely for three nights in a row, they could stop their visits. John also provided a perching stool for the bathroom for Mary to perch on at the basin when strip washing.
2. A longer-term focus in terms of what changes might be useful to maintain Mary's independence and safety longer-term once she was out of plaster.

John identified a longer-term need for grab rails in the toilet, shower, outside the front and back doors, and a second stair rail. Mary was asked if she agreed to having these fitted, as she owned the property. She was keen to have this done, and John marked all the positions of the rails and put the order in to 'Stay Put', a local organisation that undertakes minor works for elderly and disabled clients for the cost of the materials.

When Mary had fallen, she had not been able to get herself up and had lain on the floor for four-and-a-half hours. John described the local Community Alarm

Scheme to Mary and explained how it provides a way for people like her to summon help in an emergency at home. The scheme would supply Mary with:

- A small pendant that she could wear around her neck or carry with her; this has a red button, which, when pressed, sends a signal to the telephone.
- A new telephone which would replace Mary's old one. It could receive the signal sent from the pendant from anywhere in Mary's house or garden.

John explained: 'When you press your pendant's red button, the telephone automatically calls the control centre where an operator is always waiting to alert the nominated people to provide help as soon as your call comes in. Depending on the problem they can also alert the doctor or ambulance service. The operator will see on his computer screen some brief medical notes, which you supply when you join the scheme, and the names and addresses of three friends or relatives you have named. Therefore, you could put both your daughters down, for example. They will be contacted and the nearest available person on your list to come to your house with a key to deal with your problem and to let professional help in when it arrives'.

John also explained that these 'telephones also includes a clever device to make conversation much clearer for people who wear a hearing aid and, if it rings, you can answer it by pressing your pendant button, so there is no need rush to the phone'. Mary thought the Community Alarm Scheme sounded like a very good idea and agreed to having it set up.

John instructed the support worker about how to help Mary to maximise the activities that she still was able to do herself. It is an important element of the service that clients are continually encouraged to maintain their independence even though it would often be quicker for the support workers to do the task for the person.

Social Work Assessment

The social worker met with Mary's daughter Liz to undertake a carers' assessment. EASY-Care has been tested for practicability and validity for contact and overview assessments in primary care in the United Kingdom (Craig et al. 2015).

Mary was adamant she wanted to live at home but did admit that she felt a bit isolated and would enjoy getting out. Therefore, the social worker said she would try and arrange a weekly day centre place and transport to get there. This would also give Liz a day when she was free to be out all day. A revised care plan was draw up jointly by the therapists and social worker, and a review date set for the following week.

Intervention

During the next six weeks, Mary was supported by an intensive package of care involving her daughters, the Rapid Response Service, and the evening nursing service. She only needed visits during the night for four nights. She gained in confidence over the six-week intervention period, and the support workers undertook a programme of falls prevention exercises with her, which improved her strength and balance (Goodwin and Briggs 2012). The support workers advised

Kate and John about Mary's progress, and the care plan was amended three times to reflect her improving abilities.

After Mary's plaster was removed, Kate assessed her wrist and printed out a programme of home exercises to improve the ROM and muscle strength. These exercises were complemented by the work that the support workers were then doing with Mary to increase her independence in all aspects of her personal and domestic ADL. It was evident that if some of the caring pressure was to be reduced for Liz and Anne, then Mary was going to continue to need regular daily visits even when her wrist was no longer immobilised. The social worker organised Direct Payments to be made for Mary to use the local personal assistance scheme to employ a carer who lived in the village to visit twice a day for an early morning and late evening call.

The Rapid Response Team provides an intermediate care service of about six weeks' duration. As Mary had a history of falls, she was invited for a falls assessment at the local hospital. This led to Mary being offered a place on an eight-week Falls Group Service to improve her balance and mobility. The Rapid Response Team have found that over 30% of people referred to the Rapid Response Service had suffered a fall.

Falls Prevention Programme

The falls prevention programme was based on evidence obtained from the literature on fails prevention programmes. Mary attended the Day Hospital at her local community hospital where the falls prevention programme was based. First, she undertook a screening assessment to establish her suitability for the falls programme and to identify any needs requiring referral to other services, such as a podiatrist or optician (for intervention at an *impairment level*). The initial assessment included three standardised measures. The outcome measures for the group falls prevention programme were the Timed up and go test, the Performance-Oriented Mobility Assessment (Tinetti Scale), and a Four Test Balance Scale (Finnegan et al. 2018; Goodwin and Briggs 2012; NICE 2013).

Mary was considered to be a suitable candidate for the falls prevention programme, and after the assessment she was given a start date for her falls group programme. Mary received eight sessions spaced once per week at the local community hospital. At a *societal limitation level*, transport was provided via Red Cross Ambulance to enable Mary to access the falls prevention programme. The group sessions delivered interventions across several levels of function:

- At the *disability level*, Mary engaged in walking practice.
- At a *functional limitation level*, she was given training in, and advice on, how to cope if she did fall at home, including movements to use to attempt to get up off the floor and strategies to stay warm.
- At an *impairment level*, she engaged in group sessions to improve balance and strengthening exercises to increase her muscle strength and stamina.
- At a *societal limitation level*, Mary was given a booklet about safety in the home and advice on nutrition (feeding and nutrition is addressed at a *disability level*). In addition, group participants watched a video about falls and received advice and information regarding falls prevention.

During the eight-week period, two home visits are usually undertaken by the occupational therapist, to undertake a home hazard assessment, and by the physiotherapist to advise on the home exercise programme. The team felt that the exercise programme should be individually prescribed to take into account the person's home circumstances and abilities. Mary was given a printed sheet of exercises, and her daughters were instructed to encourage her to follow her exercise programme regularly. At the end of the eight sessions, Mary was again reassessed on the three outcomes. Mary improved on all three measures.

Mary was discharged to the care of her GP. Copies of her falls group baseline and follow-up scores were included in the discharge letter, and the GP was asked to re-refer if he felt Mary had deteriorated at a future date. Mary was followed up three months after discharge from the falls prevention programme for reassessment on the outcome measures, and to discover if Mary had any falls since she completed the programme. John also used this opportunity to re-check for home hazards and to promote the continuation of her exercise routine.

Source: Based on case study written by Mr David Jelly, Physiotherapist.

WORKSHEETS

Please now turn to the Worksheets. There are two versions of this: Worksheet 11.1 allows you to apply the NCMRR model (NCMRR 1992), and 11.2 allows you to apply the ICF model (WHO 2002); these are found on pp. 370 and 371. For this reflection, you will need to review the range of un-standardised and standardised assessments and outcome measures used within your occupational therapy or physiotherapy service or by your multidisciplinary team (MDT). If you are a student, reflect on the range of assessments and outcome measures that you have seen used on one of your clinical placements. Both worksheets contain a number of questions or instructions to be answered for each level/dimension:

- What data do you currently collect related to this level of function?
- What decisions do you need to make from this data?
- What assessments (standardised or un-standardised) do you currently use to collect data related to this level of function?
- Is this assessment method adequate?
- List potential assessments that you could use to collect data related to each level of function?

REVIEW QUESTIONS

11.1   Why can it be useful to apply a model of function as a framework for your assessment process?

11.2   What are the 10 levels in the *Hierarchy of Living Systems*, described by Christiansen (1991)?

11.3   How are the terms *body structures*, *body functions*, and *impairments* defined in the ICF model?

11.4   How are the terms *activity* and *participation*, and *activity limitations* and *participation restrictions*, defined in the ICF model?

11.5   What are the five levels proposed by the NCMRR model of function and dysfunction?

You will find brief answers to these questions at the back of this book on p. 445.

Reflecting on the Levels of Function AHPs Need to Consider: Applying the NCMRR Model.

Level of function/ dysfunction National Center for Medical Rehabilitation Research (NCMRR 1992)	What data do you currently collect related to this level of function?	What decisions do you need to make from this data?	What assessments (standardised or un-standardised) do you currently use to collect data related to this level of function?	Is this assessment method adequate? YES or NO	List potential assessments that you could use to collect data related to each level of function
Societal Limitation					
Disability					
Functional Limitation					
Impairment					
Pathophysiology					

Reflecting on the Levels of Function AHPs Need to Consider: Applying the ICF Model.

ICF dimension International Classification of Functioning, Disability and Health (WHO 2002)	What data do you currently collect related to this dimension?	What decisions do you need to make from this data?	What assessments (standardised or un-standardised) do you currently use to collect data related to this dimension?	Is this assessment method adequate? YES or NO	List potential assessments that you could use to collect data related to each dimension.
Body function and structure and impairments					
Activity and activity limitations					
Participation and participation restrictions					
Environmental factors					

REFERENCES

Abu-Awad, Y., Unsworth, C.A., Coulson, M., and Sarigiannis, M. (2014). Using the Australian Therapy Outcome Measures for Occupational Therapy (AusTOMs-OT) to measure client participation outcomes. *British Journal of Occupational Therapy* 77 (2): 44–49. https://doi.org/10.4276/030802214X13916969446958.

Andermann, A. (2016). Taking action on the social determinants of health in clinical practice: a framework for health professionals. *CMAJ* 188 (17–18): E474–E483. https://doi.org/10.1503/cmaj.160177.

Árnadóttir, G. (1990). *The Brain and Behavior: Assessing Cortical Dysfunction Through Activities of Daily Living (ADL)*. Mosby Incorporated.

Aron, D.C. (2020). Managing patients: evidence-based medicine meets human complexity. In: *Complex Systems in Medicine*, 63–74. Cham: Springer https://doi.org/10.1007/978-3-030-24593-1_6.

Baum, C. and Edwards, D.F. (1993). Cognitive performance in senile dementia of the Alzheimer's type: the kitchen task assessment. *American Journal of Occupational Therapy* 47 (5): 431–436. https://doi.org/10.5014/ajot.47.5.431.

Boulding, K.E. (1956). General systems theory – the skeleton of science. *Management Science* 2 (3): 197–208.

Brown, T. and Chien, C.-W. (2010). Top-down or bottom-up occupational therapy assessment: which way do we go? *British Journal of Occupational Therapy* 73 (3): 95–96. https://doi.org/10.4276/030802210X12682330090334.

Browne, J.E. and O'Hare, N.J. (2001). Review of the different methods for assessing standing balance. *Physiotherapy* 87 (9): 489–495. https://doi.org/10.1016/S0031-9406(05)60696-7.

Capra, F. (1982). *The Turning Point: Science. Society and The Rising Culture*. New York: Simon & Schuster.

Carswell, A., McColl, M.A., Baptiste, S. et al. (2004). The Canadian occupational performance measure: a research and clinical literature review. *Canadian Journal of Occupational Therapy* 71 (4): 210–222. https://doi.org/10.1177/000841740407100406.

Chard, G. (2004). International classification of functioning, disability and health. *British Journal of Occupational Therapy* 67 (1): 1–1. https://doi.org/10.1177/030802260406700101.

Christiansen, C. (1991). Occupational therapy intervention for life performance. In: *Occupational Therapy: Overcoming Human Performance Deficits* (eds. C. Christiansen and C. Baum), 3–44. Thorofare, NJ: Slack.

Christiansen, C. and Baum, C.M. (1991). *Occupational Therapy: Overcoming Human Performance Deficits*. Thorofare, NJ: Slack.

Craig, C., Chadborn, N., Sands, G. et al. (2015). Systematic review of EASY-care needs assessment for community-dwelling older people. *Age and Ageing* 44 (4): 559–565. https://doi.org/10.1093/ageing/afv050.

van Dulmen, S.A., van der Wees, P.J., Staal, J.B. et al. (2017). Patient reported outcome measures (PROMs) for goalsetting and outcome measurement in primary care physiotherapy, an explorative field study. *Physiotherapy* 103 (1): 66–72. https://doi.org/10.1016/j.physio.2016.01.001.

Enderby, P., John, A., and Petheram, B. (2013). *Therapy Outcome Measures for Rehabilitation Professionals: Speech and Language Therapy, Physiotherapy, Occupational Therapy*. Wiley.

Engel, G.L. (1981). The clinical application of the biopsychosocial model. *The Journal of Medicine and Philosophy: A Forum for Bioethics and Philosophy of Medicine* 6 (2): 101–124. Oxford University Press.

Finnegan, S., Bruce, J., Skelton, D.A. et al. (2018). Development and delivery of an exercise programme for falls prevention: the Prevention of Falls Injury Trial (PreFIT). *Physiotherapy* 104 (1): 72–79. https://doi.org/10.1016/j.physio.2017.06.004.

Fisher, A. (2003). *AMPS Assessment of Motor and Process Skills*. Colorado: Fort Collins.

Fisher, A.G. (1993). The assessment of IADL motor skills: an application of many-faceted Rasch analysis. *American Journal of Occupational Therapy* 47 (4): 319–329. https://doi.org/10.5014/ajot.47.4.319.

Goodwin, V. and Briggs, L. (2012). *Guidelines for the Physiotherapy Management of Older People at Risk of Falling*. London: AGILE. CSP https://agile.csp.org.uk/system/files/agile_falls_guidelines_update_2012_1.pdf.

Gower, G. (2013). Sustainable development and allied health professionals. *International Journal of Therapy and Rehabilitation* 20 (8): 403–408. https://doi.org/10.12968/ijtr.2013.20.8.403.

Hall, A.D. and Fagen, R.E. (1968, e-book 2017). Definition of system. In: *Systems Research for Behavioral Science*, 81–92. Routledge https://doi.org/10.4324/9781315130569.

Hammell, K.W. (2004). Deviating from the norm: a sceptical interrogation of the classificatory practices of the ICF. *British Journal of Occupational Therapy* 67 (9): 408–411. https://doi.org/10.1177/030802260406700906.

Hill, K.D., Schwarz, J.A., Kalogeropoulos, A.J., and Gibson, S.J. (1996). Fear of falling revisited. *Archives of Physical Medicine and Rehabilitation* 77 (10): 1025–1029. https://doi.org/10.1016/S0003-9993(96)90063-5.

Kielhofner, G. (1980). A model of human occupation, part 2. Ontogenesis from the perspective of temporal adaptation. *American Journal of Occupational Therapy* 34 (10): 657–663. https://doi.org/10.5014/ajot.34.10.657.

Kielhofner, G. (2002). *A Model of Human Occupation: Theory and Application*. Lippincott Williams & Wilkins.

Laver, A. J. (1994). *The development of the Structured Observational Test of Function (SOTOF)* (Doctoral dissertation, University of Surrey).

Laver, A J. & Baum, C. M. (1992). *An Assessment Model*. Unpublished, manuscript. Program in Occupational Therapy, Washington University School of Medicine, St Louis.

Laver, A.J. and Powell, G.E. (1995). *The Structured Observational Test of Function (SOTOF)*. NFER Nelson.

Law, M. and Baum, C. (2005). Measurement in occupational therapy. In: *Measuring Occupational Performance: Supporting Best Practice in Occupational Therapy* (eds. M.C. Law, C.M. Baum and W. Dunn), 3–20. Slack Incorporated.

Levine, R.E. and Brayley, C.R. (1991). Occupation as a therapeutic medium: a contextual approach to performance intervention. In: *Occupational Therapy. Overcoming Human Performance Deficits* (eds. C.M. Christensen and C. Baum), 590–631. Slack.

Madan, I. and Grime, P.R. (2015). The management of musculoskeletal disorders in the workplace. *Best Practice & Research. Clinical Rheumatology* 29 (3): 345–355. https://doi.org/10.1016/j.berh.2015.03.002.

Maslow, A.H. (1943). A theory of human motivation. *Psychological Review* 50 (4): 370–396.

Matuska, K.M. and Christiansen, C.H. (2008). A proposed model of lifestyle balance. *Journal of Occupational Science* 15 (1): 9–19. https://doi.org/10.1080/14427591.2008.9686602.

McDonald, R., Surtees, R., and Wirz, S. (2004). The international classification of functioning, disability and health provides a model for adaptive seating interventions for children with cerebral palsy. *British Journal of Occupational Therapy* 67 (7): 293–302. https://doi.org/10.1177/030802260406700703.

McDougall, J., Wright, V., and Rosenbaum, P. (2010). The ICF model of functioning and disability: incorporating quality of life and human development. *Developmental Neurorehabilitation* 13 (3): 204–211. https://doi.org/10.3109/17518421003620525.

McFadyen, A.K. and Pratt, J. (1997). Understanding the statistical concepts of measures of work performance. *British Journal of Occupational Therapy* 60 (6): 279–284. https://doi.org/10.1177/030802269706000614.

McGruder, J. (2004). Disease models of mental illness and aftercare patient education: critical observations from meta-analyses, cross-cultural practice and anthropological study. *British Journal of Occupational Therapy* 67 (7): 310–318. https://doi.org/10.1177/030802260406700705.

Nagi, S.Z. (1991). Chapter: Appendix A Disability concepts revisited; implications for prevention. In: *Disability in America: Toward a National Agenda for Prevention* (eds. A.M. Pope and A.R. Tarlov), 309–327. National Academies Press.

National Center for Medical Rehabilitation Research (1992). *Report and Plan for Medical Rehabilitation Research to Congress.* Bethesda, MD: NCMRR/US Dept of Health and Human Services, National Institutes of Health.

National Institute for Health and Care Excellence (2013) *Falls in older people: assessing risk and prevention.* Clinical guideline [CG161] NICE: 12 June 2013

Padegimas, E.M. and Osei, D.A. (2013). Evaluation and treatment of osetoporotic distal radius fracture in the elderly patient. *Current Reviews in Musculoskeletal Medicine* 6 (1): 41–46. https://doi.org/10.1007/s12178-012-9153-8.

Prodinger, B., Darzins, S., Magasi, S., and Baptiste, S. (2015). The International Classification of Functioning, Disability and Health (ICF): opportunities and challenges to the use of ICF for occupational therapy. *World Federation of Occupational Therapists Bulletin* 71 (2): 108–114. https://doi.org/10.1179/2056607715Y.0000000003.

Rimmer, J.H., Chen, M.D., and Hsieh, K. (2011). A conceptual model for identifying, preventing, and managing secondary conditions in people with disabilities. *Physical Therapy* 91 (12): 1728–1739. https://doi.org/10.2522/ptj.20100410.

Rogers, J.C. and Holm, M.B. (1989). The therapist's thinking behind functional assessment II. In: *AOTA Self Study Series Assessing Function, Assessment of function: An action guide.* Rockville, MD: AOTA.

Rogers, J.C. (1983). Eleanor Clarke Slagle Lectureship—1983; clinical reasoning: the ethics, science, and art. *American Journal of Occupational Therapy* 37 (9): 601–616. https://doi.org/10.5014/ajot.37.9.601.

Rogers, J.C. (2004). Occupational diagnosis. In: *Occupation for Occupational Therapists* (ed. M. Molineax), 17–31. Blackwell Publishing.

Royal College of Occupational Therapists (2004). *Guidance on the Use of the International Classification of Functioning, Disability and Health (ICF) and the Ottawa Charter for Health Promotion in Occupational Therapy Services.* London: RCOT.

Sherrington, C. and Tiedemann, A. (2015). Physiotherapy in the prevention of falls in older people. *Journal of Physiotherapy* 61 (2): 54–60. https://doi.org/10.1016/j.jphys.2015.02.011.

Skyttner, L. (2005). *General Systems Theory: Problems, Perspectives, Practice.* World scientific.

Stephenson, R. (2002). The complexity of human behaviour: a new paradigm for physiotherapy? *Physical Therapy Reviews* 7 (4): 243–258. https://doi.org/10.1179/108331902235002001.

Sumsion, T. (2000). A revised occupational therapy definition of client-centred practice. *British Journal of Occupational Therapy* 63 (7): 304–309. https://doi.org/10.1177/030802260006300702.

Trombly, C. (1993). Anticipating the future: assessment of occupational function. *American Journal of Occupational Therapy* 47 (3): 253–257. https://doi.org/10.5014/ajot.47.3.253.

Von Bertalanffy, L. (1968). *General System Theory: Foundations, Development, Applications.* New York: George Braziller. Inc.

World Health Organization. (1980). *International classification of impairments, disabilities, and handicaps: a manual of classification relating to the consequences of disease, published in accordance with resolution WHA29.35 of the Twenty-ninth World Health Assembly,* May 1976. World Health Organization. https://apps.who.int/iris/handle/10665/41003

World Health Organisation (2001). *International Classification of Functioning, Disability and Health (ICF),* 11. Geneva: WHO.

World Health Organisation (2002). *Towards a Common Language for Functioning, Disability and Health ICF,* 9. Geneva: WHO.

RESOURCES

EASY-Care Standard 2010 – A holistic profile of health and care needs, based on the priorities of the older person for support, information, or advice. https://www.cgakit.com/s-1-easy--care-standard-2010

International Classification of Functioning, Disability and Health (ICF)

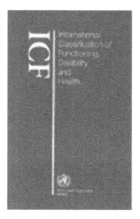

The International Classification of Functioning, Disability and Health, known more commonly as ICF, is a classification of health and health-related domains. As the functioning and disability of an individual occurs in a context, ICF also includes a list of environmental factors. https://www.who.int/standards/classifications/international-classification-of-functioning-disability-and-health

National Center for Medical Rehabilitation Research (NCMRR)

Through basic, translational, and clinical research, NCMRR aims to foster development of the scientific knowledge needed to enhance the health, productivity, independence, and quality of life of people with physical disabilities.

https://www.nichd.nih.gov/about/org/ncmrr

CHAPTER 12

Implementing the Optimum Assessment and Measurement Approach

OVERVIEW

In this chapter, we look at the factors that allied health professionals (AHPs) should consider when choosing an assessment and measurement approach for an individual, client group, or service. The chapter explores a series of goals for improving your assessment and outcome measurement practice; these are divided into goals, or challenges, to be addressed by five different groups: clinicians, managers, educators, researchers, and students. AHPs are encouraged to select some pertinent goals as the basis for identifying their own Continuing Professional Development (CPD) plans. A CPD action plan worksheet is included for this purpose, and an example of a completed CPD action plan is given.

QUESTIONS TO CONSIDER

1. How do I set about identifying appropriate standardised tests for my service?
2. How do I combine the best available evidence with my clinical experience and my knowledge of my client's preferences in order to implement the optimum assessment and measurement approach?

IMPROVING ASSESSMENT AND MEASUREMENT PRACTICE: WHERE TO BEGIN?

As we have seen throughout this book, and especially in Chapters 8, 9, and 10, knowledge of the psychometric properties of a measure is not just the concern of AHP researchers. It is also of immense relevance to any clinician who wishes to use a test to provide a baseline for treatment, a predictive or discriminative measure to guide decision making, or an outcome measure to evaluate the effects of intervention. However, the pressures of everyday practice, which for many AHPs include demanding caseloads and waiting lists, can make it challenging for AHPs to find the time to take a critical look at their assessment practice and to undertake the necessary work to make informed changes to provide a more efficient, valid, and reliable assessment process for their clients. It is a matter of balancing the gold standard of measurement with the pragmatics of real-work life situations.

To make improvements to your current assessment and measurement practice, we suggest that you follow the straightforward eight-step process outlined in Figure 12.1. The remainder of this chapter provides guidance related to the different steps in this process. Consider that even if you feel that a few clients have 'lost out' to some degree, if you take time out for CPD to work on this area, many clients should benefit from the resultant improvements in your practice in the future.

ANALYSING YOUR CURRENT ASSESSMENT PRACTICE

AHPs, as potential users of published tests, should undertake a similar process to a test developer when choosing the optimum approach for assessing their service users. AHPs should explicitly define their conceptualisation of the constructs they plan to measure, so that they can compare their definition with the description of the constructs in any test manuals they are critiquing (Chaudoir et al. 2013). They also

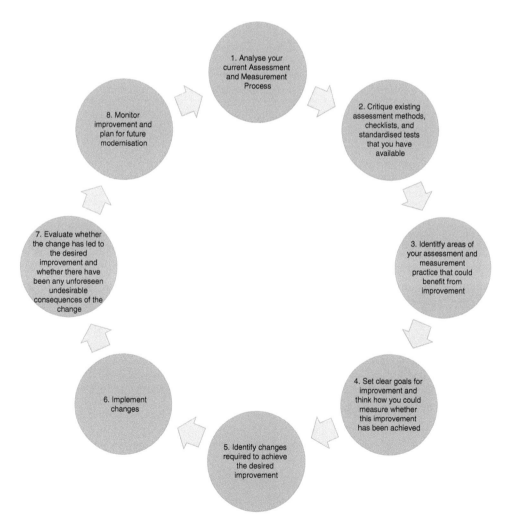

FIGURE 12.1   Improving your assessment process.

should start with a review of the relevant literature on the assessment/measurement of their client group and the constructs they wish to measure. When selecting an assessment approach for a client or group or clients, we need to consider:

- the level(s) of function to be assessed (see Chapter 11)
- the purpose(s) of the assessment (see Chapter 3)
- the data collection method(s) (see Chapter 2)
- the use of standardised versus un-standardised tools (see Chapters 7)
- the level of measurement provided by assessment methods (see Chapter 4).

In step 1, shown in Figure 11.1, you need to analyse your current assessment and measurement process. Start by reflecting on the purpose of your service. If this is not clearly articulated, then a good starting point is to develop a written statement of purpose, called a 'service specification' (see Chapter 13, and especially Figure 13.1, and Step 3). Once you are clear about the purpose of your service, review your existing assessment approaches and tests. Categorise what you currently have available (checklists, standardised tests, etc.) and the assessment methods you currently use in terms of their purposes, data source, data collection method, levels of function addressed, and levels of measurement provided. Worksheets from previous chapters will help you to do this. There are a number of simple techniques that you can use to help you structure an analysis of your current assessment process, and two frequently used methods are SWOT and mapping.

The completed test critique(s) (see Chapter 10) will assist you with both steps 1 and 5 in the 8-step process shown in Figure 12.1.

SWOT ANALYSIS

A SWOT analysis has often been used in business and industry to evaluate the internal strengths and weaknesses, and the external opportunities and threats in an organisation's environment (Sammut-Bonnici and Galea 2015). SWOT is an acronym for strengths, weaknesses, opportunities, and threats; the idea is to examine and use the results to identify priorities for action. In this chapter, we use it to enable you as an AHP to look at both internal factors (the strengths and weaknesses of your current assessment practice) and external factors (opportunities and threats) that do, or may, influence your assessment process. If you have a mission statement/vision/service specification, use these as they can be helpful as a framework for examining SWOT. The advantages to using SWOT as a starting point for examining your own/your service's current assessment practice are the following:

- SWOT is one of the most widely used strategic planning tools in current use across a range of sectors – so it familiar to the majority of staff/stakeholders and not perceived as daunting.
- It provides a good starting point.
- SWOT actively engages individuals or groups to share their views.

The disadvantages are that SWOT can often result 'in an over-long list of factors, general and often meaningless descriptions, a failure to prioritise issues and no attempt to verify conclusions . . . outputs once generated [are] rarely used' (Iles and Sutherland 2001, p. 41).

Therefore, to ensure that SWOT analyses are useful, you need to pose a second level of questions. In relation to strengths and weaknesses, you should ask the following additional questions:

- What are the causes of this strength or weakness?
- What are the consequences of this?
- Do they help or hinder us in achieving an optimum assessment process for our clients?

In relation to opportunities and threats, you should pose the following additional questions:

- What impact is this likely to have on our assessment process?
- Will it help or hinder us in achieving an optimum assessment process for our clients?
- What must we do to respond to this opportunity or threat?

(Iles and Sutherland 2001)

Refer to Worksheet 12.1 at the end of this chapter to assist you with undertaking a SWOT analysis.

MAPPING YOUR CURRENT ASSESSMENT AND MEASUREMENT PROCESS

Process mapping is one of the most powerful ways for multidisciplinary teams to understand the real problems in a service from the perspective of people using the service and their family or carers, and to identify opportunities for improvement.

Definition of Mapping

Mapping is the process by which you represent the activities and steps experienced by the client. This is a diagnostic and analytical process of discovering what actually happens. You can then use this information to find ways to improve how the patient experiences the care you deliver. (Fraser 2002, p. 4)
Source: Fraser (2002).

There are a number of advantages to mapping your assessment process (NHS Improvement 2018a) if you wish to improve your assessment and measurement practice:

- It helps you to see the whole picture of the client's journey through your assessment process: what happens now and how AHP colleagues, service users, and carers feel about the process. You might find that the service user does not understand why a particular test is given or might find a test anxiety provoking. The service user might feel that he does not receive sufficient feedback about the results of a test. AHPs might value a test because it has good reliability and validity, but may not use it regularly because it takes too long to administer and tires the client.

- It identifies where the real problems are (bottlenecks, backlogs, etc.). For example, you might discover that you have a long waiting list, but find on initial assessment that a significant number of referrals are inappropriate. If so, you might consider a trial process to triage referrals as they are received by your service. You might have only one AHP trained to administer a particular standardised assessment and have bottlenecks occurring while clients wait to receive this assessment.
- It identifies any duplication of effort (e.g. wasted time and resources). For example, the AHPs might be all collecting the same details about the person, their living situation, and the history of the presenting condition. AHPs might decide to seek informed consent from the client to share this information with the team or undertake a joint initial interview.
- It provides a baseline against which changes to your assessment process will be measured in order to evaluate whether any changes lead to a more effective and/or efficient assessment.

AHPs can use a range of methods for gathering information to help them map their clients' assessment/measurement process:

- Looking through records to see what assessment and measurement data is collected, how it is collected, and how it has been recorded.
- Physically following a person's journey (e.g. shadowing a client through an initial assessment process).
- Interviewing the client and their carer about their experience of being assessed and measured.
- Seeing key personnel to get their view (e.g. doctors who receive a summary of the assessment results, such as the client's consultant or GP).
- Getting all staff involved in the assessment process engaged in the mapping exercise, making it a team endeavour by having a stakeholder timeout to map the assessment process together, ideally involving clients and carers at this event.

There are several factors which can influence the success of your mapping exercise (Fraser 2002) and are worth considering in advance:

- You need to engage all the people who are involved in the assessment pathway as participants in the mapping process (this includes service user and carer representatives).
- It can be useful to include people who are not in your service/department but are still involved in the client process (e.g. GPs or consultants who refer clients to your service for assessment and to whom you send assessment reports).
- You need to seek agreement in advance from all stakeholders to provide required information. If you are just mapping your own assessment process, this will not be a problem but if you are part of a multidisciplinary team or provide assessment into a service, such as a memory assessment clinic for people with dementia, then looking at how your assessment fits into the whole process, for the client will require liaison with other professionals.
- Define a clear start and end point for the process you are mapping, and agree upon the level of detail from the outset. For example, your starting point might

be when the referral is received by the AHP, and the end point might be when a final report detailing outcome measurement is sent to the referral source when the person is discharged from the therapy service.

Ideally, an analysis of an assessment should not be undertaken in isolation. Many AHPs work as members of a team. Even where an AHP works in a discrete therapy service, this service is likely to be one component of a person's clinical pathway. It is helpful to engage other team members or stakeholders in the analysis of assessment processes (also see Table 12.1 below). Mapping is a good method for fostering collaboration.

Having mapped the client's assessment journey, the AHP must then begin to analyse it, for example, highlighting bottlenecks or areas of duplication. A plan-do-study-act (PDSA) cycle approach (see the section titled 'PDSA Cycle Approach' later in this chapter) can assist you to test change ideas on a small scale to see if they will bring about the improvement required (Damelio 2011; NHS Improvement 2018a).

IMPROVING YOUR ASSESSMENT PROCESS

Once you have identified the limitations in your current practice, you are ready to identify the changes required and to plan for making improvements to your assessment and measurement process. A number of service improvement models are in use across health and social care services and are helpful (McCormack et al. 2013).

TABLE 12.1   Commitment, enrolment, and compliance.

DISPOSTION	Stakeholders'/players' response to change
Commitment	Want change to happen and will work to make it happen. Willing to create whatever structures, systems and frameworks are necessary for it to work.
Enrolment	Want change to happen and will devote time and energy to making it happen within given frameworks. Act within the spirit of the frameworks.
Genuine compliance	See the virtue in what is proposed, do what is asked of them and think proactively about what is needed. Act within the letter of the frameworks.
Formal compliance	Can describe the benefits of what is proposed and are not hostile to them. They do what they are asked but no more. Stick to the letter of the framework.
Grudging compliance	Do not accept that there are benefits to what is proposed and do not go along with it. They do enough of what is asked of them not to jeopardise position. Interpret the letter of the framework.
Non-compliance	Do not accept that there are benefits and have nothing to lose by opposing the proposition. Will not do what is asked of them. Work outside framework.
Apathy	Neither in support of not in opposition to the proposal, just serving time. Don't care about the framework.

Source: Iles and Sutherland (2001). © 2001, National Coordinating Centre for the Service Delivery and Organisation. Reproduced with permission.

The following model for service improvement draws upon the work of Langley et al. (1996). This model begins with three questions:

1. *What are we trying to accomplish?*
   Step 4 in Figure 12.1, which shows the process for improving your assessment and measurement practice, requires the setting of improvement goals. You, or your multidisciplinary team, or your service, need to start with clear and focused goals for improving your assessment /measurement process.
   For example, a goal might be: *All clients will be assessed twice using a standardised, valid, reliable, and responsive outcome measure, first, when they enter our service to provide a baseline and again on discharge to provide an evaluation of the effectiveness of our intervention.*

2. *How will we know that a change is an improvement?*
   Step 7 in Figure 12.1 involves evaluating whether your changes have led to improved practice. So, this is a really important question, because not all changes lead to enhanced service, and some changes, which do provide the desired improvement, can have unexpected consequences. Your assessment process might be much more rigorous and meet your original improvement goal; however, it also takes much longer to administer, leading to slower throughput of clients through your service and increased waiting lists.
   As an example, you might measure your improvement goal by analysing whether:
   A standardised, valid, reliable, and responsive measure is identified and applied across the service. Client records show evidence of baseline data on referral and outcome data at discharge. There is no increase in waiting list numbers or waiting times for our service.

3. *What changes can we make that result in improvement?*
   This question relates to Step 5 in Figure 12.1 as it prompts the beginning of a planning cycle for change. You might already have a suitable standardised test(s) identified or a change in the current assessment process in mind. However, you might be starting from scratch and need to undertake a literature or Web-based search as a starting point.

PDSA Cycle Approach

The PDSA cycle approach to service improvement recommended by NHS Improvement (2018b) is widely used by clinical staff engaged in a range of clinical collaborations. The PDSA process will help you with stages 5, 6, 7, and 8 of the process for improving your assessment and measurement practice shown in Figure 12.1. There are four simple steps to follow in a PDSA cycle process:

1. **P = plan:** At this stage, AHPs identify what change they think will result in an improvement to their assessment process, after which they plan how they will test that change. This stage involves thinking about the 'Who, What, Where, and When' of the improvement. Deciding how to measure the improvement is critical.

2. **D = do:** At this stage, AHPs carry out their plan for improvement; this could be altering part of the assessment process or trying out a new standardised outcome measure. At this stage, AHPs need to record any unexpected events and problems, and make any useful observations. Towards the end of this

stage, AHPs should start analysing any data. For example, this could involve auditing client records to see how many clients have been given the newly adopted measure or have been assessed following the new process; reviewing data on how many AHPs have undertaken a particular training course; counting how many different clients each AHP has assessed using the new test; or analysing the qualitative feedback (e.g. questionnaires) that the AHPs have completed about clinical utility factors.

3. **S = study**: At this stage, AHPs complete the analysis of all data they have collected to evaluate whether the change has been fully implemented and whether it has resulted in the desired improvement. AHPs reflect on whether there has been a significant improvement, whether their expectations matched the reality of what actually happened when implementing the planned change, and whether, with hindsight, they would do anything differently.

4. **A = act:** At the final stage of the PDSA process, AHPs agree upon what did and did not work. They consider what further changes or amendments are required to ensure that the improvement is fully implemented and sustained. If appropriate, they plan the next PDSA cycle.

Improving your whole assessment process, including both informal and standardised assessment data collection, and assessment undertaken with all sources (client self-report, carer proxy, colleague proxy, and observational data collection methods) can be a large undertaking. To make it more achievable, we recommend breaking your assessment /measurement improvement project into small goals and undertaking a small PDSA cycle for each goal. This should mean that you divide your improvement project into 'bite-sized chunks' which feel more manageable and lead to faster results, so you can celebrate the achievement of completed goals more quickly. For example, you might:

- begin with a PDSA cycle that focuses on the quality of referral information received by your service, review how this information is used (e.g. decisions made from referral data for prioritising referrals onto a waiting list), and evaluate whether the data collected is adequate for this purpose. You might implement the use of a referral form, which provides a uniform and adequate initial assessment at referral.
- The second PDSA cycle might focus on client self-report assessment, with a particular focus on interview data gathered to provide a baseline.
- Further PDSA cycles could focus on outcome measurement.

RAID

RAID is another improvement model (Halligan et al. 2006):

- **R = review**: AHPs need to look at their current assessment process and measurement techniques, and prepare their service for change (step 1 in the 8-step process shown in Figure 12.1).
- **A = agree**: AHPs need to ensure all stakeholders (for example, clinicians, managers, other members of a multidisciplinary team, secretarial staff) are signed up to the proposed changes in the assessment process and /or measures used (an aspect of step 5 in the 8-step process shown in Figure 12.1).

- **I = implement**: AHPs then put in place the proposed changes; for example, they purchase a standardised test, attend the related training course, and implement it with clients (step 6 in the 8-step process shown in Figure 12.1).
- **D = demonstrate**: At this stage, the AHPs need to show that the changes made have led to improvements. For example, they now have individual client and group data that shows a standardised measure is being used, and that enables the service to review whether interventions have had the desired / anticipated outcome, both on an individual client and service population basis (step 7 in the 8-step process shown in Figure 12.1).

The step of agreement is essential if any change is to be adopted wholeheartedly by stakeholders and is to lead to a sustainable change. There are different levels of agreement (Iles and Sutherland 2001) that differentiate between commitment, enrolment, and compliance. It is preferable to have considerable commitment for change from all stakeholders, but it is not always 'necessary for everyone to be as fully-signed up at this' (p. 47). The different levels of agreement or resistance to change are defined in Table 12.1. It is useful to rate each of your stakeholders against these criteria if you can, so that you are aware of the levels of support and resistance you might experience from colleagues when implementing your planned change.

LINKING IMPROVING YOUR ASSESSMENT PRACTICE TO CONTINUING PROFESSIONAL DEVELOPMENT (CPD)

AHPs working in the United Kingdom have to be registered with the Health & Care Professions Council (HCPC). The HCPC has standards for AHPs around the undertaking and recording of CPD. HCPC look for evidence of a range of CPD activities, which include: CPD (HCPC 2020, see https://www.hcpc-uk.org/cpd/)

These activities might include (HCPC 2020, see https://www.hcpc-uk.org/cpd/your-cpd/cpd-activities):

- **Work-based learning**. For example, reflecting on experiences at work, considering feedback from service users, or being a member of a committee.
- **Professional activity**. For example, being involved in a professional body or giving a presentation at a conference.
- **Formal education**. For example, going on formal courses or carrying out research.
- **Self-directed learning**. For example, reading articles or books.

A number of these activities are helpful when undertaking a review of your current assessment practice and when critiquing the evidence to improve areas of your practice where you cannot demonstrate that the current methods you are using are the most effective and efficient available.

To begin setting yourself some personal development plans (PDP) for improving your assessment practice, we have included a Worksheet (see Worksheet 12.2) and a series of goals for AHPs related to assessment and measurement.

ASSESSMENT AND OUTCOME MEASUREMENT GOALS FOR EFFECTIVE PRACTICE

AHPs working in a wide variety of roles (clinician, researcher, manager, educator, therapy consultant, or student) can all play a part in service improvement by working to reduce barriers and facilitate the implementation of evidenced-based, effective, and efficient assessment processes with the administration of valid and reliable outcome measures at the heart of therapy practice. This will require changes in attitudes, knowledge, skills, and behaviour. We suggest you identify the role(s) you undertake and select from the goals as the basis for identifying your own CPD to improve your assessment practice. A worksheet (Worksheet 12.2) is provided for this purpose, and an example of a completed CPD action plan is provided in Table 12.2 below.

TABLE 12.2   Continuing Professional Development (CPD) goals for improving assessment practice: an example.

CPD goal	Action plan	Comments/ideas	Date accomplished
Example: **As a clinician I need to increase my application of standardised outcome measures**	1. Contact the Special Interest Group (SIG) for AHPs in my area, and ask about appropriate standardised outcome measures for my client group. 2. Borrow/obtain at least two of the recommended measures, and review the manuals and materials. 3. Pilot with at least five clients to evaluate clinical utility and face validity. 4. Use the Test Critique Worksheet to summarise my findings from Actions 2 and 3 5. If I find a suitable test that requires funding, make a business case for required resources. Time scale: 1 year. Review progress at my next annual appraisal.	1. I have copied a number of journal articles on potential assessments and placed in my CPD file – make time to read them! 2. Perhaps we could set up a journal club for our department or within my MDT?	1. Received emails from SIG members with recommendations for tests. March 2019 2. Borrowed test from neighbouring hospital for a weekend and reviewed manual. April 2004. Appears appropriate for our service. 3. Organised to have sample test from publisher for two weeks and tried out with three patients. June 2004. 4. Completed test critique. June 2019. 5. Made business case to manager for funding to purchase two copies of the test for our department. August 2019. Test purchased. December 2019. Provided in-house training on test administration for colleagues. January 2020.

GOALS FOR CLINICIANS

- Clinicians need to increase their application of standardised outcome measures.
- Clinicians need to follow standards laid down for test users.
- Clinicians need to use the outcome data gathered to improve service provision for users and carers.
- Clinicians need to work with other AHPs (clinicians and researchers) to identify limitations in assessment practice and outcome measures, and identify the need for improved measures.
- Clinicians need to share information on standardised tests and outcomes with other AHPs and professionals working with similar client groups.
- Clinicians should become 'lifelong learners' who seek opportunities to attend courses or conferences where they can learn more about assessment and allocate CPD time for reading in order to stay up to date with the growing literature on standardised outcome measures for their client group.
- If you supervise students on practice placement, explain your rationale for your assessment process, share your clinical reasoning, and encourage students to critique the standardised tests used within your service.

GOALS FOR THERAPY MANAGERS

For managers, Cole et al. (1995) identified five major challenges, which we have expanded into the following goals for service improvement:

- Managers need to value outcome measurement as an integral part of providing an effective service. They must explicitly articulate this attitude to staff and encourage staff still using predominately non-standardised assessment to change their attitudes and behaviour and embrace evidenced-based assessments.
- Managers need to ensure that AHPs have received the appropriate training to administer the specific standardised assessments used in their service and ensure that the staff, under their management, maintain the appropriate standards of test administration.
- Managers should encourage the sharing of data within departments and across services including the shared electronic systems.
- Managers should formulate a well-articulated case to educate service leaders/managers and funding agencies that the information obtained from evidenced-based outcome measures is essential for making informed decisions about competing resource allocation.
- Managers should take responsibility for collating service-wide data and providing information obtained from evidenced-based outcome measures in a readily useable form.
- Managers should become 'lifelong learners' who seek opportunities to attend courses or conferences where they can learn more about assessment and allocate CPD time for reading in order to stay up to date with the growing literature on standardised outcome measures for their service user population.

GOALS FOR EDUCATORS

- Educators need to ensure that a significant emphasis is placed in the curriculum for developing AHP students' attitudes, knowledge, and skills related to assessment and outcome measurement, and highlight that competence in assessment and evaluation is an essential part of providing high-quality services.
- Educators should teach AHP students how to undertake test critiques and provide role modelling by disseminating critical reviews of outcome measures.
- Educators need to encourage AHP students to engage in projects/assignments that examine the evidence base for published tests and for existing assessment processes which they observe in practice.
- Educators are needed to contribute to the identification of areas where practice can be improved and further development of measures is needed.

GOALS FOR AHP RESEARCHERS

- Researchers need to contribute to the identification of areas where practice can be improved and further development of measures is needed.
- Researchers need to undertake research to build up on the body of evidence for existing outcome measures, for example, by conducting further validity and reliability studies, or obtaining normative data for different populations.
- Researchers need to take lead roles in the adaptation of existing measures and/or the development of new measures in areas where practice can be improved and further development of measures is needed to provide clinically useful, evidenced-based outcome measures.

GOALS FOR AHP STUDENTS

- Students must understand and apply the principles of robust assessment and strive to base their assessment practice on the application of well-evidenced procedures and outcome measures.
- Students should strive to become 'lifelong learners' who stay up to date with the growing literature on standardised outcome measures for the client groups they interact with in practice, and once qualified, to continue a quest for knowledge and stay up to date on outcome measures for their client group.
- As AHPs of the future, students should become proactive agents for change in the services where they undertake practice placements. When you qualify and start work, you should share knowledge and skills, particularly in services where the application of outcome measures is not common practice, perhaps by running an in-service training event for colleagues or by implementing the use of standardised measures with your own caseload.

CONCLUSION: ACHIEVING AN EFFECTIVE AND EFFICIENT ASSESSMENT

The role of assessment is of paramount importance to AHP practice. Assessment enables the AHP to:

- describe the person's functional problems in the form of a therapy diagnosis;
- formulate a prognosis;
- use the diagnosis and prognosis as a baseline for treatment planning;
- monitor the person's responses during treatment; and
- evaluate the effectiveness of the intervention (Law and Letts 1989).

The practice setting and the nature of the AHP service will place parameters around the type of assessment that is possible. AHPs need to be pragmatic in their choices, but also should lobby for improvements when restrictions place unacceptable limitations on the quality of the assessment that can be undertaken; a rushed, one-time assessment, for example, is rarely a sufficient baseline from which to plan effective treatment. No assessment of human functioning can be entirely objective, and AHPs need to make careful observations, hypotheses, and judgements that could be open to some degree of error. Therefore, in order to ensure that their assessments are as valid and reliable as possible, AHPs should endeavour to use standardised assessments where available. Health and social care professionals need to continue the shift from the use of non-standardised 'AHP-constructed' assessments to well-researched, clinically useful, standardised measures.

In an environment that places increasing emphasis on quality, clinical governance, and evidenced-based practice, a greater use of standardised assessments should assist AHPs to present more objective and precise findings and to evaluate their interventions in a reliable and sensitive manner. AHPs need to make time to examine critically all non-standardised assessments used within their service. Where these non-standardised assessments are found to be unsuitable for future practice, AHPs need to review and trial potential standardised measures to replace them.

In summary, when selecting assessments for a service, care should be taken that a potential test has good face validity and clinical utility, in addition to thorough standardisation, established validity, and acceptable levels of reliability. It should be remembered that a good test administration can be rendered useless if the results are not documented adequately and the results are not shared with the client and other relevant personnel; so, when planning an assessment, sufficient time should be allowed for scoring, interpretation, report writing, and feedback.

Assessment should never be viewed in isolation, for it is not an end in itself.

Assessment always should be at the heart of the initial interaction with a client and then should be interwoven as an important component of the whole intervention process, right through to a final evaluation when the client is discharged from the AHP service.

It is critical that we continue to review our assessment process and measurement tools on a regular basis. New research might be available that could strengthen or reduce the rationale for using a particular test. A recently published measure might be more reliable or responsive or have better face validity and clinical utility, making it a better choice for your client group. Your service might change; for example, a different intervention approach could be implemented, leading to the requirement for the measurement of different outcomes. It is very helpful to set a date for the next review of assessment and measurement and to identify a lead clinician who will prompt others when this review is due and facilitate the review process. For your service to thrive and to continually offer best practice, you need to develop a culture where it is acceptable – and indeed, desirable – for everyone to question practice and to present and debate ideas. A question from a client, or a suggestion from a student or new member of staff could lead you another step along the path of evidence-based practice. We *wish you every success in this journey!*

SUGGESTED TASKS

1. Give an example of:
    a. a standardised self-report assessment
    b. a standardised proxy assessment
    c. a standardised observational assessment that would be appropriate for your client group and practice setting.
2. Use Worksheet 12.1 to analyse your current assessment process through a SWOT analysis.
3. Review the goals for improving assessment practice, select at least three goals of relevance to you, and then complete Worksheet 12.2.

WORKSHEET 12.1   Analysing Your Current Assessment Process – SWOT Analysis

Strengths	Weakness
Opportunities	Threats

WORKSHEET 12.2   Continuing Professional Development Goals for Improving Assessment Practice

CPD goal	Action plan	Comments / ideas	Date accomplished

REFERENCES

Chaudoir, S.R., Dugan, A.G., and Barr, C.H. (2013). Measuring factors affecting implementation of health innovations: a systematic review of structural, organizational, provider, patient, and innovation level measures. *Implementation Science* 8 (1): 22. https://doi.org/10.1186/1748-5908-8-22.

Cole, B., Finch, E., and Gowland, C. (1995). *Physical Rehabilitation Outcome Measutres*, 24–78. Canada: A Waverly Company.

Damelio, R. (2011). *The Basics of Process Mapping*, 2e. CRC Press.

Fraser, S.W. (2002). *The Patient's Journey: Mapping, Analysing and Improving Healthcare Processes.* Kingsham Press Ltd [Paperback] Paperback – 15 Jun. 2002.

Halligan, A., Cullen, R., and Rogers, P.G. (2006). RAID methodology: the NHS Clinical Governance Team's approach to service improvement. *Clinical Governance: An International Journal* 11 (1): 69–80. https://doi.org/10.1108/14777270610647047.

Health & Care Professions Council (HCPC) – Standards of Continuing Professional Development https://www.hcpc-uk.org/standards/standards-of-continuing-professional-development

Iles, V. and Sutherland, K. (2001). *Managing Change in the NHS. Organisational Change: A Review for Health Care Managers, Professionals and Researchers.* National Co-ordinating Centre for NHS Service Delivery & Organisation R & D (NCC SDO). https://www.healthknowledge.org.uk/sites/default/files/documents/publichealthtextbook/5c/5c2_review.pdf.

Langley, G., Nolan, K., Nolan, T. et al. (1996). *The Improvement Guide: A Practical Approach to Enhancing Organizational Performance.* San Francisco: Calif Jossey-Bass.

Law, M. and Letts, L. (1989). A critical review of scales of activities of daily living. *American Journal of Occupational Therapy* 43 (8): 522–528. https://doi.org/10.5014/ajot.43.8.522.

McCormack, B., Manley, K., and Titchen, A. (eds.) (2013). *Practice Development in Nursing and Healthcare.* Wiley.

NHS Improvement (2018a). *Process mapping - a conventional model.* Online library of Quality, Service Improvement and Redesign tools. https://improvement.nhs.uk/documents/2143/conventional-process-mapping.pdf

NHS Improvement (2018b). *Plan, Do, Study, Act (PDSA) cycles and the model for improvement*, Service Improvement and Redesign tools. https://improvement.nhs.uk/resources/pdsa-cycles

Sammut-Bonnici, T. and Galea, D. (2015). *SWOT analysis. Wiley Encyclopedia of Management, Wiley Online Library*, vol. 12, 1–8. John Wiley & Sons, Inc. https://doi.org/10.1002/9781118785317.weom120103.

RESOURCES

NHS Improvement Quality, service improvement and redesign (QSIR) tools – https://www.england.nhs.uk/quality-service-improvement-and-redesign-qsir-tools/

CHAPTER 13

Using Assessment and Outcome Measures in Service Evaluation

OVERVIEW

In this chapter, we will explore what service evaluation is and why it is important for improving service. We will consider the purpose of evaluation, the data and resources needed, and the need for outcome measures in an evaluation process. We conclude with consideration of how you need to implement your findings and disseminate them to all relevant stakeholders. At the end of the chapter, we present two case studies to illustrate the processes and need for service evaluation and outcome measures, and the importance of stakeholder views.

QUESTIONS TO CONSIDER

1. What is evaluation?
2. Why is evaluation important?
3. What is service improvement?
4. Why are outcome measures needed in service evaluation and improvement?
5. Who are the stakeholders in your service?

WHAT IS EVALUATION?

An evaluation has to be specifically designed to address the questions being asked and the nature of the intervention being evaluated. This means using different methods, working in different settings, with varied populations and data, under specific constraints of time, expertise and resources, both human and financial.

(Heath Foundation 2015, p. 4)

Robust evaluation tells us not only whether an intervention (the term we will use throughout to refer to a quality improvement project, programme or initiative) worked, but also why and how – allowing us to learn lessons for spreading successful interventions and developing new ones. Evaluation that is done inadequately, or not done at all, can render an intervention at best a wasted effort, with improvements only realised at local level. At worst, evaluation can lack credibility, especially if there is a bias towards emphasising success and ignoring failure, which can undermine efforts to improve patient care.

(The Health Foundation 2015, p. 5)

Evaluation has been defines as 'the process of judging or calculating the quality, importance, amount, or value of something' (https://dictionary.cambridge.org/dictionary/english/evaluation). In this chapter, the evaluation of a health and or social care service is described. Evaluation should become not just an essential component of clients' care or therapy, but should also be regularly undertaken to monitor and review your service. According to Corr (2003), evaluation should be undertaken to 'assess the effects and effectiveness of a policy, practice or service' and to 'establish whether the effects of a service can really be attributable to the service or whether they result from some other factors' (p. 235). Undertaking a service evaluation can lead to 'recommendations for change, which ultimately shape and focus a service' (p. 235). In addition to using measurement to explore individual client outcomes, allied health professionals (AHPs) can apply the same or different measures to explore group outcomes and evaluate various aspects of their service. Outcome measures can be used to address important questions related to service provision, funding issues, and healthcare policy. For example, functional outcomes may be used to determine eligibility criteria for a particular service or to evaluate the performance of a service to decide upon future service provision. Unless we evaluate our services, we cannot know whether we are truly meeting our aims and objectives. Even if we can demonstrate we are meeting the clinical aims and objectives outlined in our service specification, we might be unable to demonstrate that our service is efficient and offering best value for money.

Measures of service outcome (Austin and Clark 1993, p. 21) are useful because they can serve to:

- show that the intervention offered by the service is appropriate and effective;
- indicate areas where service development might be required or additional resources deployed;
- enable changes that lead to an improvement in consumer satisfaction;
- show that a contracted service has been provided; and
- indicate effective use of health resources.

What Is a Service Evaluation?

A *Service Evaluation* is designed and conducted to solely define or judge current care. The choice of treatment, care or services is that of the care professional and patient/service user according to guidance, professional standards and/or patient/service user perspectives. This usually involves analysis of existing data but may also include administration of interview (s) or questionnaires(s)/outcome measures. Source: Modified from HRA (2017).

What Is Service Improvement?

NHS Improvement (2017) defines *Service Improvement* as using initiatives leading to increased quality and patient/service user experience at lower cost. A systematic approach that uses specific techniques to deliver and measure sustained improvement in quality. Source: Based on The Health Foundation (2013).

PLANNING A SERVICE EVALUATION

The Evidence Works (West of England Academic Health Science Network, BNSSG Research and Evidence Team and NIHR CLAHRC West 2016) website provides useful information on health service evaluation (http://www.nhsevidencetoolkit.net). A summary of the process outlined by the West of England group is given below. The group suggest a five-step process as shown in Figure 13.1. We will follow these steps as we discuss service evaluation and the importance of outcome measures in process. Once you have read the chapter, Worksheet 13.1 (p. 407) will help you work through the steps of the evaluation cycle.

STEP 1: IDENTIFY AND UNDERSTAND – BEGINNING A SERVICE EVALUATION

Shown in the box below are a number of questions that you need to ask yourself to identify and understand your service, such as who your key stakeholders are and what is the evidence. First, you need to define the service you wish to evaluate. It helps to have a service specification. If you do not have a specification for your service, the following headings are a useful guide:

- Overview: business need and vision
- Scope: purpose and description
- Service Delivery: models used and operational information
- Performance and Quality Measures: standards, monitoring, and data

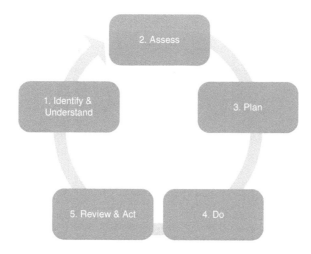

FIGURE 13.1   The evaluation cycle. *Source*: Adapted from West of England Academic Health Science Network, BNSSG Research and Evidence Team and NIHR CLAHRC (2016).

Step 1: Identify and Understand Questions

1. Who are my stakeholders?
2. What is the evidence base?
3. What will/does the service do?
4. How will/does the service work?

Once you have a clear description of the service or the part of a service (e.g. a time-limited treatment group, such as a falls prevention programme, pain management programme, anxiety management group, or reminiscence group). Then you need to outline clearly the parameters of the evaluation by answering the questions:

- *What do we want/need to know/measure about this service? (Steps 2 and 3)*
- *In order to obtain this information/measurement, what information do we need to collect? (Step 4)*
- *What decisions will be made from this information? (for example, whether to continue with a pilot intervention approach, or might this form the evidence for bid for additional funding to spread the treatment programme to another part of the service or for funding for an additional AHP?) (Step 5)*
- *What is the benefit for the stakeholders (e.g. service users, AHPs, referral sources, managers, funding agencies) from undertaking this service evaluation? (all steps)*

When setting objectives for service evaluation as part of service improvement, it is helpful to write these using a SMART format (Griffiths and Schell 2002, p. 232):

S = Specific

M = Measurable

A = Achievable

R = Realistic

T = Time bound

STEP 2: ASSESS – THE NEED FOR THE EVALUATION

To evaluate AHP services, we need to measure both process and service outcomes (also called programme outcomes). 'Process outcomes' is a term used to describe measures of the intervention itself (Robertson and Colborn 2000, p. 541). *Process outcomes* (Robertson and Colborn 2000) are based on feelings, client, and AHP perspectives, reactions to doing tasks, and analysis of what facilitated function. However, these constructs can be complex to measure.

Research that focuses on clinical reasoning can help you to understand the process of assessment and intervention (see Chapter 6). Robertson and Colborn (2000) state: 'If outcomes research mandates clear distinctions regarding specific services and subsequent outcomes, then finding strategies to directly link treatment and performance is the central goal of today's outcomes research in occupational therapy. The major challenges facing us are (a) what process variables should be measured, (b) what the best way to measure them is, and (c) how process and outcome can be linked in a treatment session'.

It is useful to examine our process outcomes for a number of reasons:

- to understand what we are currently achieving;
- to understand how stakeholders such as the service user, and/or the carer, experience the process;
- to understand what causes staff to be frustrated; and
- to understand what we need to improve.

Process measurement can include examination of the:

- Process time or cycle times
- Satisfaction
- Errors
- Utilisation.

Hughes (2008) recognised the need to use the framework of quality first proposed by Donabedian, in 1980, to consider the structure, process, and outcome of a service. The five-step process outlined in Figure 13.1 supports this framework, Steps 1 and 2 being structure, Steps 3 and 4 being the process, and Step 5 being the outcomes. The case studies at the end of the chapter illustrate aspects of these steps.

Service outcomes is a term applied to measures of the overall AHP service's efficiency and effectiveness. If you are undertaking a service evaluation, it is vital to define the global service outcomes, and the range of individual client outcomes, which the service aims to achieve. The outcome measures you select for the service evaluation must be matched to the intended goals of your service. The service level predetermined outcome(s) may be articulated in your service specification and/or in clinical guidelines, pathways, protocols, or standards. Individual client/AHP outcome goals are negotiated within the framework of the above for each service user and should be documented in the client's notes. Service outcomes provide information about the overall therapy service, and quantitative data about your service can include:

- the number and patterns (e.g. referral sources) of referrals during a defined time period
- length (range, mean, and standard deviation) of waiting times during a defined time period
- caseload numbers (range, mean, and standard deviation) for AHPs and therapy support staff during a defined time period
- for therapy services that operate a maximum caseload and use a caseload weighting system to decide on an optimum and maximum caseload, factors used to calculate caseload weighting can be analysed
- frequency and duration of contact with clients
- how many treatments were provided
- AHPs' client-contact/treatment hours versus non-client-contact hours
- how many clients were discharged to independent living situations
- how many clients were able to return to work following intervention
- delayed transfers of care, for example, how many patients were ready for discharge but were awaiting aids and adaptations or the start of another service before they could be discharged safely from your service
- discharge destinations.

STEP 3: PLAN – THE PURPOSE AND RESOURCES

When undertaking a service evaluation, try not to re-invent the wheel; where possible, use available data collected routinely as part of your normal service process. Review all the current information you have about your service, for example:

- referral criteria;
- any printed information for service users, carers, referral sources (e.g. service users' leaflet about the service, information about how to use a piece of equipment, instructions for exercises);
- forms used for assessment, care planning, documenting client notes;
- standardised tests used, especially outcome measures; and
- any data that is routinely recorded (e.g. waiting list numbers, referral and discharge rates per month, patient contacts, and caseload sizes).

You can also use data from national standards, examples of good practice, and public health data to help provide a benchmark for comparison. In the absence of ongoing continuous data about an aspect of your service, take a snapshot of data gathering to provide you with a baseline. Then in future ensure that measuring is an ongoing part of the new process.

Once you have identified your service evaluation parameters, formulate some specific questions. The nature of the question will lead you towards your evaluation method. Weigh up the pros and cons of the possible methods. Involving representatives from your key stakeholder groups is an important aspect of helping you to design, deliver, and disseminate your evaluation and the associated findings. Batalden et al. (2016) stated: 'Healthcare is not a product manufactured by the healthcare system, but rather a service, which is co-created by healthcare professionals in relationship with one another and with people seeking help to restore or maintain health for themselves and their families' (p. 515). Figure 13.2 outlines their conceptual model of healthcare service coproduction.

Service inputs are those factors that are required to deliver the entire service, including staffing costs, the service environment, equipment, materials, and

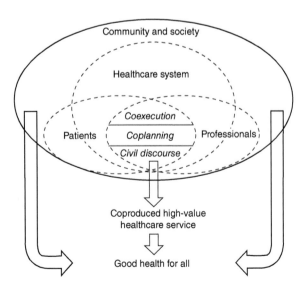

FIGURE 13.2   Conceptual model of healthcare service coproduction. *Source*: Batalden et al. (2016). © 2017, BMJ Publishing Group Limited.

other overheads (such as mileage costs for travelling to home visits and out-reach clinics).

If you wish to measure service inputs, you could consider:

- Staff input requirements, including professional staff, assistants/technician/support staff, and administrative staff (e.g. receptionist, secretary).
- Service environment department/service accommodation and overheads, such as clinic space rented from other service providers, for example, to run a pain assessment and management clinic at a health centre.
- Equipment; this might be equipment needed to perform a test (such as standardised test materials, tape measure, stopwatch, digital goniometer), and equipment that is used to assess the client's potential improvement using a piece of equipment, such as a walking frame or stick or a raised toilet seat.
- Materials; these are often consumable and may need replacing (e.g. stationery, test forms, food for a kitchen assessment, disposable gloves).

STEP 4: DO – COLLECTING AND ANALYSING THE DATA AND OUTCOME MEASURES

Where possible, combine methods of measurement and/or sources of data, and triangulate results to increase the reliability and validity of your findings. In Chapter 2, we looked at how self-report, proxy, and observational data can be triangulated to provide a comprehensive assessment of an individual client. This same process can be applied to service evaluation. To do this, you could divide the outcomes you evaluate into categories. These might be related to the stakeholder focus (see Table 13.1).

The first case study on p. 401 at the end of this chapter by Kathryn Moyse, from the Royal College of Speech & Language Therapists (RCSLT), gives an example of the importance of outcomes to assist data collection and analysis, with the aim of supporting the profession by delivering quality services.

The second case study (p. 404) by Dr Sue Pemberton, Yorkshire Fatigue Clinic, illustrates 10 tips for commissioning a specialist service, considering aspects of the five-step evaluation process and the importance of outcome measurement.

Financial data is often analysed as part of a service evaluation; this might include analysis of the cost of service inputs (such as staffing costs, mileage for making home assessment visits, cost of equipment and materials). Financial analysis might also involve a comparison of costs and outcomes of different models of service delivery. For example, you might compare the cost of a proxy report of the home environment versus an AHP observational assessment undertaken at a home visit with an outcome of readmission rates following discharge. The hypothesis might be that although the observational assessment is more expensive (AHP's time and travel costs), it leads to a more accurate assessment of risk and requirements for aids and adaptations to ensure a safe discharge.

Another way to categorise is by source of data, for example, client-focused measures versus staff-focused measures. Client-focused measures might include:

- the number of handovers of care a client experiences between AHPs, members of the multidisciplinary team (MDT), or between qualified and unqualified staff members;
- waiting times and delays experienced; and
- use of expert, professional, versus assistant staff time.

TABLE 13.1   Concepts of outcome and outcome measurement: the different perspectives of stakeholders.

Stakeholder	Perspective related to service outcomes
Client, carer	• Relief of distress and discomfort • Reduced disability • Increased satisfaction with their health and abilities • Appropriate and timely information about their condition, the assessment, and intervention process • Redress when initial outcome is unsatisfactory • Safety during care • Value for money in terms of charges paid • Equity and personalised service
AHP, clinician	• To measure the direct results of their interventions with clients • Assisting client to achieve optimal level of ability • The client's satisfaction with the process and intervention
Manager	• Resources used to provide an effective and efficient service • Referral rates, waiting times, discharges, of clients through the service within a specific time frame • Caseload numbers and weighting • Staff skill mix • Sickness, vacancies • Number and nature of compliments and complaints
Commissioner/ funding agency	• Improving the collective health status of the population • Population-wide indicators of the level of the service (mortality rates, morbidity indicators, waiting times, readmission rates) • Number and nature of compliments and complaints
Consumer groups, charities, voluntary sector	• Advocate for better services • Provide information on rights, benefits, and services available • Identify unmet needs and provide services to supplement statutory provision
Population	• People treated as individuals and given choice, respect, and dignity • Access to services

Source: Adapted from Austin and Clark (1993).

Staff-focused measures could be used with AHPs, managers, admin staff, support staff, and members of the MDT. These might include:

- a staff satisfaction questionnaire;
- sickness and absence data; and
- staffing levels, unfilled vacancies, and the use of agency staff.

Measures can also be categorised in terms of *direct* and *indirect service outcomes*. Direct measures of service outcome will include data from standardised tests, questionnaires, and client/patient records. 'Indirect measures are measures which, by inference, should indicate performance' (Austin and Clark 1993, p. 23). They include data such as 'weekly/monthly work analysis surveys, records of staff turnover, client throughput, waiting lists and readmission rates' (p. 23) and less easily measured variables such as 'opportunity for staff to become involved in continuing education and research, the cooperation with of staff with outside agencies, professional identity and confidence. These reflect aspects of a working environment which one assumes to be conducive to the delivery of a quality service' (p. 23). Caution needs to be exercised in supposing a direct relationship between these measures and the quality of a service. For example, one AHP might see more clients than another AHP. This provides a valid measure of throughput in a given time period and might be used to consider efficiency, but it will not provide any indication of whether the first or second AHP is providing a more effective service. A direct measure to evaluate whether clients were achieving their predefined/desired outcomes would be needed to measure the effectiveness of the service.

STEP 5: REVIEW AND ACT – IMPLEMENTATION AND DISSEMINATION

Service evaluation should lead to plans for improvement, which in turn should be evaluated following implementation, thus leading to a continuous cycle of service improvement. The dissemination of your findings should be targeted for the specific audiences (Gagnon 2011). Thinking back to the co-productive model introduced in Figure 13.1 (Batalden et al. 2016), you need to ensure that you collaborate with your stakeholders to develop an implementation approach that is appropriate to your audience (Gagnon 2011), which might be your service users, organisation, other AHPs, and/or commissioners.

This first case study illustrates the importance of data collection and analysis with the aim of supporting the profession by delivering quality services.

Case Study: RCSLT Online Outcome Tool

By **Kathryn Moyse**, Royal College of Speech & Language Therapists (RCSLT)

Background

The RCSLT is undertaking a programme of work on data collection and analysis with the aim of supporting the profession by delivering quality services. Although health and social care policies across the United Kingdom reference the importance of data information and technology in delivering care (Health and Social Care Board 2016; NHS England 2019a, 2019b; Scottish Government 2018; Welsh Government 2015), there remain numerous barriers for speech and language therapists (SLTs). This includes the absence of tools to support data collection and analytics. In response to this challenge, the RCSLT Online Outcome Tool (ROOT) has been developed to support the speech and language therapy profession by collecting, analysing, and reporting on outcome measures data.

The Approach

Choosing an Outcome Measure

Members of the speech and language therapy profession were consulted on the important properties of an outcome measure for the collection of consistent outcome measures data to enable services to monitor local performance as well as contributing to a national dataset that could potentially be used for benchmarking and increasing the impact of the profession. Key criteria were identified (Powell and Lowenthal 2014), and the RCSLT then commissioned a review of the existing outcome measurement tools available to SLTs against these criteria. Therapy Outcome Measures for Rehabilitation Professionals (TOMs) (Enderby and John 1997, 2015, 2019a, b; Enderby et al. 2006) data was selected from 63 candidate measures following a synthesis and Delphi consensus approach (Fink et al. 1984).

TOMs is based on the domains of the International Classification of Functioning (ICF) introduced by the World Health Organisation (WHO 1980, 2001), and also includes domains for 'patient well-being' and 'carer well-being', as the management of emotions, concern, and anxiety is frequently an objective of therapeutic interventions. The dimensions of impairment, activity, participation, patient well-being, and carer well-being are rated on an ordinal 11-point rating scale, at the start and end of an episode of care.

The adoption of TOMs by SLTs was acknowledged to be an 'opt-in' process, and it was made clear that this should not prevent SLTs using a broad range of tools as appropriate to their clinical management.

Developing a Digital Solution

The ROOT was developed to enable SLTs to record and monitor outcomes of individual patients/clients. SLTs submit de-personalised data on individuals referred for speech and language therapy intervention to the online database, including data on individuals' age, gender, diagnoses, and TOMs ratings at the beginning and end of an episode of care. The ROOT generates reports that show change over time in association with intervention and aggregates data from a team/service and generates descriptive statistical reports; Figures 13.3 and 13.4). These reports are tailored for different purposes and audiences (e.g. SLTs, commissioners, service managers, cli-

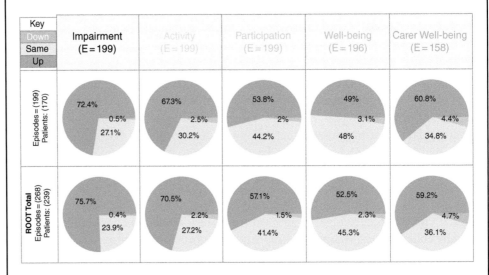

FIGURE 13.3   Direction of change in TOMs between start and final ratings across each domain of the TOMs (Impairment, Activity Participation, Well-being and Carer Well-being) for children and young people with phonological disorder. The report shows data for one service (anonymised) and that from across all contributing services ('ROOT Total'). Provided for illustration purposes only. Source: Kathryn Moyse, Royal College of Speech & Language Therapists (RCSLT).

	Improvement in Five Domains	Improvement in Four or More Domains	Improvement in Three or More Domains	Improvement in Two or More Domains	Improvement in One or More Domains	No Improvement in Any Domain
	0%	21.43%	21.43%	42.86%	85.71%	14.29%
ROOT total	0%	24.14%	37.93%	51.72%	82.76%	17.24%

FIGURE 13.4   Percentage of individuals with dysphagia whose TOMs scores have improved across 0–5 domains of the TOMs. The report shows data for one service (anonymised) and that from across all contributing services ('ROOT Total'). Provided for illustration purposes only. Source: Kathryn Moyse, Royal College of Speech & Language Therapists (RCSLT).

ents, and the professional body). Optional filters drill reports down to specific groups as required for more detailed data analysis.

Following an initial pilot, the ROOT is now being rolled out across the speech and language therapy profession. In April 2020, this national database held the outcomes of 37 000 individuals who have received speech and language therapy from 39 organisations.

Value

The speech and language therapy services using the ROOT report that it is easy and efficient, compared with existing methods in use, offering both a time and cost saving. Feedback indicates that the reports generated by the ROOT are useful in monitoring the outcomes in association with SLT interventions, both for individual service users and across clinical groups. They have been using the reports generated by the ROOT to support a number of functions, including:

- Supporting individual clinicians with their clinical decision making
- Providing information about the impact of speech and language therapy to key stakeholders, including funders and commissioners
- Supporting service improvement and planning

Initial reviews of the data (Enderby and Moyse 2018; Enderby et al. 2018; Moyse et al. 2020) have exposed variation in outcomes associated with different service provision, which is aligned with national policies focusing on understanding warranted and unwarranted variation in services. For example, some services having an increased impact on social participation and well-being, whereas other services have a greater impact on impairment and independence (Enderby and Moyse 2018; Enderby et al. 2018).

In the longer term, as the number of speech and language therapy services using the ROOT expands, the vision is to be able to identify services that are delivering the best outcomes and sharing examples of best practice to improvement the delivery of quality speech and language therapy across the profession.

Source: Kathryn Moyse, Royal College of Speech & Language Therapists (RCSLT).

This second case study illustrates 10 tips for commissioning a specialist service, considering aspects of the five-step evaluation process and the importance of outcome measurement.

Dr Sue Pemberton, Yorkshire Fatigue Clinic, York, United Kingdom

Commissioning a Specialist Rehabilitation Service for Chronic Fatigue Syndrome/Myalgic Encephalomyelitis (CFS/ME)

This case study presents the development of a local rehabilitation service for adults and young people with the condition Chronic Fatigue Syndrome/Myalgic Encephalomyelitis (CFS/ME) in collaboration between an independent provider and three Clinical Commissioning Groups. CFS/ME is a disabling condition that significantly impacts an individuals' ability to live their daily life (NICE 2007).

1. **Recognise the rehabilitation you already commission.**

Service provision for this condition nationally is inconsistent, with many geographical areas lacking any service provision. From 2004 to 2006, the government launched the CFS/ME Investment Programme with the aim of addressing gaps in service provision across England and supported the development of 13 centres of expertise, 36 adult, and 11 specialist children's local multidisciplinary teams (Pinching and Noons 2006). However, when the funding was devolved to local areas, some services were closed, and many areas still lacked local provision. In this example, the specialist service available was based in a city outside of the local commissioners' areas and involved patients having to travel for up to two hours. Therefore, the commissioners were aware of the rehabilitation available, but knew that this did not meet the local needs.

2. **Have ambition for your services and the people they serve**

Consequently, when a specialist occupational therapist with considerable experience in this condition discussed with them the concept of developing more local services, they were willing to encourage this development. They enabled the service to grow slowly by permitting the general practitioners to choose between the established provider at a distance, and the local option. They maintain control over the process by allocating funding through the Individual Funding Panel and authorising treatment on a case-by-case basis. They were then able to look at the evidence of service outcomes and patient experience after a year to gain the confidence to support the local rehabilitation team as the preferred provider.

3. **Make your services join up and have some common key principles in your service specifications**

After two years, the demand for the local service had grown to the point that authorising funding individually had become too time consuming for the commissioners, and they decided to offer the service on an NHS contract through the procurement process. At this time, they drew up a service specification which outlined the expected pathway through the rehabilitation process, and specific outcome measures by which the contract would be assessed. The tendering process wanted prospective providers to outline how they would link with other local services, such as community mental health services, education, and local communities.

4. **Rehabilitation should not be an extra or an add-on – it should be considered throughout each person's journey**

Rehabilitation is currently the only treatment approach for CFS/ME as no pharmacological treatments are available (NICE Guidelines 2007). In addition, no specific biomedical tests will identify the condition, although investigations in primary care are necessary to exclude other possible causes. Consequently, rehabilitation in this situation was central to the commissioning process.

5. **Consider what outcomes you want; identify some common measures and ask your services to work together**

In this case, the commissioners utilised the clinical measures that had been collected as part of the Investment Programme which had been referred to as the Minimum Data Set (Pinching and Noons 2006). Initially, all the Minimum Data Set measures were specified and collected; however, as the purpose of the data set had previously been researched, over time the commissioners and service agreed to reduce the requirement and focus on Clinical Global Impressions Scale, physical functioning, and self-efficacy. Patient experience was felt to be a vital indicator, and a questionnaire was devised that patients could complete anonymously online when they are discharged from the service. The results of this are available to the commissioners and used by the service to make improvements.

6. **Consider the range of settings where your services are delivered, especially community settings, the third sector, and care homes (including respite care)**

The specific needs of this patient group were considered, as travelling can increase their symptoms and could cause a relapse in their health. Consequently, a range of options were developed which would be suitable for the different levels of severity. Outpatient and group options are delivered in the most populated city within the area, as this is cost-efficient for those who are able to travel. Home-based rehabilitation, where the AHP travels to the patients' own home, was made available to those who are house-bound or bed-bound. Access was also increased by providing the option for telephone or videoconferencing sessions, alongside support through direct email access to an AHP.

7. **Take a strategic view on what you invest to save.**

There are increasing costs to the NHS as the number of people with long-term conditions continues to rise (House of Commons Health Committee 2014). Accessing rehabilitation services can lead to increased daily function and improved symptom management. In this service, 40% of patients reported feeling very much better or much better at one year after starting treatment (Collin and Crawley 2017). As rehabilitation can take longer than one year, the local results showed a further increase in patients who reported feeling very much better or much better at discharge.

8. **Cross-check your local services against the rehabilitation model to identify gaps or duplication and outcomes being achieved.**

As there are three Clinical Commissioning Groups involved, there is a contract manager who liaises with the provider, and any gaps or areas of duplication can be discussed. A pathway form was developed to ensure that the correct patients are seem by the service, and those patients whose needs could be met in other services are redirected, such as rheumatology or mental health services.

9. **Ask for advice and support if necessary: what forums do you use to share good practice locally, regionally, and nationally?**

The commissioners can access information about the service and the referral pathway on the local electronic resource for GPs. Patients submit feedback through the local Health Watch Website in addition to through the service directly.

10. **Ask your providers and service users how improvements could be made and what can be done differently to improve outcomes for people**

Through the quarterly meetings between the lead clinician and contract manager, ideas for improving the service can be discussed and developed. The feedback given through the anonymous online patient survey is available to inform ways to improve outcomes, in addition to feedback through social media.

Source: Dr Sue Pemberton, Yorkshire Fatigue Clinic, York, UK.

Worksheet 13.1 will help you work through the evaluation cycle.

Steps	Questions to ask	Your responses	Comments
Step 1 – Identify and Understand	Who are my stakeholders? What is the evidence base? What will/does the service do? How will/does it work?		
Step 2 – Assess	Do I need to do an evaluation? What will I measure? What is/are the benefit(s)? Am I doing an evaluation?		
Step 3 – Plan	What is the purpose of my evaluation? What are my SMART goals? What approach should I take? What are the potential outcomes? What resources do I need?		
Step 4 – Do	How will I collect the data? How will I measure? How will I analyse the data?		
Step 5 – Review and Act	What decisions will be made from this information? How will I implement my findings? How will I share and present (disseminate) my findings?		

Source: Adapted from Evaluation Works ,West of England Academic Health Science Network, BNSSG Research and Evidence Team and NIHR CLAHRC West (2016).

REFERENCES

Austin, C. and Clark, C.R. (1993). Measures of outcome: for whom? *British Journal of Occupational Therapy* 56 (1): 21–24. https://doi.org/10.1177/030802269305600107.

Batalden, M., Batalden, P., Margolis, P. et al. (2016). Coproduction of healthcare service. *BMJ Quality & Safety* 25 (7): 509–517. https://doi.org/10.1136/bmjqs-2015-004315.

Collin, S.M. and Crawley, E. (2017). Specialist treatment of chronic fatigue syndrome/ME: a cohort study among adult patients in England. *BMC Health Services Research* 17: 488. https://doi.org/10.1186/s12913-017-2437-3.

Corr, S. (2003). Evaluate, evaluate, evaluate. *British Journal of Occupational Therapy* 66 (6): 235–235. https://doi.org/10.1177/030802260306600601.

Donabedian, A. (1980). *The Definition of Quality and Approaches to Its Assessment and Monitoring*, vol. I. Ann Arbor: Health Administration Press.

Enderby, P. and John, A. (1997). *Therapy Outcome Measures: Speech-Language Pathology*. San Diego, London: Singular Publishing Group, Inc.

Enderby, P. and John, A. (2015). *Therapy Outcome Measures for Rehabilitation Professionals*, 3rde. Croydon: J & R Press Ltd.

Enderby, P. and John, A. (2019a). *Therapy Outcome Measures for Rehabilitation Professionals*, 4the. Croydon: J & R Press Ltd.

Enderby, P. and John, A. (2019b). *User Guide: Therapy Outcome Measures*. Croydon: J & R Press Ltd.

Enderby, P. and Moyse, K. (2018). International classification of functioning—an approach to outcome measurement. *Perspectives of the ASHA Special Interest Groups* 3 (17): 99–108. https://doi.org/10.1044/persp3.SIG17.99.

Enderby, P., John, A., and Petheram, B. (2006). *Therapy Outcome Measures for Rehabilitation Professionals: Speech and Language Therapy, Physiotherapy, Occupational Therapy, Rehabilitation Nursing & Hearing Therapists*, 2nd Ed. Chichester: Wiley.

Enderby, P., Moyse, K., Bedwell, M., and Guest, P. (2018). Getting to the ROOT of outcomes. *RCSLT Bulletin* 791: 13–15. https://www.rcslt.org/speech-and-language-therapy/guidance-for-delivering-slt-services/outcome-measurement/outcome-tool-overview/.

Fink, A., Kosecoff, J., Chassin, M., and Brook, R.H. (1984). Consensus methods: characteristics and guidelines for use. *American Journal of Public Health* 74 (9): 979–983. https://ajph.aphapublications.org/doi/abs/10.2105/AJPH.74.9.979.

Gagnon, M.L. (2011). Moving knowledge to action through dissemination and exchange. *Journal of Clinical Epidemiology* 64 (1): 25–31. https://doi.org/10.1016/j.jclinepi.2009.08.013.

Griffiths, S. and Schell, D. (2002). Professional context. In: *Occupational Therapy and Physical Dysfunction: Principles, Skills and Practice* (eds. A. Turner, M. Foster and S.E. Johnson), 211–252. Elsevier Health Sciences.

Health and Social Care Board (2016). *eHealth and Care Strategy for Northern Ireland*. Health and Social Care Board. Available from: https://www.health-ni.gov.uk/publications/ehealth-and-care-strategy [Accessed 13 May 2021].

Health Research Authority (HRA). (2017) Defining Research available from http://www.hra-decisiontools.org.uk/research/docs/DefiningResearchTable_Oct2017-1.pdf [Accessed 13 May 2021].

House of Commons Health Committee (2014) Managing the care of people with long-term conditions Second Report of Session 2014–15 available on the Committee website at https://publications.parliament.uk/pa/cm201415/cmselect/cmhealth/401/40102.htm

Hughes, R.G. (2008). Tools and strategies for quality improvement and patient safety. In: *Patient Safety and Quality: An Evidence-Based Handbook for Nurses.* Agency for Healthcare Research and Quality (US).

Moyse, K., Enderby, P., Chadd, K. et al. (2020). Outcome measurement in speech and language therapy: a digital journey. *BMJ Health & Care Informatics* 27 (1): e100085. https://doi.org/10.1136/bmjhci-2019-100085.

National Institute for Health and Care Excellence (2007) Chronic fatigue syndrome/ myalgic encephalomyelitis (or encephalopathy): diagnosis and management (NICE Guideline 53). Available at: www.nice.org.uk/Guidance/CG53 [Accessed 18 September 2019].

NHS England. (2019a) *A Digital Framework for Allied Health Professionals.* NHS England. Available from: https://www.england.nhs.uk/publication/a-digital-framework-for-allied-health-professionals/ [Accessed 13 May 2021].

NHS England. (2019b) *The NHS Long Term Plan.* NHS England. Available from: https://www.england.nhs.uk/long-term-plan/ [Accessed 13 May 2021].

NHS Improvement (2017) *Quality, Service Improvement and redesign* NHS Improvement https://www.england.nhs.uk/qsir-programme/

NHS Improvement (2018) *Service specification template Corporate services productivity programme* July 2018 NHS Improvement. https://www.england.nhs.uk/commissioning/spec-services/key-docs/

Pinching, AJ, Noons PA (2006) CFS/ME service investment programme report 2004–2006. Programme report. *Plymouth: University of Exeter*

Powell, G. and Lowenthal, D. (2014). Outcomes and outcome measures. *RCSLT Bulletin* 749: 22–24.

Robertson, S.C. and Colborn, A.P. (2000). Can we improve outcomes research by expanding research methods? *American Journal of Occupational Therapy* 54 (5): 541–543.

Scottish Government. (2018) *Scotland's Digital Health and Care Strategy: enabling, connecting and empowering.* Scottish Government. Available from: https://www.gov.scot/publications/scotlands-digital-health-care-strategy-enabling-connecting-empowering/ [Accessed 13 May 2021].

The Health Foundation (2013). *Quality Improvement Made Simple. What Everyone Should Know About Health Care Quality Improvement.* The Health Foundation https://www.health.org.uk/publications/quality-improvement-made-simple.

The Health Foundation (2015). *Evaluation: What to Consider.* London: Health Foundation https://www.health.org.uk/publications/evaluation-what-to-consider.

Welsh Government. (2015) *Informed Health and Care: A Digital Health and Social Care Strategy for Wales.* Welsh Government. Available from: https://gov.wales/sites/default/files/publications/2019-03/informed-health-and-care-a-digital-health-and-social-care-strategy-for-wales.pdf [Accessed 13 May 2021].

West of England Academic Health Science Network, BNSSG Research and Evidence Team and NIHR CLAHRC West (2016) Evaluation Toolkit. https://nhsevaluationtoolkit.net/what-is-evaluation/

World Health Organization (1980). *The International Classification of Impairments, Disabilities and Handicaps.* Geneva: World Health Organization https://apps.who.int/iris/handle/10665/41003 [Accessed 13 May 2021].

World Health Organization (2001). *The International Classification of Functioning, Disability and Health.* Geneva: World Health Organization https://www.who.int/standards/classifications/international-classification-of-functioning-disability-and-health [Accessed 13 May 2021].

RESOURCES

Evaluation Works – https://nhsevaluationtoolkit.net/what-is-evaluation/. All resources and graphics on this website are © West of England Academic Health Science Network, BNSSG Research and Evidence Team and NIHR CLAHRC West 2016. We are happy for you to reuse any of these materials so long as it is not for commercial purposes and you include credits to all three organisations with links back to the originating page(s) on this website. For further information, please email info@nhsevidencetoolkit.net

The Health Foundation – https://www.health.org.uk/what-we-do/supporting-health-care-improvement

SECTION 4

DEVELOPING AND EVALUATING ASSESSMENTS AND OUTCOME MEASURES

CHAPTER 14

Test Development

OVERVIEW

In this chapter, we consider the process for developing and standardising an assessment for use in allied health professional (AHP) practice. The chapter also explores the features of criterion-referenced tests, Guttman scaling, and Rasch analysis. We discussed normative/norm-referenced tests in Chapter 7. The process for undertaking a norming study is summarised.

QUESTIONS TO CONSIDER

1. Is there an outcome measure already able?
2. What are my test construction decisions?
3. What are the features of a criterion-referenced test?

CONSIDERATIONS FOR TEST DEVELOPMENT

Test development is a time-consuming, complex, and iterative process of construction, evaluation, revision, and re-evaluation. Therefore, it is important to investigate the outcome measures and tests already available. There are useful resources to identify the standardised outcome measures and tests already available such as:

- The COnsensus-based Standards for the selection of health Measurement INstruments (COSMIN – https://www.cosmin.nl). COSMIN aims to improve the selection of outcome measurement instruments both in research and in clinical practice by developing methodology and practical tools for selecting the most suitable outcome measurement instrument.

- The Royal College of Speech and Language Therapists Online Outcome Tool discussed in the case study in Chapter 13 (https://www.rcslt.org/speech-and-language-therapy/guidance-for-delivering-slt-services/outcome-measurement/outcome-tool-overview/)
- The American Psychiatric Association, Online Assessment Measures (https://www.psychiatry.org/psychiatrists/practice/dsm/educational-resources/assessment-measures)
- The Cicely Saunders Institute of Palliative Care, Policy & Rehabilitation, Kings College London lists a number of rehabilitation outcome measures (https://www.kcl.ac.uk/cicelysaunders/research/outcome/rehabilitation/Rehab-outcome-measures)

Explore these databases before you decide to develop a further outcome measure or standardised test.

As the process of rigorous test construction is complex, it is not our intention to provide detailed guidance in this chapter. Several authors describe and discuss the process of test construction and would provide a sensible starting point for any AHP considering embarking on test development; for example, see: Anastasi (1988); Pett et al. (2003); and Kline (2015). When embarking on the development of the Structured Observation Test of Function (SOTOF; Laver 1994; Laver and Powell 1995), the views of others in test development were considered. Pynsent (2004) also advises 'that designing a new instrument is a complex task not to be undertaken lightly' (p. 2). He provides a 'design pathway' for the process of developing an outcome measure. This is shown in Figure 14.1. (Note: Some of the psychometric terms in this figure are defined in Chapters 8 and 9.)

As we explored in the section titled 'Standardisation' in Chapter 7, standardisation is a process of taking an assessment and developing a fixed protocol for its administration and scoring, and then conducting psychometric studies to evaluate whether the resulting assessment has acceptable levels of validity and reliability. There are two ways in which assessments can be standardised: either in terms of procedures, materials, and scoring or in terms of normative standardisation (de Clive-Lowe 1996). The first method of standardisation involves the provision of detailed descriptions and directions for the test materials; method of administration; instructions for administration; scoring; and interpretation of scores (Jones 1991). Standardisation 'extends to the exact materials employed, time limits, oral instructions, preliminary demonstrations, ways of handling queries from test takers, and every other detail of the testing situation' (Anastasi 1988, p. 25). Manuals are recommended to establish a standardised patient instruction method (Zandbelt et al. 2001). If a test is published in its entirety in a professional journal, information on the method should be included in the description of the test.

To standardise the *test materials*, the exact test materials should be listed or included. Some tests provide materials as part of a standardised test battery. If the AHP has to collect the materials together for the test, then precise details of how to construct the test (with exact sizes, colours, fabric of materials, etc.) are required.

To standardise the *method of administration*, the test conditions should be described in detail. The number of people tested at any one time should be specified (i.e. individual or group assessment, size of group). Information about the time required for

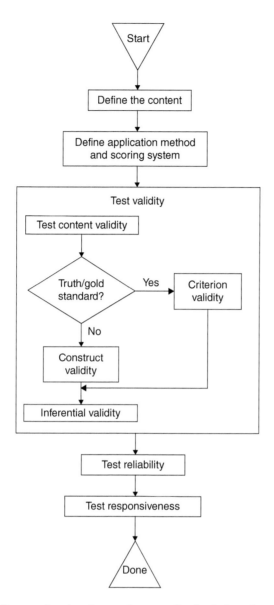

FIGURE 14.1   Flow diagram showing the requirements for the design of an outcome measure. *Source*: Pynsent (2004). © 2004, Taylor & Francis.

administration should be given. The *Manual for the Comprehensive Health Assessment Tool* (CHAT) by The Offender Health Research Network (2013) provides a useful example of a manual (http://www.ohrn.nhs.uk/OHRNResearch/CHATManualV32013.pdf, Chitsabesan et al. 2014). The manual outlines the background, development and validation of CHAT, details on how to complete the CHAT, and additional guidance.

In order to produce standardised instructions for administration by an AHP, detailed written instructions should be provided. The exact wording for any instructions to be given to the test taker are required. To maintain standardisation, AHPs should be told to follow all instructions exactly. In the following box is an example of test instructions taken from the Gross Motor Function Measure (GMFM) Test Manual (Russell et al. 1993, pp. 41 and 42).

Example Test Instructions from the GMFM

Lying and Rolling

This dimension includes 17 items in the prone and supine positions.
These items include the child's ability to:

- Roll from prone or supine
- Perform specific tasks while maintaining supine or some variation of prone

Item 1. Supine, Head in Midline: Turns Head with Extremities Symmetrical

1. Does not maintain head in midline
2. Maintains head in midline one to three seconds
3. Maintains head in midline, turns head with extremities asymmetrical
4. Turns head with extremities symmetrical

Starting Position

Position the child with head in midline and, if possible, the arms at rest and symmetrical (but not necessarily at the side). This will make it easier to determine the appropriate score.

Instructions

Instruct the child to turn the head from side to side or follow an object from one side to the other.

The child can be instructed to keep the arms still, or, in the case of a younger child who may try to reach for the object, observe whether the upper extremity movements are 'symmetrical' or 'asymmetrical'.

For a score of 2 (extremities 'asymmetrical'), there should be very obvious asymmetry that is dominated by the head position.

To standardise the *scoring system*, clear guidelines need to be provided for scoring. The person's performance on the test should be evaluated on the basis of empirical data. Scoring methods vary from test to test and may include the use of raw scores, which may then be converted to another type of score. If scores are being added, subtracted, divided, or multiplied, then make sure the level of measurement allows the numbers to be handled in that way (see Chapter 4). Information should be included to guide the AHP in the interpretation of scores. AHPs should be aware that a number of factors may influence the person's performance on the test, including test anxiety, fatigue, interruptions, and distractions.

In addition to basic administration details, other subtle factors might affect a person's test performance. For example, when giving oral instructions, 'rate of speaking, tone of voice, inflection, pauses, and facial expression' all may influence how a person responds (Anastasi (1988), pp. 25–26).

CONSTRUCTING A STANDARDISED TEST

AHPs may find that they cannot obtain a published measure that measures exactly what they want, either with the group of clients they treat and/or in the setting that they practice, so they sometimes decide to design their own measure.

However, it is important to ensure you have checked if there is an already validated assessment tool and/outcome measures available (see the section titled 'Considerations for Test Development' earlier in this chapter).

The AHP Outcome Measures UK Working Group, a cross-disciplinary group representing a number of professional bodies, has developed a checklist called 'Key Questions to Ask When Selecting Outcome Measures: A Checklist for Allied Health Professionals, 2019' to assist individual AHPs and teams with selecting outcome measures. The checklist is intended to guide discussions and support decision making. It contains some key questions to ask when considering which outcome measure is most suitable for your area of practice. The checklist is available to download from the Royal College of Speech and Language Therapists (RCSLT) website (https://www.rcslt.org/outcome-measures-checklist/).

Even if you do not intend to attempt to develop a test yourself, it is useful for any student or clinician to have a basic understanding of the test development process, so that they can establish whether a potential measure for their service has been rigorously developed. Crocker and Algina (1986) summarise the test construction process as a series of 10 steps.

A 10-Step Test Construction Process

1. Identify the primary purpose(s) for which test scores will be used.
2. Identify behaviours that represent the construct or define the domain.
3. Prepare a set of test specifications, delineating the proportion of items that should focus on each type of behaviour identified in step two.
4. Construct an initial pool of items.
5. Have items reviewed (and revise as necessary).
6. Hold preliminary try-outs (and revise as necessary).
7. Field-test the items on a large sample representative of the examinee population for whom the test is intended.
8. Determine the statistical properties of item scores and, when appropriate, eliminate items that do not meet pre-established criteria.
9. Design and construct reliability and validity studies for the final form of the test.
10. Develop guidelines for test administration, scoring, and for the interpretation of test scores (e.g. prepare norm tables and suggest recommended cutting scores or standards for performance).

Source: Crocker and Algina (1986). © 1986, Houghton Mifflin Harcourt.

The psychometric literature focuses on the scientific aspects of test construction, such as item analysis and factor analysis (Hubley and Zumbo 2013). Other aspects, such as item writing, have 'remained private, informal, and largely undocumented ... typically the test developer will conceptualize one or more incidents, direct observations, expert judgement and the development of instruction objectives' (Crocker and Algina 1986, p. 67). A critical part of test development is identifying the primary purpose and then defining relevant content and selecting specific test items for a measure. This will help ensure that a clinically useful measure is produced; 'clarifying the major purposes for which test scores will be used and establishing priorities among these probable uses greatly increases the likelihood that this final form of the test will be useful for the most important purpose it is to serve' (p. 67). This is more challenging when the focus of the measure is a psychological construct, as opposed to an observable behaviour or functional ability. In this case, a very thorough understanding of the theory underlying the construct is the starting point for test development. Stanley and Hopkins (1972, as cited by Royeen 1989) described a four-step process for developing a measure of a construct and then establishing the measure's validity:

1. Develop a set of tasks or items based on the rational analysis of the construct.
2. Derive testable predictions regarding the relationship between the construct and other variables; for example, if the test measures anxiety, we should expect to find some relationship between test scores and clinical ratings of anxiety.
3. Conduct empirical studies of these theoretical predictions.
4. Eliminate items or tasks that operate contrary to theory (or revise the theory), and proceed again with steps 2 and 3 (Royeen 1989, p. 57).

Crocker and Algina (1986) suggested that 'to broaden, refine, or verify the view of the construct to be measured, the test developer should engage in one or more of the following activities:

1. *Content analysis:* With this method, open-ended questions are posed to subjects about the construct of interest, and their responses are sorted into topical categories ...
2. *Review of research*: The behaviours that have been most frequently studied by others are used to define the construct of interest ...
3. *Critical incidents:* A list of behaviours is identified that characterises extremes of the performance continuum for the construct of interest ...
4. *Direct observations:* The test developer identifies the behaviours by direct observation ...
5. *Expert judgement:* The test developer obtains input from one or more individuals who have first-hand experience with the construct ...
6. *Instruction objectives:* Experts in a subject are asked to review instructional materials and develop a set of instructional objectives when an achievement test is being developed. An instructional objective specifies an observable behaviour that [people] should be able to exhibit after a course of instruction ...' (p. 68)

If you do decide to attempt to develop a test yourself, then for a comprehensive and detailed breakdown of the procedures and sequence of content validation needed for robust test development, see Haynes et al. (1995), Appendix A of their article 'Content Validity in Psychological Assessment: A Functional Approach to Concepts and Methods'. They state that content validation is a multi-method, quantitative, and qualitative process that is applicable to all elements of a test. The reason test developers need to focus on content validation during initial test development is 'to minimize potential error variance associated with an assessment instrument and to increase the probability of obtaining supportive construct validity indices in later studies' (p. 243).

When developing an assessment that will be used to measure outcomes, the test developer needs to consider a number of issues. The sensitivity of an outcome measure to the type and amount of change anticipated to occur during a therapeutic intervention is one of the most important considerations. Many functional assessments measure a narrow range of functions with scales that have large increments between each recorded ability level. Such scales produce summary scores that often do not have the sensitivity to detect small improvements in function (Fisher 2003). A scale comprising more increments of change is likely to be more sensitive, and longer scales make it easier to measure change over a wider range of functional ability (Fisher 2003; Fisher and Merritt 2012).

When developing a test, there are a number of decisions to be made because the type of information collected and the proposed purpose of the new test can influence its construction. The elements of a test 'are all the aspects of the measurement process that can affect the obtained data. For example, the elements of questionnaires include individual items, response formats, and instructions. The elements of behavioural observation include observation codes, time sampling parameters, and the situations in which observation occurs' (Haynes et al. 1995, p. 238). When developing a test, all these elements need to be considered. This means that many decisions have to be made during a test development process.

TEST CONSTRUCTION DECISIONS

This list is drawn from on a number of publications such as Law et al. 1990, Royeen 1989, Thorborg et al. 2011, and Velozo et al. 2012.

- What level of data is involved (nominal, ordinal, interval, or ratio)? (Note: See Chapter 4 for definitions and descriptions of data at each of these measurement levels.)

- What will the results be used for? (Note: See Chapter 3 for a discussion about the different requirements AHPs have for making measurements.)
- Should you use a scale, index, or typology? (Note: See the *Introduction* for definitions of scale, index, and typology.)
- What types of statistical analysis would be useful?
- Should you use a comparative scale or a non-comparative scale?

- How many scale divisions or categories should be used (e.g. 1 to 10; 1 to 7; −3 to +3)?
- Should there be an odd or even number of scale divisions? (An odd number of divisions gives a neutral centre value, whereas an even number of divisions forces respondents to take a non-neutral position).
- What should the nature and description of the scale labels be?
- What should the physical form or layout of the scale be, for example, graphic, simple linear, vertical, or horizontal?
- Should a response to each item be forced or should it be left optional, for example, by providing a not-applicable or not-tested option?

Examples of comparative scaling techniques used in some AHP assessments include:

- **Paired comparison scale**: The client is presented with two items at a time and, asked to select one (for example: do you prefer to be alone or to socialise with friends?)
- **Rank-order scale**: The client is presented with several items simultaneously and asked to rank them (for example: Rate the following leisure activities from 1 to 10 with 1 = the activity that you enjoy doing the most and 10 = the activity that you enjoy the least). This is an ordinal level scaling technique.

Examples of non-comparative scaling techniques used in some AHP assessments include:

- **Continuous rating scale** (also called the graphic rating scale): The client is asked to rate the test item, for example, the degree of pain experienced when undertaking a particular movement, by placing a mark on a line. The line is usually labelled at each end (e.g. 'no pain' at one end and 'unbearable pain' at the other). There are sometimes a series of numbers, called scale points (e.g. 0–10) under the line.
- **Likert scale:** With this type of scaling, people are asked to specify their level of agreement to each of a list of statements. This form of scale was named after Rensis Likert, who invented the scale in 1932. Clients have to indicate the amount of agreement or disagreement they have with each test item statement (from 'strongly agree' to 'strongly disagree'). This is usually presented on a 5- or 7-point scale. The same format is used for multiple test items. For example, in a measure of carer burden, carers might be asked to rate the following type of item: 'owing to the amount of time spent caring for my loved one I do not have enough time to socialise with other family'. They would then answer this by circling one of the following responses:
  1. Strongly disagree
  2. Disagree
  3. Neither agree nor disagree
  4. Agree
  5. Strongly agree

Royeen (1989) provided a checklist for instrument development; this takes the form of a series of questions related to different psychometric properties. Validation is undertaken by a test developer to collect evidence to support the types of inferences that are to be drawn from the results of an assessment (Crocker and Algina 1986). Although validity can be quantified, it can be related to the robustness of the theoretical underpinnings of a test, and therefore evaluation of test validity may involve qualitative and subjective methods. Cronbach (1960) suggested that test developers should not validate their test, but rather explore validity in terms of an interpretation of data arising from a specified procedure.

Royeen (1989) noted that 'the validity question is always specific: how well does this instrument assess the characteristic, construct, or behaviour the user desires to measure?' (p. 54). Royeen suggested that to establish whether a measure has acceptable levels of validity, the following questions should be addressed (note: information pertaining to these areas should be provided by test developers in a test manual and/ or in research articles in professional journals):

If *content validity* is claimed, answers are needed to these questions:

- Source(s) of items?
- Panel of content experts used?
- Statistical techniques(s) used (e.g. factor analysis)?
- Item-total correlation (r and N)?

If *criterion validity* is claimed, answers are needed to these questions:

- Outside criterion used?
- Standardisation (validity) group used? (describe characteristics, size, etc.)
- Correlation with criterion?

If *construct validity* is claimed, answers are needed to these questions:

- Theoretical basis? (described)
- Source(s) of items?
- Panel of experts used?
- Statistical technique(s) used (e.g. convergent-divergent)?
- Item-total correlation (r and N)?

(Note: For definitions of the different types of validity, see Chapter 8. In terms of the abbreviations used by Royeen, r refers to Pearson 'r' coefficient of correlation (1989, p. 61), and N is traditionally the abbreviation used to represent the total number of items).

Standardised assessments provide for measurement against a criterion or norm and can be divided into two main types: norm-referenced or criterion-referenced tests. The following sections will describe each of these types.

CRITERION-REFERENCED TESTS

A criterion-referenced test is a test that examines performance against predefined criteria and produces raw scores that are intended to have a direct, interpretable meaning (Crocker and Algina 1986). The person's score on this type of test is interpreted by comparing the score with a pre-specified standard of performance or against specific content and/or skills (Rikli and Jones 2013). The AHP uses this type of test to judge whether the person has mastered the required standard (for example, to judge whether the person has sufficient independence to be safe to be discharged to live alone at home). The person's performance is not compared to the ability of other people; it is evaluated only against the defined criterion (whereas norm-referenced assessments evaluate performance against the scores of a normative sample; see below).

Criterion assessments usually have one of two main purposes:

- estimation of the domain score, i.e. the proportion of items in the domain which the subject can pass correctly; or
- mastery allocation.

In mastery allocation, the domain score is divided into a number of mutually exclusive mastery categories, which are defined by cut scores. The observed test results are used to classify people into the mastery categories. 'The most commonly cited example has one cut score and two categories, master and non-master' (Crocker and Algina 1986). This is useful for AHPs who are often involved with examining a person's competence or level of mastery. Criterion-referenced tests are important because AHPs are concerned with desired outcomes, such as specified levels of ability in activities of daily living (ADL) tasks, range of movement (ROM), or mobility. In an AHP assessment, a score representing 'master' might be labelled *able* or *independent* or *observed;* whereas a score representing 'non-master' might be labelled *unable* or *dependent* or *not observed.*

With a criterion-referenced measure, it is essential to have a detailed and unambiguous definition of the criteria against which the person is to be judged. For example, if the desired outcome is independence in getting dressed, then the test should describe exactly what the person should be able to do in order to be assessed as being competent in dressing. Depending on the activity to be assessed, different criteria might be necessary for people of different gender, age, or cultural backgrounds. In some cases, a time limit might form part of the criteria.

An example of a criterion-referenced measure is the Severe Impairment Battery (SIB; Panisset et al. 1994). This test was developed to evaluate severe cognitive deficits. The test has 40 items, 38 of which use mastery scoring with a three-point scale (p. 5):

2 = correct
1 = partially correct, an approximate or closely related answer
0 = incorrect

The test developers state that 'there is, of course, no cut off for normal as the test should only be used with patients known to be severely impaired' (Saxton et al. 1993, p. 5).

THE PROCESS FOR UNDERTAKING A NORMING STUDY

As discussed in the section titled 'Normative Data' in Chapter 7, norm-referenced test and normative data are used interchangeably in this book and in the literature. The second method of standardisation involves conducting a *norming study*. In a norm-referenced test, a person's performance is considered against the 'normal' performance by comparing their score to a range of scores obtained from a representative group of people; this is known as the normative sample or normative group (Lenhard et al. 2019). The scores are placed in norm tables within the test manual. These tables give the distribution, or spread, of scores that the normative group obtained (de Clive-Lowe 1996). Crocker and Algina (1986) described nine basic steps for conducting a norming study which they state are recommended irrespective of whether norms are intended for local or wider use.

Nine Steps for Conducting a Norming Study

1. Identify the population of interest (e.g. people with a particular diagnosis or service users eligible for a particular health service, or people of a specified age, geographical, or socio-economic background).

2. Identify which statistics are to be produced on the normative sample data (e.g. mean, standard deviation, and percentile ranks).

3. Decide what amount of sampling error can be tolerated for any of the statistics identified (a common example is the sampling error associated with the mean).

4. Develop a method for sampling from the population of interest (this might involve random sampling, stratified sampling, or seeking volunteers).

5. Estimate the minimum sample size needed to keep the sampling error within the specified limits.

6. Obtain the sample, administer the test, and collect data. The test developers should record any reasons for attrition, and if a substantial num-

ber of people pull out of the sample, it may be necessary to continue to implement the sampling method to obtain additional people from the population to ensure the desired sample size.

7. Calculate all the statistics of interest.

8. Identify the normative scores that are needed from the data, and develop normative score conversion tables for the test.

9. Write up the norming procedure in the test manual, and prepare guidelines for the interpretation of the normative scores.

The Brief Infant Sleep Questionnaire – Revised (BISQ-R) is an example of an age-based norm-referenced scoring system (Mindell et al. 2019). Janssen et al. (2019) provide a useful descriptive of population norms for the EQ-5D-3L through a cross-country analysis of population surveys for 20 countries.

GUTTMAN SCALING

Guttman scales can be helpful because they are constructed in a way that enables the AHP to administer only those items which fall at the outer boundaries of the client's ability and provide a useful indicator of the maximum level of difficulty that the person can master. Guttman (1941, as cited in Crocker and Algina 1986) described a response-scaling method called scalogram analysis. Items are worded to increase in strength/severity/demand so that once a respondent agrees with one item statement, he should also agree with all the statements that express weaker/less severe/less demanding items (Abdi 2010). In a Guttman scale, if the client passes an item high on the scale, the implication is that he will also be able to pass less demanding items lower down on the scale (McDowell and Newell 1987).

On these types of scales, the AHP will often be directed to start testing at the test items level they consider the client can manage. They will test up the scale items until the person has three consecutive failures and will test down the scale to achieve three consecutive passes. AHPs have been using Guttman scaling methods for many years. The Physical Self-maintenance Scale (PSMS), developed by Lawton and Brody back in 1969, was founded on the theory that a person's functional ability could be ordered in a hierarchy ranging from physical self-maintenance, instrumental ADL, to behaviours related to motivation and social interaction (Lawton and Brody 1969). The PSMS comprises 5-point scales, which range from total dependence to total independence, and are used to rate six test items that fall on a Guttman scale. The six domains are Toileting; Feeding; Dressing; Grooming; Physical Ambulation; and Bathing (see McDowell and Newell 1987, pp. 66–68, for test items.

Another example of a Guttman Scale is the Arthritis Impact Measurement Scale (AIMS, Meenan et al. 1982), which is a patient self-report measure. It covers the domains of physical, social, and emotional well-being and was developed as an outcome measure for intervention with people with arthritis. The AIMS comprises 45 items grouped into nine scales (mobility; physical activity; dexterity; household activity; social activity; ADL; pain; depression; and anxiety) comprising five items each. Items for each scale were selected using Guttman analyses and internal consistency correlations. Items are listed in hierarchical order of difficulty based on the Guttman order, and as experienced by people with arthritis, for each of the nine scales. Therefore, a person indicating disability on one question would also be expected to indicate disability on the items below it (see McDowell and Newell 1987, pp. 271–276, for the test items and a critique of the AIMS).

RASCH ANALYSIS

A limitation of many AHP observational assessments is that they produce ordinal level raw scores. The unit of measurement needs to be at an interval level so that comparisons of how much more or how much less the person exhibits of the construct or behaviour can be made (Bond and Fox 2015). In the past decade or so, AHP researchers have turned to Rasch analysis to help develop a more robust form of functional measurement. The Rasch measurement model enables a test developer to produce a unidimensional linear measure that is based on additive numbers. It can be applied to convert ordinal scores into linear (also referred to as additive) level measures and is useful for developing criterion-referenced hierarchical scales (Fisher 2003). Test developers use Rasch analysis to transform observed counts of ordinal data (raw scores) into an approximately equal-interval number line (linear continuum or scale representing the variable; Bond and Fox 2015).

Rasch analysis provides goodness-of-fit statistics that are used to undertake construct validity analyses of a scale by, first, exploring hypotheses about what should occur when a particular sample is given the test and, second, confirming whether or not the test items fit the hypothesised model (Fisher 2003). In this approach, the test developer begins by defining the construct or performance variable to be measured as a continuous, unidimensional construct or behaviour, which people possess to varying degrees. The construct should have the potential to be visualised as falling along a vertical line. This vertical line represents the measure of a person's ability, i.e. ability to participate (on the left side of the vertical line) and item difficulty, i.e. most difficult items (on the right side of the vertical line; Souza et al. 2017). A measurement developed to evaluate this construct should cover the full range. For example, a measure of some domain of function, such as mobility, should encompass all levels of that function from minimal through moderate to maximal level of performance. Different people measured against this construct would be placed at various points along the line depending on how much or little they demonstrated the trait/ability/behaviour being measured.

'Rasch analysis allows for the comparison of a person to other individuals, one item to other items, and individuals to items. Furthermore, the Rasch model can be used to build new scales, to suggest improvements to existing scales and to estimate the stability of item difficulty estimates among different groups, thus allowing for comparisons of homogeneous measures' (Souza et al. 2017, p. 2). Árnadóttir and Fisher (2008) used Rasch analysis methods to explore the *A-ONE* (**A**DL-focused **O**ccupation-based **N**eurobehavioral **E**valuation) validity and reliability. The greater the person's level of ability, the more test items they should pass. Therefore, when test items are ordered in terms of difficulty, we are able to hypothesise where a person will be positioned along the line and then to determine their exact location after they have been rated on all the test items. Dye et al. (2013) showed, using Rasch analysis, the viability of the Dynamic Gait Index (DGI) for people attending a balance disorders clinic.

Another example of an AHP measure that has been developed using the Rasch analysis model is the Assessment of Motor Process Skills (AMPS; Fisher 2003). Its test developer, Anne Fisher, was one of the first AHPs to recommend this approach to scaling. The AMPS is based on two linear scales: the AMPS motor skill scale and the AMPS process skill scale. Rasch analysis has been used to calibrate the challenge presented by ADLs that are observed for the test, the difficulty of the skill items on the linear scales, and the severity of the AHP raters who administer the test. The software most commonly cited for Rasch analysis is WINSTEPS, a two-facet model and, FACETS, a many-faceted model.

SUMMARY

In this chapter, we have explored the considerations and requirements for test development. We have asked you to reflect on whether a further test or outcome measure is required. The following review questions will help you reflect on the chapter and the requirements for test development. The following case study provides an overview of one outcome measure used by AHPs. The case study describes what Australian Therapy Outcome Measures (AusTOMs) is, how it can be used, and insights into some of the research supporting its psychometric properties.

Case Study: Australian Therapy Outcome Measures (AusTOMs)
By Professor Carolyn Unsworth

Introduction

This case study presents information on a free outcome measure that is used internationally by allied health professionals (AHPs), called the AusTOMs. Scales have been developed for use by occupational therapists (OTs) Unsworth and Duncombe (2014), physiotherapists (PTs) (Morris et al. 2014), and speech pathologists (SPs) (Perry and Skeat 2014), (see Figure 14.2) although other AHPs may also work with these disciplines to score clients using AusTOMs.

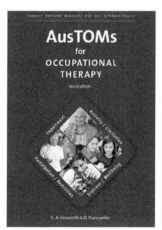
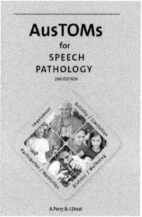
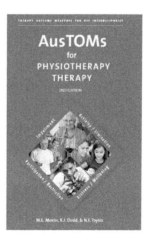

FIGURE 14.2   AusTOMs manuals.

What Is AusTOMs?

The AusTOMs are scales that AHPs score with clients of all diagnoses and all ages. The AusTOMs measures the outcome of interventions and can be used with clients who are expected to improve as well as clients who may deteriorate due to degenerative conditions. AHPs select the AusTOMs scales that best reflect the goals they set with the client, and scores are recorded related to a person's function, participation, and well-being at the start and conclusion of a therapy goal. The AusTOMs-OT have been translated into Swedish, Arabic, and Japanese, and Chinese and Turkish translations are underway.

How Was This Outcome Measure Developed?

The AusTOMs were based on the Therapy Outcome Measures (TOMs) from the United Kingdom (Enderby and John 1997; Enderby et al. 1998) and the International Classification of Function (ICF) (WHO 2001). As the TOMs were designed for the UK reimbursement system, they were not mapped to the ICF at that time. Scales are focused around client diagnoses; a research team in Australia set about developing scales specifically for use by OTs, PTs, and SPs that mapped directly to ICF, reflected a client's function and impairments, and could be used internationally (Skeat et al. 2003). The research team worked on the AusTOMs from 2001 to 2004, and hundreds of AHPs contributed to the development and testing process through Delphi surveys (Perry et al. 2004; Skeat and Perry 2004). The scales and manual were published in 2004, and the manuals updated in 2014. More than 30 peer-reviewed articles have been published supporting the use of the AusTOMs.

How Do I Score a Client or Patient on the AusTOMs?

An AHP selects the scale that best matches the goal set with the client, from the 12 AusTOMs-OT scales, 9 AusTOMs-PT scales, and 6 AusTOMs-SP scales (as detailed in Table 14.1). For example, an SP working on improving the rate and continuity of speech with a child who stutters would select the 'Fluency' scale to rate. Since an AHP is usually only working on a small number of goals at any one time, only a small number of scales would be selected at any one time.

TABLE 14.1   AusTOMs scales for occupational therapy, physiotherapy, and speech pathology.

AusTOMs-OT Scales	AusTOMs-PT Scales	AusTOMs-SP Scales
1. Learning and Applying Knowledge	1. Balance and Postural Control	1. Speech
2. Functional Walking and Mobility	2. Cardiovascular System Related Functions	2. Language
3. Upper Limb Use	3. Musculoskeletal Movement Related Functions	3. Voice
4. Carrying Out Daily Life Tasks and Routines	4. Neurological Movement Related Functions	4. Fluency
5. Transfers	5. Pain	5. Swallowing
6. Using Transport	6. Respiratory System Functions	6. Cognitive – Communication
7. Self-Care	7. Sensory Functions	
8. Domestic Life – Home	8. Skin Functions	
9. Domestic Life – Managing Resources	9. Urinary and Bowel Continence	
10. Interpersonal Interactions and Relationships		
11. Work, Employment, and Education		
12. Community Life, Recreation, Leisure, and Play		

Source: Professor Carolyn Unsworth.

All outcome measures must have an initial and final score to measure change over time. For clients who may be with a service for extended periods, interim scores can be recorded. The AusTOMs initial score is recorded following an initial interview and administration of any routine assessments (e.g. Functional Independence Measure or Timed Up and Go). The selected scales are scored on the client's admission (or goal start) and discharge (or goal end). Every AusTOMs scale has four domains: (i) impairment, (ii) activity/limitation, (iii) participation/restriction, and (iv) distress/well-being. All are scored on an 11-point ordinal scale between 0 (low) and 5 (high), with half points possible. The AusTOMs scales can be scored in under five minutes. AHPs can bring AusTOMs scores to team meetings to discuss client progress, or score clients together during meetings. The domains of participation/restriction and distress/well-being are universal across all scales and disciplines and are ideal for different disciplines to rate together.

Once AHPs have begun collecting AusTOMs data, it is important to analyse this on a regular basis and use the findings to improve services. Aggregated outcome data is vital to demonstrate to clients, managers, and funders that AHP practice is achieving worthwhile outcomes across the domains of impairment, activity limitation, participation, and well-being. AusTOMs outcome data can guide service prioritisation and staffing levels or identify gaps in service provision. An excellent example of how to use AusTOMs outcome data for these purposes is detailed in Unsworth (2017).

Are There Any Examples of Implementing AusTOMs in Practice?

Selecting and implementing an outcome measure requires careful evaluation of a range of measures against criteria developed to meet the needs of the specific service. Livesey and Crosbie (2016) provide an example of the process used by one health service in the United Kingdom to evaluate a range of measures and then describe their selection and implementation of AusTOMs. In another example, occupational therapy services were benchmarked using AusTOMs to compare outcomes of clients who experienced upper limb problems following stroke from two rehabilitation facilities (Unsworth et al. 2009).

What Research Underpins This Outcome Measure?

A variety of studies have been published detailing the reliability and standard error of measurement (Fristedt et al. 2013; Morris et al. 2005; Scott et al. 2006; Unsworth et al. 2018); validity (Abu-Awad et al. 2014, Unsworth et al. 2004); sensitivity (Chen and Eng 2015; Frowen et al. 2010; Unsworth 2005; Wenke et al. 2008); and minimal clinically important difference (Unsworth et al. 2015) of the AusTOMs. AusTOMs have also been used in case control and randomised controlled trials to investigate intervention effectiveness (Timmer et al. 2019; Wenke et al. 2008). All publications demonstrate that AusTOMs are performing well to produce valid and reliable estimations of client performance in areas that matter to AHP practice. In a study currently underway, a team of Australian podiatry researchers are investigating if AusTOMs-PT scales are reliable when used to measure podiatry outcomes.

Where Can I Find Out More About This Outcome Measure?

Further information on the AusTOMs (and free download), can be found on the website https://austoms.com.

Source: Professor Carolyn Unsworth.

REVIEW QUESTIONS

14.1   What are the features of a criterion-referenced test?
14.2   What is Guttman scaling?
14.3   What is Rasch analysis?

You will find brief answers to these questions at the back of this book on p. 445.

REFERENCES

Abdi, H. (2010). Guttman scaling. In: *Encyclopedia of Research Design* (ed. N. Salkind), 558–560. Thousand Oaks, CA: Sage.

Abu-Awad, Y., Unsworth, C.A., Coulson, M., and Sarigiannis, M. (2014). Using the Australian Therapy Outcome Measures for Occupational Therapy (AusTOMs-OT) to measure client participation outcomes. *British Journal of Occupational Therapy* 77 (2): 44–49. https://doi.org/10.4276/030802214X13916969446958.

Anastasi, A. (1988). *Psychological Testing*, 5e. New York, NY: Macmillan.

Árnadóttir, G. and Fisher, A.G. (2008). Rasch analysis of the ADL scale of the A-ONE. *American Journal of Occupational Therapy* 62 (1): 51–60. https://doi.org/10.5014/ajot.62.1.51.

Bond, T.G. and Fox, C.M. (2015). *Applying the Rasch Model: Fundamental Measurement in the Human Sciences*, 3e. Routledge.

Chen, Z. and Eng, J.Y. (2015). Use of the Australian Therapy Outcome Measures for Occupational Therapy (AusTOMs-OT) in an early supported discharge programme for stroke patients in Singapore. *British Journal of Occupational Therapy* 78 (9): 570–575. https://doi.org/10.1177/0308022614562582.

Chitsabesan, P., Lennox, C., Theodosiou, L. et al. (2014). The development of the comprehensive health assessment tool for young offenders within the secure estate. *The Journal of Forensic Psychiatry & Psychology* 25 (1): 1–25. https://doi.org/10.1080/14789949.2014.882387.

de Clive-Lowe, S. (1996). Outcome measurement, cost-effectiveness and clinical audit: the importance of standardised assessment to occupational therapists in meeting these new demands. *British Journal of Occupational Therapy* 59 (8): 357–362. https://doi.org/10.1177/030802269605900803.

Crocker, L. and Algina, J. (1986). *Introduction to Classical and Modern Test Theory*. New York: Holt, Rinehart and Winston.

Cronbach, L.J. (1960). *Essentials of Psychological Testing*, 2e. New York.

Dye, D.C., Eakman, A.M., and Bolton, K.M. (2013). Assessing the validity of the dynamic gait index in a balance disorders clinic: an application of Rasch analysis. *Physical Therapy* 93 (6): 809–818. https://doi.org/10.2522/ptj.20120163.

Enderby, P. and John, A. (1997). *Therapy Outcome Measures: Speech-Language Pathology Technical Manual*. London: Singular.

Enderby, P., John, A., and Petherham, B. (1998). *Therapy Outcome Measures Manual: Physiotherapy, Occupational Therapy, Rehabilitation Nursing*. San Diego: Singular.

Fisher, A. (2003). *AMPS Assessment of Motor and Process Skills*. Fort Collins, Colorado.

Fisher, A.G. and Merritt, B.K. (2012). Conceptualizing and developing the AMPS within a framework of modern objective measurement. *Assessment of Motor and Process Skills*

1: 14–11. https://www.innovativeotsolutions.com/wp-content/uploads/2018/07/ampsChapters14-15.pdf.

Fristedt, S., Elgmark, E., and Unsworth, C.A. (2013). The inter-rater and test-retest reliability of the self-care and transfer scales and intra-rater reliability of all scales of the Swedish translation of the Australian Therapy Outcome Measures for Occupational Therapy (AusTOMs-OT-S). *Scandinavian Journal of Occupational Therapy* 20: 182–189. https://doi.org/10.3109/11038128.2013.777940.

Frowen, J., Cotton, S., Corry, J., and Perry, A. (2010). Impact of demographics, tumor characteristics, and treatment factors on swallowing after (chemo) radiotherapy for head and neck cancer. *Head & Neck* 32 (4): 513–528. https://doi.org/10.1002/hed.21218.

Guttman, L. (1941). An outline of the statistical theory of prediction. In: *The Prediction of Personal Adjustment*, vol. 48 (ed. P. Horst), 253–318. New York: Social Science Research Council.

Haynes, S.N., Richard, D.C.S., and Kubany, E.S. (1995). Content validity in psychological assessment: a functional approach to concepts and methods. *Psychological Assessment* 7 (3): 238–247. https://doi.org/10.1037/1040-3590.7.3.238.

Hubley, A.M. and Zumbo, B.D. (2013). Psychometric characteristics of assessment procedures: an overview. In: *APA Handbooks in Psychology®. APA Handbook of Testing and Assessment in Psychology, Vol. 1. Test Theory and Testing and Assessment in Industrial and Organizational Psychology* (eds. K.F. Geisinger, B.A. Bracken, J.F. Carlson, et al.), 3–19. American Psychological Association https://doi.org/10.1037/14047-001.

Janssen, M.F., Szende, A., Cabases, J. et al. (2019). Population norms for the EQ-5D-3L: a cross-country analysis of population surveys for 20 countries. *The European Journal of Health Economics* 20 (2): 205–216. https://doi.org/10.1007/s10198-018-0955-5.

Jones, L. (1991). The standardised test. *Clinical Rehabilitation* 5 (3): 177–180. https://doi.org/10.1177/026921559100500301.

Kline, P. (2015). *A Handbook of Test Construction (Psychology Revivals): Introduction to Psychometric Design*. Routledge.

Laver, A. J. (1994). *The Development of the Structured Observational Test of Function (SOTOF)* (Doctoral dissertation, University of Surrey). The Development of the Structured Observational Test of Function (SOTOF). - Surrey Research Insight Open Access

Laver, A.J. and Powell, G.E. (1995). *The Structured Observational Test of Function (SOTOF)*. NFER Nelson.

Law, M., Baptiste, S., McColl, M. et al. (1990). The Canadian occupational performance measure: an outcome measure for occupational therapy. *Canadian Journal of Occupational Therapy* 57 (2): 82–87. https://doi.org/10.1177/000841749005700207.

Lawton, M.P. and Brody, E.M. (1969). Assessment of older people: self-maintaining and instrumental activities of daily living. *The Gerontologist* 9 (3_Part_1): 179–186. https://doi.org/10.1093/geront/9.3_Part_1.179.

Lenhard, A., Lenhard, W., and Gary, S. (2019). Continuous norming of psychometric tests: a simulation study of parametric and semi-parametric approaches. *PLoS One* 14 (9) https://doi.org/10.1371/journal.pone.0222279.

Livesey, C., & Crosbie, V (2016). *Outcome measure feature: Say it, do it, show it, prove it.* OTnews, 24 (12), 26–27.

McDowell, I. and Newell, C. (eds.) (1987). General health measurements. In: *Measuring Health: A Guide to Rating Scales and Questionnaires*, 285–290. New York: Oxford University Press.

Meenan, R.F., Gertman, P.M., Mason, J.H., and Dunaif, R. (1982). The arthritis impact measurement scales. Further investigations of a health status measure. *Arthritis & Rheumatism: Official Journal of the American College of Rheumatology* 25 (9): 1048–1053. https://doi.org/10.1002/art.1780250903.

Mindell, J.A., Gould, R.A., Tikotzy, L. et al. (2019). Norm-referenced scoring system for the brief infant sleep questionnaire–revised (BISQ-R). *Sleep Medicine* 63: 106–114. https://doi.org/10.1016/j.sleep.2019.05.010.

Morris, M., Perry, A., Unsworth, C. et al. (2005). Reliability of the Australian therapy outcome measures for quantifying disability and health. *International Journal of Therapy and Rehabilitation* 12 (8): 340–346. https://doi.org/10.12968/ijtr.2005.12.8.19536.

Morris, M.E., Dodd, K.J., and Taylor, N.F. (2014). *AusTOMs for Physiotherapy*, 2e. La Trobe University, Melbourne. ISBN 9781921915352.

Offender Health Research Network (2013) *Manual for the Comprehensive Health Assessment Tool (CHAT)*. http://www.ohrn.nhs.uk/OHRNResearch/CHATManualV32013.pdf (accessed 13 May 2021).

Panisset, M., Roudier, M., Saxton, J., and Boiler, F. (1994). Severe impairment battery: a neuropsychological test for severely demented patients. *Archives of Neurology* 51 (1): 41–45. https://doi.org/10.1001/archneur.1994.00540130067012.

Perry, A. and Skeat, J. (2014). *AusTOMs for Speech Pathology*, 2e. Melbourne: La Trobe University. ISBN 9781921915369.

Perry, A., Morris, M., Unsworth, C. et al. (2004). Therapy outcome measures for allied health practitioners in Australia: the AusTOMs. *International Journal for Quality in Health Care* 16 (4): 285–291. https://doi.org/10.1093/intqhc/mzh059.

Pett, M.A., Lackey, N.R., and Sullivan, J.J. (2003). *Making Sense of Factor Analysis: The Use of Factor Analysis for Instrument Development in Health Care Research*. Sage.

Pynsent, J. (2004). Choosing an outcome measure. In: *Outcome Measures in Orthopaedics and Orthopaedic Trauma*, 2e (eds. P. Pynsent, J. Fairbank and A. Carr), 1–7. London: Arnold.

Rikli, R.E. and Jones, C.J. (2013). Development and validation of criterion-referenced clinically relevant fitness standards for maintaining physical independence in later years. *The Gerontologist* 53 (2): 255–267. https://doi.org/10.1093/geront/gns071.

Royeen, C.B. (ed.) (1989). *Clinical Research Handbook: An analysis for the service professions*. Slack Incorporated.

Russell, D.J., Rosenbaum, P.L., Gowland, C. et al. (1993). *Manual for the Gross Motor Function Measure*. Hamilton: McMaster University.

Saxton, J., McGonigle-Gibson, K.L., Swihart, A.A., and Boller, F. (1993). *The Severe Impairment Battery (SIB) Manual*. Pittsburgh, PA: Alzheimer's Disease Research Center. Pearson: 9780749131777.

Scott, F., Unsworth, C.A., Fricke, J., and Taylor, N. (2006). Reliability of the Australian Therapy Outcome Measures for Occupational Therapy (AusTOMs – OT) self-care scale. *Australian Occupational Therapy Journal* 53: 265–276. https://doi.org/10.1111/j.1440-1630.2006.00584.x.

Skeat, J. and Perry, A. (2004). Outcomes in practice: lessons from AusTOMs. *Acquiring knowledge in Speech, language and Hearing* 6 (3): 123–126.

Skeat, J., Perry, A., Morris, M. et al. (2003). The use of the ICF framework in an allied health outcome measure: Australian Therapy Outcome Measures (AusTOMs). In: *Australian Institute of Health and Welfare, ICF Australian user guide. Version 1.0*, 77–81. Canberra: Australian Institute of Health and Welfare.

Souza, M.A.P., Coster, W.J., Mancini, M.C. et al. (2017). Rasch analysis of the participation scale (P-scale): usefulness of the P-scale to a rehabilitation services network. *BMC Public Health* 17 (1): 934. https://doi.org/10.1186/s12889-017-4945-9.

Stanley, J. C., & Hopkins, K. D., (1972). *Hopkins. Educational and Psycho logical Measurement and Evaluation. Englewood Cliffs, New Jersey: Prentice-Hall, 11.*

Thorborg, K., Hölmich, P., Christensen, R. et al. (2011). The Copenhagen Hip and Groin Outcome Score (HAGOS): development and validation according to the COSMIN checklist. *British Journal of Sports Medicine* 45 (6): 478–491. https://doi.org/10.1136/bjsm.2010.080937.

Timmer, A.J., Unsworth, C.A., and Browne, M. (2020). Occupational therapy and activity pacing with hospital associated deconditioned older adults: a randomised controlled study. *Disability and Rehabilitation* 42 (12): 1727–1735. https://doi.org/10.1080/09638288.2018.1535630.

Unsworth, C.A. (2005). Measuring outcomes using the Australian Therapy Outcome Measures for Occupational Therapy (AusTOMs – OT): data description and tool sensitivity. *British Journal of Occupational Therapy* 68 (8): 354–336. https://doi.org/10.1177/030802260506800804.

Unsworth, C.A. (2017). Analysing and interpreting outcomes data to support evidence-based practice using the example of AusTOMs-OT. *British Journal of Occupational Therapy* 80 (10): 631–637. https://doi.org/10.1177/0308022617722480.

Unsworth, C.A. and Duncombe, D. (2014). *AusTOMs for Occupational Therapy*, 3e. Melbourne: La Trobe University. ISBN 9781921915345.

Unsworth, C., Duckett, S., Duncombe, D. et al. (2004). Validity of the AusTOM scales: a comparison of the AusTOMs and EuroQol-5D. *Health and Quality of Life Outcomes* 2: 1–12. https://doi.org/10.1186/1477-7525-2-64.

Unsworth, C.A., Bearup, A., and Rickard, K. (2009). Benchmark comparison of outcomes for clients with upper limb dysfunction following stroke using the Australian Therapy Outcome Measures for Occupational Therapy (AusTOMs-OT). *American Journal of Occupational Therapy* 63 (6): 732–774. https://doi.org/10.5014/ajot.63.6.732.

Unsworth, C.A., Coulson, M., Swinton, L. et al. (2015). Determination of the minimum clinically important difference on the Australian Therapy Outcome Measures for Occupational Therapy (AusTOMs-OT). *Disability and Rehabilitation* 37 (11): 997–1003. https://doi.org/10.3109/09638288.2014.95245.

Unsworth, C.A., Timmer, A., and Wales, K. (2018). Reliability of the Australian Therapy Outcome Measures for Occupational Therapy (AusTOMs-OT). *Australian Occupational Therapy Journal* 65 (5): 375–386. https://doi.org/10.1111/1440-1630.12476.

Velozo, C.A., Seel, R.T., Magasi, S. et al. (2012). Improving measurement methods in rehabilitation: core concepts and recommendations for scale development. *Archives of Physical Medicine and Rehabilitation* 93 (8): S154–S163. https://doi.org/10.1016/j.apmr.2012.06.001.

Wenke, R.J., Theodoros, D., and Cornwell, P. (2008). The short-and long-term effectiveness of the LSVT® for dysarthria following TBI and stroke. *Brain Injury* 22 (4): 339–352. https://doi.org/10.1080/02699050801960987.

World Health Organization (2001). *International Classification of Functioning, Disability and Health (ICF)*. Geneva: WHO.

Zandbelt, M.M., Welsing, P.M.J., Van Gestel, A.M., and Van Riel, P.L.C.M. (2001). Health assessment questionnaire modifications: is standardisation needed? *Annals of the Rheumatic Diseases* 60 (9): 841–845. https://ard.bmj.com/content/60/9/841.

RESOURCES

- **The Allied Health Professions (AHP) Outcome Measures UK Working Group**, a cross-disciplinary group representing a number of professional bodies has developed a checklist, ***Key questions to ask when selecting outcome measures: a checklist for allied health professionals,*** 2019, to assist individual AHPs and teams with selecting outcome measures. https://www.rcslt.org/outcome-measures-checklist/

- **COnsensus-based Standards for the selection of health Measurement INstruments (COSMIN)** COSMIN aims to improve the selection of outcome measurement instruments both in research and in clinical practice by developing methodology and practical tools for selecting the most suitable outcome measurement instrument. https://www.cosmin.nl

- **The Royal College of Speech and Language Therapists Online Outcome Tool** discussed in the first case study in Chapter 13 (https://www.rcslt.org/speech-and-language-therapy/guidance-for-delivering-slt-services/outcome-measurement/outcome-tool-overview/ [Accessed 13 May 2021])

- **The American Psychiatric Association**, Online Assessment Measures (https://www.psychiatry.org/psychiatrists/practice/dsm/educational-resources/assessment-measures [Accessed 13 May 2021])

- **The Cicely Saunders Institute of Palliative Care, Policy & Rehabilitation**, Kings College London lists a number of rehabilitation outcome measures (https://www.kcl.ac.uk/cicelysaunders/research/outcome/rehabilitation/Rehab-outcome-measures [Accessed 13 May 2021])

CHAPTER 15

Conducting Psychometric Studies

In this final chapter, we consider the process of conducting psychometric studies. We will refer to a number of chapters within the book, in particular, to Chapters 8–10. The chapter concludes with a case study to illustrate the face validity of the Structured Observational Test of Function (SOTOF) from the perspective of people with a neurological diagnosis.

PSYCHOMETRIC PROPERTIES

Psychometric properties can include scale construction, standardisation, reliability (internal consistency, retest, and inter-rater), validity (content, concurrent, and construct) and responsiveness (Carlon et al. 2010). These psychometric characteristics (validity, reliability, and responsiveness) are the factors that determine the measure as clinically useful (Vianin 2008). Allied health professionals (AHPs) often want to use test scores to draw inferences about the person's functioning in situations that are beyond the scope of the assessment session. For example, an AHP might need to use the person's test scores on a mobility assessment to predict his mobility in the community. In order to do this, the AHP must be able to justify any inferences drawn, by having a coherent rationale for using the test score in this way.

AHPs also need clear reasons for selecting a particular test instead of other available assessments. An essential part of such justification involves an understanding of the validity and reliability of test scores (Crocker and Algina 1986). Good test design is related strongly to reliability and validity (Kline 2000). It is particularly important that students and clinicians can establish whether a measure has acceptable levels of validity and reliability, and so these two areas are covered in some depth in Chapters 8 and 9. Chapter 10 provides further advice on test critique and on how to locate and select appropriate standardised tests for therapy service. In construct validity, 'the focus is on assessing relationships among the tool's items and determining if items are consistent with the theory as operationally defined' (Gélinas et al. 2008, p. 121), and is crucial to establishing the psychometric property of a test.

CLASSICAL TEST THEORY

When conducting psychometric studies, *classical test theory* (CTT) is commonly used (DeVellis 2006). CTT 'comprises a set of concepts and methods that provide a basis for many of the measurement tools currently used in health research' (DeVilis, p. S50). *Factor analysis* is the procedure associated with CTT. See the section titled 'Factorial Validity' in Chapter 8 for more details on factor analysis.

Factor analysis is a statistical method used to describe variability among observed, correlated variables in terms of a potentially lower number of unobserved variables called factors (Lawley and Maxwell 1962). The purpose of factor analysis is to summarise the data to understand the relationships and patterns across the variables and enable interpretation (Yong and Pearce 2013). Variables are 'grouped' for analysis. A factor would usually have at least three variables (Yong and Pearce).

ITEM RESPONSE THEORY

Item response theory (IRT) is suggested to have a number of potential advantages over CTT in assessing self-reported health outcomes (Hays et al. 2000). Hays and colleagues state that 'IRT also facilitates evaluation of differential item functioning, inclusion of items with different response formats in the same scale, and assessment of person fit and is ideally suited for implementing computer adaptive testing' (p. II28). *Differential item functioning* (DIF; https://uk.sagepub.com/en-gb/eur/book/differential-item-functioning) informs test validity and is a method for studying measurement equivalence (Osterlind and Everson 2009; Walker, 2011). Teresi and Fleishman (2007) suggested that 'inaccurate assessment may lead to incorrect estimates of effects in research, and to suboptimal decisions at the individual, clinical level' (p. 33)

ESTABLISHING THE OVERALL VALIDITY OF A TEST

If a test is to be used for a range of purposes, then several types of validity may need to be examined. Anastasi (1988, p. 162) provides an excellent example of how an arithmetic test could be used for four different purposes, each of which would require a different validity study:

1. If the test was to be used as a maths test in a primary school and the purpose was to identify how much a pupil had learnt about maths up to this point, then the validity study required would be a content validity study.
2. If the arithmetic test was being used as an aptitude test to predict which pupils would be good at maths in secondary school, and the purpose was to judge

how well a pupil might learn maths in the future, then criterion-related validity is required, and evidence of predictive validity will be needed.

3. If this same arithmetic test is also to be used for diagnosing people with learning disability by identifying specific areas where a person is not performing at maths to a level expected for his age, then again criterion-related validity will be required, but this time concurrent validity and discriminant validity studies will be undertaken.

4. Finally, if the arithmetic test is to be used as a measure of quantitative reasoning and the AHP wishes to assess a person's cognitive processes, then construct-related validity would be required.

As there is no single recognised measure of validity, it is usual for researchers to conduct a range of studies to examine its different aspects (Bartram 1990). For example, Baum and Edwards (1993) undertook four analyses to examine aspects of the validity of the Kitchen Task Assessment (KTA):

1. Correlation analysis was used to examine the relationship among the six variables in the measure; 'correlation coefficients of .72 –.84 suggested that one dimension might exist . . . and that the cognitive domains selected for the KTA all contribute to the measurement of the cognitive performance of the task' (p. 433).

2. Factor analysis was undertaken to identify common relationships among the variables, to determine the internal structure of the variables and to establish the KTA as a unidimensional instrument.

3. Correlation analysis was undertaken with other published valid and reliable tests, three neuropsychological, and two functional assessments to determine the construct validity of the KTA. Results indicated that 'the KTA, as a test of practical cognitive skills, is related to the cognitive skills measured by [the other three] neuropsychological tests' (p. 435).

4. The fourth investigation involved an analysis of variance to examine performance of subjects on the KTA compared to stages of Senile Dementia of the Alzheimer Type (SDAT). The results showed that 'the KTA differentiates performance across all stages of the disease' (p. 435).

The developers of the Life Satisfaction Index – Parents (LSI-P; Renwick and Reid 1992) have undertaken several studies to examine different aspects of the validity of their test. Studies have been conducted to examine the construct validity, concurrent validity, and discriminant validity of the LSI-P. The initial version consisted of 18 items for each of the five domains. These items went through two review processes. First, three occupational therapy clinical experts reviewed items. Second, 23 reviewers used a 4-item criteria for review across five Canadian provinces to examine the content validity of each item. A criterion level of reviewer agreement was set for the inclusion of items in the final version of the test. The discriminant and concurrent validity of the LSI-P were examined with a sample comprising 17 parents of a child with Duchenne muscular dystrophy (DMD) and 39 parents of children without physical disabilities. The LSI-P was administered to both groups of parents in their own homes. Parents also completed the concurrent measure (the Satisfaction with Life Scale and the Questionnaire on Resources and Stress).

Bartram (1990) has presented several arguments for ensuring good face validity. First, good face validity can have indirect effects on the outcome of a person's performance 'by facilitating rapport between the test and the test-taker which may, in turn, increase reliability' (p. 76). Second, engaging a person's motivation to engage in an assessment to the best of his ability is critical to obtaining valid and reliable test results, and 'people are more likely to take seriously activities which seem reasonable and which they feel they understand' (p. 76).

Face validity is particularly important when a test developed for one population is used with a different client group. For example, many neuropsychological tests were originally developed for child populations. Some of these tests were later standardised for an older adult population; however, the content of the tests often remained unchanged. Thus, the test content was not necessarily meaningful and relevant for older adults, who might perceive test materials as childish and demeaning. A person's perception of the relevance of test materials affects his/her motivation to undertake the test and therefore impacts the reliability of test results. If the tasks selected as the basis of a neuropsychological test do not relate to the tasks the person would be undertaking in everyday life, then the client may not understand the relevance of a test to his own life and situation. For example, an older adult will rarely need to construct a three-dimensional block design from a diagram or model, nor be required to copy geometric shapes as part of his everyday activities. The more contrived a test content is from the everyday activities of the person being tested, the more important it is to consider face validity. Therapists should always explain the purpose of an assessment procedure to the client prior to testing, but this is especially important where face validity is not strong.

When reviewing potential tests, therapists may have to conduct their own face validity studies because there is a 'paucity of available research on face validity, despite its probable contribution to prevalent attitudes towards tests' (Anastasi 1988, p. 145). Face validity studies are critical to client-centred practice, and service users and carers must be engaged to 'play an active and integral part in the validation process' if measures are 'to be truly valid' (Wolf 1997, p. 364). An example of a face validity study is provided by Laver (1994), who demonstrated that the SOTOF (Laver and Powell 1995) had high face validity with a sample of 40 patients with stroke. Following the administration of SOTOF, patients were given a structured interview that comprised both open and closed questions. For example, patients were asked:

- 'What did you think this assessment was for?'
- 'Were these tasks something you would normally do?'
- 'Did you mind being asked to do these tasks?'
- 'What did you think of the assessment?'

Patients were also given questions related to their experience of being tested:

- 'Did you find the assessment . . . easy, upsetting, enjoyable, difficult, boring, stressful, useful, interesting, relaxing, irrelevant'?

This question format presented the possibility of a negative testing experience and enabled subjects to give an affirmative answer to a negative concept; this is particularly important when conducting research with older populations, who tend to be acquiescent, polite, and affirmative in their responses. When seeking feedback from clients on their experience of a test or conducting a face validity study, it is preferable to have the client interviewed by a different AHP than the one who undertook the assessment as some clients find it more difficult to provide negative feedback to the person who has given the test.

Bowman et al. (2009) developed the Clinician Readiness for Measuring Outcomes Scale (CReMOS). The paper is a useful example of the range of psychometric properties that required testing to develop an outcome measure. They conducted scale development and psychometric testing of the CReMOS through a series of studies:

1. Content validity testing – to test the extent to which the items on a test are representative of the entire domain the test seeks to measure.
2. Construct validity testing – to test the extent to which the measure actually tests the theory [construct] it is trying to measure.
3. Internal consistency reliability – to estimate how much total test scores would vary if slightly different items were used.
4. Temporal reliability (or stability) – to examine the correlation of the measure when administered to the same sample on two different occasions. Sometimes referred to as test–retest.

The following case study illustrates the face validity of the SOTOF from the perspective of people with a neurological diagnosis.

Designing a Face Validity Research Study: The Face Validity of the Structured Observational Test of Function (SOTOF) from the Perspective of Patients with a Neurological Diagnosis

Eden Marrison, BHSc(OT), York Teaching Hospital NHS Foundation Trust

Introduction

I examined the face validity (Marrison 2020) of the SOTOF (2nd edition; Laver-Fawcett and Marrison 2016) after the changes were made from the first edition developed in 1994 (Laver and Powell 1995). Patients with neurological diagnoses were assessed using the SOTOF and then interviewed to gather their experiences, views, and opinions of undertaking the assessment. The SOTOF was developed for older adults (age 60+) with possible neurological disturbance (Laver and Powell 1995). The SOTOF is a standardised test that provides a detailed description of occupational performance in activities of daily living (*ADL*) and neuropsychological deficits that impact the performance of personal ADL tasks. A literature-based first stage content validity study (Marrison and Laver-Fawcett 2016) led to further development of SOTOF's dynamic assessment component. Face validity and content validity were previously evaluated (Laver and Powell 1995), and a further study was required following the changes made for the 2nd edition.

There are limited face validity studies on assessment tools, and many studies focus on the patients' perspectives of undertaking interventions/rehabilitation programmes. However, there are very few studies on patients' perspectives of undertaking a standardised assessment (Casserley-Feeney et al. 2008; Cooper et al. 2008; Hills and Kitchen 2007; Hook and Andrews 2005; MacDonald et al. 2002; May 2001).

(continued)

(continued)

STUDY DESIGN

This study used a mixed-method, cross-sectional design. A cross-sectional design was chosen as participants would be selected based on inclusion and exclusion criteria, and this study was a one-time measurement of exposure and outcome. This type of design is used for population-based surveys (Setia 2016). The mixed-method research design combined both qualitative and quantitative data to add depth and breadth of understanding to the study and to expand and strengthen the study's conclusions (Greene 2007; Johnson et al. 2007). Complex research questions are better understood when using a mixed-method approach (Creswell and Plano Clark 2011).

The design involved a semi-structured interview; this was chosen using a qualitative, phenomenological design. This design was used to allow the researcher to understand the meaning of another persons' description of undertaking the SOTOF and to hear their experiences and meanings described through language (Davidsen 2013; Giorgi and Giorgi 2003). Phenomenology is most useful when the researcher wishes to find out about an individuals' experience of an event (Aveyard and Sharp 2013). An interview approach has been shown to be useful and effective for face validity studies previously (Barnett et al. 2015). A semi-structured approach allows a researcher to gather richer and more detailed data, as participants have freedom to express themselves, and it gives the researcher an opportunity to probe participants to expand on their answers (French et al. 2001).

The interview questions used in this study were based on Laver's face validity study on SOTOF (1st edition) to allow comparison of results. Laver used quantitative, dichotomous, closed questions relating to the participants' potential experience of being tested, providing them with negative suggestions to allow the opportunity for them to express an adverse experience. Further questions were added to the interview questions, as this was a phenomenological study. The researcher was aiming to get more detailed data regarding a person's lived experience. Prompts were added to some of the questions to enable the researcher to probe deeper into the person's perspectives and encourage participants to elaborate on their answers. For this study, the same dichotomous closed questions were to be used with some additional pairs of words added. However, following feedback from a statistician on the Research ethics panel, these were converted into Likert scales. To enable researchers to compare samples with the first edition face validity SOTOF study and plan for future studies, demographic data was collected for gender; age; highest level of education; ethnicity; participants' health conditions; and diagnosis.

Patients' Questionnaire for Semi-structured Interview

'Hello, my name is . . .
What would you prefer I called you . . .?
Thank you for completing the assessment with your occupational therapist. We are going to ask you a few questions about what you thought about the assessment and how you found doing it'.

If needed, describe the SOTOF assessment to help the person remember which assessment you are talking about: the assessment had an eating task, pouring a drink, washing hands, and putting on an item of clothing.

If necessary, remind the person about the consent process, and show him/her a copy of their signed consent form.

'Are you still happy to take part in the interview?'

1. What did you think of the assessment?
2. How did you feel when you were doing the assessment?
3. When the therapist was giving instructions, how did you find following these instructions? Prompt: Were you able to follow them easily? Were they difficult to follow?
4. What do you think the purpose of the assessment is? Prompt: Did you know what your occupational therapist was assessing/trying to find out during the test?
5. Have you recently been involved in any other assessments while you have been staying on the ward? If yes, how did this assessment compare to the other one(s)?
6. Were the four tasks familiar activities to you? Prompt: The assessment had an eating task, pouring a drink, washing hands, and putting on an item of clothing. What other everyday tasks would be important to you while in hospital?
7. I am now going to give you some words, which might describe how a person might experience doing the assessment. Please tell me whether you strongly agree, agree, are neutral, disagree, or strongly disagree with the statements. Note: The format of the next set of closed questions used a Likert scale, and participants were asked to indicate their level of agreement or disagreement with each statement using a 5-point scale from 'strongly agree' to 'strongly disagree'. As well as having these questions read to the participant by the interviewer, we also used an enlarged, laminated version of the questions and the rating scale:
8. I found doing the assessment . . .

'Strongly agree', 'Agree', 'Neutral', 'Disagree', 'Strongly disagree'

I found doing the assessment . . .	Strongly agree	Agree	Neutral	Disagree	Strongly disagree
Boring					
Easy					
Useful					
Upsetting					
Relaxing					
Difficult					
Interesting					
Stressful					
Irrelevant					
Enjoyable					
Tiring					
Encouraging					
Distressing					
Straightforward					
Complicated					
Motivating					
Confusing					
Simple					

(continued)

(*continued*)

9. What do you think about the time it took to complete the assessment? Prompt: How long do you think it took? Did you think it was long? Quick? Do you think it took longer than you would have liked an assessment to take?

10. Were you offered any breaks between the assessment activities, e.g. between the eating and the pouring a drink tasks? Did you feel you needed a break during the assessment?

11. Is there anything you did not like about the assessment? Prompt: Did you dislike any parts/elements of each task and/or what the occupational therapist asked you to do?

12. Do you have any additional comments about the assessment and/or your experience of doing the assessment that you would like to add?

SAMPLE

This study used a convenience and purposive sampling method of inpatients on a ward that was accessible to the researcher. Participants were all undertaking the SOTOF test after a recent stroke or had other neurological diagnoses. This method was cost-effective, time-efficient, and targeted the ideal population of patients with neurological diagnosis in an inpatient setting.

The study required a minimum of 10 participants, and recruitment was undertaken until data saturation was considered to have been achieved, up to a maximum of 35 patients. A minimum of 10 was decided upon owing to the World Health Organisation's (WHO 2017) suggestion that qualitative research studies should have at least 10 participants. The Consensus-based Standards for the selection of health Measurement Instruments (COSMIN) Checklist Manual (Mokkink et al. 2012, p. 31) states that no standards were developed for assessing face validity because 'face validity requires a subjective judgement'. The COSMIN checklist (Terwee et al. 2012) states that sample sizes below 30 for psychometric studies are poor. However, sample sizes for qualitative studies using interview and focus group data collection methods tend to be smaller than those for quantitative psychometric studies (Dickerson 2006).

DATA COLLECTION

Occupational therapists identified potential participants from their caseloads to the lead researcher. They were screened for inclusion/exclusion criteria and given a participants' information sheet with 24 hours to consider participation in the study with support from family members or appropriate others if needed. Informed consent was then obtained following answers to any further questions. The occupational therapists working on the ward then completed the SOTOF with each participant. The semi-structured interview was conducted by an independent research assistant or research supervisor, who did not work on the ward, within 48 hours of completion of the SOTOF. *A research assistant or the research supervisor, rather than the occupational therapist who completed the SOTOF assessments, conducted the participant interviews.* This increased trustworthiness, reduced potential bias, and allowed the participant to be honest about their experiences.

DATA ANALYSIS

The research assistant transcribed interviews verbatim. Descriptive statistics were used to analyse the closed questions rating on the 5-point agreement scale. The qualitative data was analysed using thematic analysis. Thematic analysis is useful when trying to gain information about people's experiences and for analysing transcribed focus groups and interviews (Clarke and Braun 2013). The data was analysed following the six stages outlined by Braun and Clarke (2006). Thematic analysis is a widely used qualitative data analysis method. It is one of a cluster of methods that focus on identifying patterned meaning across a dataset. Patterns are identified through a rigorous process of data familiarisation, data coding, and theme development and revision (Braun and Clarke 2006; French et al. 2001). It suits research questions related to people's experiences and views; it is a flexible approach while still providing detailed and rich data (King 2004).

The researchers' co-supervisor checked analysis from the patient interview transcripts to introduce independent verification and increase trustworthiness. The researcher completed a reflective process prior to analysing the data to try to put aside beliefs and prior knowledge about the SOTOF assessment (Carpenter 2007).

Ethics approval was obtained via the UK National Health Service (*NHS*) Health Research Authority (*HRA*), Research Ethics Committee (*REC*), and from the university where the researcher (EM) was studying for an MSc by Research.

Source: Eden Marrison, BHSc(OT), York Teaching Hospital NHS Foundation Trust.

REVIEW QUESTIONS

15.1   What are the psychometric properties of a test?

You will find brief answers to these questions at the back of this book on p. 445.

REFERENCES

Anastasi, A. (1988). *Psychological Testing*, 5e. New York, NY: Macmillan.

Aveyard, H. and Sharp, P. (2013). *A beginner's Guide to Evidence-Based Practice in Health and Social Care*, 2e. Maidenhead: McGraw-Hill/Open University Press.

Barnett, L.M., Ridgers, N.D., Zask, A., and Salmon, J. (2015). Face validity and reliability of a pictorial instrument for assessing fundamental movement skill perceived competence in young children. *Journal of Science and Medicine in Sport* 18 (1): 98–102. https://doi.org/10.1016/j.jsams.2013.12.004.

Bartram, D. (1990). *Reliability and Validity. Testing People. A Practical Guide to Psychometrics*. Windsor: NFERNELSON.

Baum, C. and Edwards, D.F. (1993). Cognitive performance in senile dementia of the Alzheimer's type: the Kitchen task assessment. *American Journal of Occupational Therapy* 47 (5): 431–436. https://doi.org/10.5014/ajot.47.5.431.

Bowman, J., Lannin, N., Cook, C., and McCluskey, A. (2009). Development and psychometric testing of the clinician readiness for measuring outcomes scale. *Journal of Evaluation in Clinical Practice* 15 (1): 76–84. https://doi.org/10.1111/j.1365-2753.2008.00957.x.

Braun, V. and Clarke, V. (2006). *Using Thematic Analysis in Psychology. Qualitative Research in Psychology* 3 (2): 77–101. https://doi.org/10.1191/1478088706qp063oa. Available from http://eprints.uwe.ac.uk/11735/2/thematic_analysis_revised [Accessed 28 November 2017].

Carlon, S., Shields, N., Yong, K. et al. (2010). A systematic review of the psychometric properties of quality of life measures for school aged children with cerebral palsy. *BMC Pediatrics* 10 (1): 81. https://doi.org/10.1186/1471-2431-10-81.

Carpenter, D.R. (2007). Phenomenology as method. In: *Qualitative Research in Nursing: Advancing the Humanistic Imperative* (eds. H.J. Streubert and D.R. Carpenter), 75–99. Philadelphia, PA: Lippincott.

Casserley-Feeney, S.N., Phelan, M., Duffy, F. et al. (2008). Patient satisfaction with private physiotherapy for musculoskeletal pain. *BMC Musculoskeletal Disorders* 9: 50. https://doi.org/10.1186/1471-2474-9-50.

Clarke, V. and Braun, V. (2013). Teaching thematic analysis: overcoming challenges and developing strategies for effective learning. *The Psychologist* 26 (2): 120–123.

Cooper, K.S., Smith, B.H., and Hancock, E. (2008). Patient centredness in physiotherapy from the perspective of the low back pain patient. *Physiotherapy* 94: 244–252. https://doi.org/10.1016/j.physio.2007.10.006.

Creswell, J.W. and Plano Clark, V.L. (2011). *Designing and Conducting Mixed Methods Research*, 2e. Thousand Oaks: Sage Publications.

Crocker, L. and Algina, J. (1986). *Introduction to Classical and Modern Test Theory*. New York: Holt, Rinehart and Winston.

Davidsen, A.S. (2013). Phenomenological approaches in psychology and health sciences. *Qualitative Research in Psychology* 10 (3): 318–339. https://doi.org/10.1080/14780887.2011.608466.

DeVellis, R.F. (2006). Classical test theory. *Medical Care*: S50–S59. https://www.jstor.org/stable/41219505?seq=1.

Dickerson, A.E. (2006). Securing samples for effective research across research designs. In: *Research in Occupational Therapy Methods of Inquiry for Enhancing Practice* (ed. G. Kielhofner). Philadelphia: FA Davies.

French, S., Reynolds, F., and Swain, J. (2001). *Practical Research: A Guide for Therapists*, 2e. Oxford: Reed Educational and Professional Publishing.

Gélinas, C., Loiselle, C.G., LeMay, S. et al. (2008). Theoretical, psychometric, and pragmatic issues in pain measurement. *Pain Management Nursing* 9 (3): 120–130. https://doi.org/10.1016/j.pmn.2007.12.001.

Giorgi, A. and Giorgi, B. (2003). Phenomenology. In: *Qualitative Psychology* (ed. J.A. Smith), 25–50. London: Sage.

Greene, J.C. (2007). *Mixed Methods in Social Inquiry*. San Francisco: Jossey-Bass.

Hays, R.D., Morales, L.S., and Reise, S.P. (2000). Item response theory and health outcomes measurement in the 21st century. *Medical Care* 38 (9 Suppl): II28. https://www.ncbi.nlm.nih.gov/pmc/articles/PMC1815384.

Hills, R. and Kitchen, S. (2007). Satisfaction with outpatient physiotherapy: focus groups to explore the views of patients with acute and chronic musculoskeletal conditions. *Physiotherapy Theory and Practice* 2: 1–20. https://doi.org/10.1080/09593980601023705.

Hook, A. and Andrews, B. (2005). The relationship of non-disclosure in therapy to shame and depression. *British Journal of Clinical Psychology* 44 (3): 425–438. https://doi.org/10.1348/014466505X34165.

Johnson, B.R., Onwuegbuzie, A.J., and Turner, L.A. (2007). Toward a definition of mixed methods research. *Journal of Mixed Methods Research* 1: 112–133. https://doi.org/10.1177/1558689806298224.

King, N. (2004). Using templates in the thematic analysis of text. In: *Essential Guide to Qualitative Methods in Organizational Research* (eds. C. Cassell and G. Symon), 257–270. London, UK: Sage.

Kline, P. (2000). *The Handbook of Psychological Testing*. Psychology Press.

Laver, A. J. (1994). The Development of the Structured Observational Test of Function SOTOF(Doctoral dissertation, University of Surrey).

Laver, A.J. and Powell, G.E. (1995). *The Structured Observational Test of Function (SOTOF)*. Windsor: NFER-Nelson.

Laver-Fawcett, A.J. and Marrison, E. (2016). *Structured Observational Test of Function (SOTOF)*, 2e. York: York St John University.

Lawley, D.N. and Maxwell, A.E. (1962). Factor analysis as a statistical method. *Journal of the Royal Statistical Society. Series D (The Statistician)* 12 (3): 209–229. https://doi.org/10.2307/2986915.

MacDonald, C.A., Cox, P.D., and Bartlett, D.J. (2002). Productivity and client satisfaction: a comparison between physical therapists and student-therapist pairs. *Physiotherapy Canada* 54: 92–101.

Marrison E (2020) *Face and content validity and clinical utility of the Structured Observational Test of Function (SOTOF) from the perspective of patients with a neurological diagnosis and a stroke rehabilitation multi-disciplinary team*. Masters by Research Degree thesis. York St John University, School of Sciences, Technology and Health. York.

Marrison, E., Laver Fawcett, A., (2016) Contributing to the improvement of the dynamic aspect of the Structured Observational Test of Function (SOTOF). In: COTEC-ENOTHE 2016, 15-19 June 2016, Galway, Ireland.

May, S.J. (2001). Patient satisfaction with management of back pain. *Physiotherapy* 87: 4–20. https://doi.org/10.1016/S0031-9406(05)61186-8.

Mokkink LB, Terwee CB, Patrick DL, Alonso J, Stratford PW, Knol DL, Bouter LM and de Vet HCW (2012) COSMIN checklist manual. Available at: https://fac.ksu.edu.sa/sites/default/files/cosmin_checklist_manual_v9.pdf

Osterlind, S.J. and Everson, H.T. (2009). *Differential item functioning*, vol. 161. Sage Publications. https://uk.sagepub.com/en-gb/eur/book/differential-item-functioning.

Renwick, R.M. and Reid, D.T. (1992). Life satisfaction of parents of adolescents with Duchenne muscular dystrophy: validation of a new instrument. *The Occupational Therapy Journal of Research* 12 (5): 296–312. https://doi.org/10.1177/153944929201200503.

Setia, M.S. (2016). Methodology series module 3: cross-sectional studies. *Indian Journal of Dermatology* 61 (3): 261–264. http://doi.org/10.4103/0019-5154.182410 (accessed 21 August 2018. https://www.ncbi.nlm.nih.gov/pmc/articles/PMC4885177.

Teresi, J.A. and Fleishman, J.A. (2007). Differential item functioning and health assessment. *Quality of Life Research* 16 (1): 33–42. https://doi.org/10.1007/s11136-007-9184-6.

Terwee, C.B., Mokkink, L.B., Knol, D.L. et al. (2012). Rating the methodological quality in systematic reviews of studies on measurement properties: a scoring system for the COSMIN checklist. *Quality of Life Research* 21 (4): 651–657. https://doi.org/10.1007/s11136-011-9960-1.

Vianin, M. (2008). Psychometric properties and clinical usefulness of the Oswestry disability index. *Journal of Chiropractic Medicine* 7 (4): 161–163. https://doi.org/10.1016/j.jcm.2008.07.001.

Walker, C.M. (2011). What's the DIF? Why differential item functioning analyses are an important part of instrument development and validation. *Journal of Psychoeducational Assessment* 29 (4): 364–376. https://doi.org/10.1177/0734282911406666.

Wolf, H. (1997). Assessments of activities of daily living and instrumental activities of daily living: their use by community-based health service occupational therapists working in physical disability. *British Journal of Occupational Therapy* 60 (8): 359–364. https://doi.org/10.1177/030802269706000809.

World Health Organisation (WHO) (2017) *Essential Medicines and Health Products Information Portal: World Health Organisation Resource* [Internet]. Available from http://apps.who.int/medicinedocs/en/d/Js6169e/7.6.html [Accessed 26th August 2018].

Yong, A.G. and Pearce, S. (2013). A beginner's guide to factor analysis: focusing on exploratory factor analysis. *Tutorial in Quantitative Methods for Psychology* 9 (2): 79–94. https://doi.org/10.20982/tqmp.09.2.p079.

Brief Answers to Chapter Review Questions

There are review questions at the end of some of the chapters, in other chapters there are suggested tasks to complete. This section provides some brief answers to the review questions.

CHAPTER 2: METHODS OF ASSESSMENT AND SOURCES OF ASSESSMENT DATA

1. What is meant by direct and indirect assessment methods?

   Direct measures involve observations, standardised assessment and person self-report. In direct methods can include referral information, person's healthcare records, and reports from the person's carer or family members or form other professionals or service providers who are working with the client.

2. What three categories of sources for gathering assessment data?

   Three sources for gathering assessment data are:
   - *Self-report from the person*
   - *Proxy/informant report*
   - *Direct observation undertaken by the AHP*

3. What methods could you use for collecting self-report data?

   Self-report data can be collected by interview, by asking the client to keep a journal and or the use of standardised and unstandardised checklists and questionnaires.

4. List the types of informants or proxies might an AHP use?
   - *The person's primary carer*
   - *Other member of the AHP's multidisciplinary team*
   - *Other health professionals involved in the person's care*
   - *Other professionals working with the person*

5. What methods could you use for collecting proxy or informant report data?

   Methods of collected proxy/informant report data include interviewing the proxy face to face in person, or by video conferencing, or by telephone, through case conferences, ward rounds, team meetings or via written data (letters, standardised or unstandardised checklists and questionnaires, referrals, healthcare notes, and assessment reports).

---

6. What are the three main phases of an interview?

The three phases of an interview are initiation, development and, closing.

7. What factors might influence the outcome of an interview?

The factors that might influence the outcome of an interview are;
- *perceptual factors, such as how sensory stimuli affect the way the other person is perceived;*
- *conceptual factors (which include the AHP's knowledge base);*
- *role issues (which include the way each person perceives the role they play in the interview);*
- *self-esteem issues (which involve the way each person feels about themselves);*
- *environmental factors;*
- *the influence of the AHP;*
- *the influence of the person, and;*
- *the nature of the dynamic interactions between AHP and the person.*

8. Give an advantage and a disadvantage for using self-report data.

An advantage of collecting self-report data is that you gain insight into the person's perspectives, values, beliefs, and priorities. These help you develop meaningful, person-centred goals and plans.

A disadvantage of collecting self-report data is that this approach is not ideal for those people with communication difficulties or those who lack insight.

CHAPTER 3: PURPOSES OF ASSESSMENT AND MEASUREMENT

1. What factors should you consider when selecting a discriminative assessment for your service?

When selecting a discriminative assessment you need to consider the quality of the normative data and the relevance of the normative sample to your population/ health condition group, in order for you to generalise with confidence from the normative data in the test manual. Also, do review the test manual for evidence of associated literature and evidence of discriminative validity.

2. Define predictive assessment.

Predictive assessment is undertaken by AHPs to predict the future ability of a person or to predict a specific outcome in the future.

3. Why do AHPs undertake evaluative assessment and why should they use standardised outcome measures for this purpose?

AHPs need to be able to detect change in ability over time, and evaluative assessments undertaken to monitor a person's progress during rehabilitation, reablement and or intervention, to determine the effectiveness of the approach. It is critical to use objective and sensitive measures of outcome to avoid subjective, unreliable estimates of ability.

4. Why should AHPs evaluate their service?

AHPs need to undertake evaluations of their services to monitor that the service offered is appropriate to and effective.

CHAPTER 4. WHAT IS MEASUREMENT?

1. Describe the similarities and differences between nominal and ordinal scales.

   Both nominal and ordinal scales assign numbers to categorical data; however, with ordinal sales the categories can be assigned to some sort of rank order. This means that a nominal scale is sufficient to measure the proportion of the population who has a particular characteristic or who achieves a particular outcome, while an ordinal scale can describe how one test score compares with another.

2. What property does a ratio scale have that is not present in the other three types of scale?

   A ratio scale has a fixed origin or absolute zero point. This means that a ration scale can be used to tell us how proportionally different one test score is from another test score.

3. Define an interval scale.

   In an interval scale, scores are classified by both order and by a known and equal interval points. This means an interval scale has rank order and the distances between the numbers have meaning with respect to the property being measured. An interval scale enables us to define how one test score differs from another.

CHAPTER 6: THE IMPORTANCE OF CLINICAL REASONING AND REFLECTIVE PRACTICE IN EFFECTIVE ASSESSMENT

1. What is clinical reasoning?

   Clinical reasoning plays a critical role in enabling an AHP to connect practice based on best evidence with practice that is client centred and centred upon a person's unique presentation of problems and needs. External clinical evidence is used to inform clinical decisions, but should not replace individual clinical expertise. Clinical reasoning is the process through which clinical expertise is applied to individual client problems; the AHP engages in clinical reasoning to decide whether available external evidence applies to the individual client's presentation. When the clinician decides external evidence does apply, clinical reasoning is required to establish how this evidence should be applied in this particular case and underlies clinical decision making around how the evidence should be integrated into this client's assessment, management and / or intervention.

2. What type of questions do AHPs attempt to answer through pragmatic reasoning?

   Pragmatic reasoning is how the AHP obtains an understanding about how the personal context and the practice setting impact the assessment and treatment processes she implements. The types of questions an AHP might ask include
   - *Who referred this client for therapy and, why was this referral made?*
   - *Who is paying for this treatment, and what are their expectations of the outcome of therapy?*
   - *What family / carer support does the client have, what are these people's expectations and abilities, can they provide resources (practical support, physical help, encouragement, finances) to assist with the client's intervention?*
   - *How much time will I have available to work with this client?*
   - *What clinical and client based environments are available for therapy and what standardised tests, equipment and adaptations can I access to support the therapeutic process?*

- *What are the expectations of my manager, supervisor and multi-disciplinary colleagues?*
- *What are my clinical competencies and will these be sufficient to provide the client with the therapy they need?*

3. What are the four components of diagnostic reasoning?

The four components of diagnostic reasoning are cue acquisition, hypothesis generation, cue interpretation, and hypothesis evaluation.

4. How could you document your reflections on your practice?

Reflections can be documented as diary entries, reflective journal, significant incident analysis, case analysis, stories, and notes from supervision, mentorship or peer reflection sessions. These should be kept in a portfolio of continuing professional development (CPD).

CHAPTER 7: STANDARDISATION

1. What makes a test standardised?

Standardisation is a process of taking an assessment and developing a fixed protocol for its administration and scoring and then conducting psychometric studies to evaluate whether the resultant assessment has acceptable levels of validity and reliability. A standardised test is a measurement tool that is, published and developed, for a specific purpose and, for use with a particular population or health condition group.

2. What is a norm-referenced test?

A norm referenced test determines a person's placement on a normal distribution curve. It is used often in education and students / pupils compete against each other on this type test, this is sometimes referred to as 'grading on a curve'. In therapy, it is a test that is used to evaluate performance of a person against the scores of a peer group whose performance has been described using a normative sample. Types of scoring on normative tests can include: developmental norms; within group norms (standard scores, percentiles); and fixed reference group norms.

3. What is standard deviation and how is it used in measurement?

Standard Deviation (σ) is a measure of the spread or extent of variability of a set of scores around their mean. It is the average amount a score varies from the average score in a series of scores. An important attribute of the standard deviation as a measure of spread is that if the mean and standard deviation of a normal distribution are known, it is possible to compute the percentile rank associated with any given score. In a normal distribution, about 68% of the scores are within one standard deviation of the mean and about 95% of the scores are within two standard deviations of the mean. The standard deviations from the mean indicate the degree to which a person's performance on the test is above or below average.

CHAPTER 8: VALIDITY AND CLINICAL UTILITY

1. Describe one method to examine the content validity of a test.

The use of an expert panel is one method to examine content validity of a test.

2. Define construct validity.

Construct validity involves the extent to which an assessment can be said to measure a theoretical construct or constructs.

3. List one type of criterion-related validity and describe a method for evaluating this type of criterion-related validity.

One type of criterion-related validity is concurrent validation undertaken by comparing two or more measures that have been designed to measure the same or similar content or constructs. Criterion-related validity looks at the effectiveness of a test in predicting an individual's performance in specific activities, this is measured by comparing performance on the test with a criterion, which is a direct and independent measure of what the assessment is designed to predict. Another type is predictive validity; this type refers broadly to the prediction from the test to any criterion performance, or specifically to prediction over a time interval.

4. What is predictive validity and why is it important to AHPs?

Predictive validity is "the accuracy with which a measurement predicts some future event, such as mortality. This is critical to AHPs because in clinical practice they often need to make predictions. For example, AHPs may need to predict a client's function in a wide range of activities from observation of just a few activities. AHPs frequently have to predict functioning in the future, such as upon discharge. AHPs often need to predict the person's ability in a different environment.

5. What is face validity and why should AHPs consider it?

Face validity is the extent to which a test is viewed subjectively as covering the concept it purports to measure. A test with face validity will have a clear purpose. AHPs should consider face validity as a person's perception of whether the test is relevant and meaningful is critical.

6. What factors would you examine if you wanted to evaluate a test's clinical utility?

Clinical utility is the overall usefulness of an assessment in a clinical situation and covers aspects of a test such as reasonable cost, acceptability, training requirements, administration time, and interpretation of scores, portability, and ease of use.

CHAPTER 9: RELIABILITY

1. What is reliability?

Reliability of a test refers to how stable its scores remain overtime and across different examiners.

2. What is the difference between int<u>er</u>-rater reliability and int<u>ra</u>-rater reliability?

Inter-rater reliability refers to the agreement between or among different AHPs (raters) administering the test. Intra-rater reliability refers to the consistency of the judgements made by the same AHP (test administrator / rater) over time.

3. Define test-retest reliability.

Test-retest is a term used to describe the properties of measurement tools evaluated twice on different time occasions. Stability is an important concept for AHPs as we need to know whether a behaviour or level of function is stable or has changed over time.

4. What would be an acceptable correlation coefficient for test-retest reliability?

An acceptable correlation coefficient for test-retest reliability is considered to be 0.70 or above.

5. What is responsiveness and why is it important if you want to measure outcomes?

Responsiveness to change can also be considered a fundamental characteristic of the evaluation instruments, designed to measure longitudinal change through time. The responsiveness of a test is critically important to AHPs because they often need to measure changes in aspects of people's functioning, for example when evaluating the impact of intervention or monitoring the effects of medication. When using evaluative measures, the AHP should ensure that the test used is responsive to picking up both the type and amount of change in behaviour or function that is anticipated, or desired, as the result of intervention.

CHAPTER 11: APPLYING MODELS TO ASSESSMENT AND OUTCOME MEASUREMENT

1. Why can it be useful to apply a model of function as a framework for your assessment process?

   An explicit application of a model of function can help an individual AHP, an AHP service or a MDT to review their assessment practice and facilitate communication about assessment, outcome measurement and intervention.

2. What are the 10 levels in the *Hierarchy of living systems*, described by Christiansen (1991)?

   The 10 levels in the Hierarchy of living systems are: Atom, Molecules, cells, organs, person, family group, organisation, societies, homo sapiens, biosphere.

3. How are the terms body structures, body functions and impairments defined in the ICF model?

   - *Body Functions are physiological functions of body systems (including psychological functions).*
   - *Body Structures are anatomical parts of the body such as organs, limbs and their components.*
   - *Impairments are problems in body function or structure such as a significant deviation or loss.*

4. How are the terms activity and participation, and activity limitations and participation restrictions, defined in the ICF model?

   - *Activity is the execution of a task or action by an individual.*
   - *Participation is involvement in a life situation.*
   - *Activity Limitations are difficulties an individual may have in executing activities.*

5. What are the five levels proposed by the NCMRR model of function and dysfunction?

   - *Pathophysiology*
   - *Impairment*
   - *Functional limitation*
   - *Disability*
   - *Societal Limitation*

CHAPTER 14: TEST DEVELOPMENT

1. What are the features of a criterion-referenced test?

   Criterion-referenced tests compare a person's knowledge or skills against a predetermined standard, learning goal, performance level, or other criterion. With criterion-referenced tests, each person's performance is compared directly to the standard, without considering how other students perform on the test. AHPs use criterion-referenced tests to judge whether a person has mastered the required standards (e.g. to judge whether the pet son has sufficient ability to be safe to be discharged home to live alone).

2. What is Guttman scaling?

*A **Guttman scale** (also known as cumulative **scaling** or scalogram analysis) is an ordinal **scale** type where statements are arranged in a hierarchical order so that someone who agrees with one item will also agree with lower-order, easier, less extreme items.*

The purpose of Guttman scaling is to establish a one-dimensional continuum for a concept you wish to measure.

3. What is Rasch analysis?

*Rasch analysis allows us to convert observed counts of ordinal data (raw scores) into approximately equal-interval number line. This enables as to compare how much more or less the person exhibits of the construct or behaviour being measured. Therefore, **Rasch analysis** allows researchers to use a respondent's raw test or scale scores and express the respondent's performance on a linear scale that accounts for the unequal difficulties across all test items.*

CHAPTER 15: CONDUCTING PSYCHOMETRIC STUDIES

1. What are the psychometric properties of a test?

Psychometric properties are characteristics of tests and other measures of human characteristics that identify and describe attributes of an instrument, such as its reliability, validity or appropriateness for use in a particular circumstance. Such as face validity, test-retest reliability, and responsiveness.

Index

Page numbers in **bold** indicate tables.